DOCTOR OF SOCIETY

THE WELLCOME INSTITUTE SERIES IN THE HISTORY OF MEDICINE

Edited by W.F. Bynum and Roy Porter
The Wellcome Institute

Medical Fringe and Medical Orthodoxy 1750–1850
W.F. Bynum and Roy Porter

Florence Nightingale and the Nursing Legacy
Monica Baly

Social Hygiene in Twentieth Century Britain
Greta Jones

Problems and Methods in the History of Medicine
Roy Porter and Andrew Wear

Vivisection in Historical Perspective
Nicolaas A. Rupke

Abortion in England, 1900–1967
Barbara Brookes

The Hospital in History
Edited by Lindsay Granshaw and Roy Porter

Women as Mothers in Pre-industrial England
Edited by Valerie Fildes

Birth Control in Germany, 1871–1933
James Woycke

The Charitable Imperative
Colin Jones

Medicine at the Courts of Europe, 1500–1837
Edited by Vivian Nutton

Mad Tales from the Raj
Waltraud Ernst

British Medicine in an Age of Reform
Edited by Roger French and Andrew Wear

DOCTOR OF SOCIETY

THOMAS BEDDOES AND THE SICK TRADE IN LATE-ENLIGHTENMENT ENGLAND

Roy Porter

ROUTLEDGE

London and New York

First published in 1992
by Routledge
11 New Fetter Lane, London EC4P 4EE

Simultaneously published in the USA and Canada
by Routledge
a division of Routledge, Chapman and Hall Inc.
29 West 35th Street, New York, NY 10001

Typeset by LaserScript Limited, Mitcham, Surrey
Printed and bound in Great Britain by Biddles Ltd, Guildford and
King's Lynn

British Library Cataloguing in Publication Data
Porter, Roy *1946–*
Doctor of society: Thomas Beddoes and the sick trade in
late enlightenment England.
1. England. Medicine, history. Beddoes, Thomas *1760–1808*
I. Title II. Series
610.942

Library of Congress Cataloging in Publication Data
Porter, Roy, 1946–
Doctor of society: Thomas Beddoes and the sick trade in late
enlightenment England/Roy Porter.
p. cm. – (The Wellcome Institute series in the history
of medicine)
Includes bibliographical reference and index.
1. Beddoes, Thomas, 1760–1808. 2. Physicians – England
Bibliography.
3. Medicine – England – History – 18th century. I. Title.
II. Series.
[DNLM: 1. Beddoes, Thomas, 1760–1808. 2. History of Medicine,
18th Cent. – England. WZ 100 B399P]
R489.B4P67 1991
610′.92 – dc20
[B]
DNLM/DLC
for Library of Congress 91-3415
CIP

ISBN 0–415–04850–8

To Michael Neve

Contents

	Acknowledgements	ix
1.	Introduction	1
2.	Life	11
3.	The eighteenth-century medical milieu	22
4.	The advancement of scientific medicine	37
5.	The problem patient	58
6.	Enlightenment and pathology	86
7.	Cashing in on vulgar errors	119
8.	Reforming the profession	140
9.	Instructing the people	154
10.	Conclusion	183
	Bibliography	195
	Index	227

Acknowledgements

Why Beddoes?

Surely it is natural that a medical historian specializing in the eighteenth century, fascinated by the social history of medicine, and concerned with getting to grips with the Enlightenment, should find Thomas Beddoes a source of perpetual interest, puzzlement and pleasure.

Putting it in those terms, however, masks the very personal stimuli which have led to my own personal interest. Thanks first and foremost to Michael Neve. It was he who first conveyed to me, in the early 1970s – not least on long summer walks through Clifton – the excitement and importance of the circle of Bristol radicals of whom Beddoes was the centre, their experiments in living no less than in medicine and science, their commitment to the politics of knowledge and the knowledge of politics. As any reader of this book will see, I have profited more than I can document from his researches, analyses, suggestions, and insights into Beddoes and the Bristolian intellectual environment.

My thanks also to numerous other scholars who have worked on Beddoes and his friends, colleagues, and times. Above all, to Dorothy Stansfield, whose enviable recent biography, *Thomas Beddoes M.D. 1760–1808, Chemist, Physician, Democrat* (1984) confirmed my conviction that Beddoes was a quite extraordinary man, raised my knowledge and understanding of Beddoes's life to a new pitch, and yet left me believing that there were more, or at least, other things, to be said. But my gratitude extends to many others besides: to Trevor Levere, F.F. Cartwright, W.D.A. Smith and others who have vastly enhanced my grasp of Beddoes the man of science; and to Mary Fissell, who, together with Michael Neve, has illuminated the Bristol medical background.

More recently, I have been grateful for the forebearance of friends and seminar audiences, repeatedly willing to tolerate a colleague who had Beddoes in his bonnet, and was cultivating what must often have seemed to them – and probably still does seem – a self-indulgent involvement with a bloody-minded and long-winded provincial medicine man, whose importance and interest was somewhat less than he imagined.

Dorothy Porter has sometimes looked askance at my obsession with Beddoes; but her consistent commitment to a demanding, sociologically-informed, theoretically-aware social history of medicine, and her unfailingly astringent criticisms have made this a less sloppy work than it would otherwise have been. In earlier books, we together worked out the general interpretative framework within which this book moves. I hope she will not find it a travesty of some of her views and approaches.

The inspiration has been theirs, the mistakes are mine.

I am further grateful to Gill Davies at Routledge for the encouragement she has given this project. At the Wellcome Institute, Marika Antoniw sat typing with remarkable speed, accuracy and cheerfulness when normal people would have been doing their Christmas shopping; and Andy Foley, gallantly as ever, manned the xerox machine. Jean Runciman was, as always, the perfect copy editor and indexer.

Roy Porter
January 1991

1

Introduction

> It has been said that a man of genius can discourse on anything.
>
> (Peacock, *Gryll Grange*)

This book may seem neither fish, flesh, nor foul. It is a study of Thomas Beddoes (1760–1808), in my view, alongside Erasmus Darwin, the most challenging and original medical man active in England in the era of the French Revolution. But it is not a scholarly biography, an archive-based investigation of his development and doings, his family and friends, his circle and influence, his chequered career and its legacy. Nor is it a day-to-day analysis of Beddoes's labours at the bedside and in the laboratory, his projects and achievements in chemistry, mineralogy, geology, physiology, meteorology, and many other -ologies. Nor is it even a systematic survey of the subjects upon which he so prodigally wrote: pedagogics, hygiene, language, philosophy, politics. Readers seeking illumination on these and many other aspects of Beddoes's life and works must look elsewhere – above all, to Dorothy Stansfield's thoroughly researched, and admirably balanced and sympathetic biography, to F.F. Cartwright's older study, and also to a stream of papers that have appeared in recent years, especially those by Trevor Levere.[1]

My aims are narrower and different. I am interested in Beddoes's opinions (and, goodness knows, he was a man of opinions!). I address Beddoes's writings – principally his publications, but also his correspondence – primarily to tease out his views about the meaning of health and medicine, and the light they will shed, directly and obliquely, upon the 'sickness culture' of late-Enlightenment England. In Beddoes's breast there breathed a scientist. As a young researcher, he regarded disease as an enemy which laboratory science could conquer, indeed would rapidly and gloriously vanquish. It was not to be. His early Promethean visions were dashed, the frustrations of daily medical practice ground him down, and he grew oppressed by the unpalatable realities of life in wartime England, darkened by alarm, repression, and bigotry. Another Beddoes then became dominant, one who recognized that there was more to sickness, more to pain and suffering, and more to the doctor's role, than had first been thought of in his philosophy.

Beddoes was to recognize that illness was not simply an adventitious foe. It was more like a familiar, integral to sufferers' lives: wealth-specific, class-specific, gender-specific, *mores*-specific. Its incidence was an index of certain social realities: it spoke about absolute and relative distributions of plenty and poverty, of power and oppression, of education and ignorance, succour and neglect. The attentive doctor could thus be a diagnostician of social pathology in the body politic. To such a doughty political radical as Beddoes, the techniques of medicine could thereby underpin the causes of popular rights and citizenship, of liberty, equality and fraternity.

But while conducting this 'gross anatomy' of society, Beddoes also grew fascinated, if exasperated, with sickness on far more personal and experiential planes. Sickness, he discovered – and, in his books, explored with an *engagé* and often idiosyncratic blend of pique and prejudice – was also part of the thick texture of individual and community lives. It was a mode, sometimes very negative, of self-experience; it could be a form of group identity, a currency of social exchange, providing negotiating counters for interpersonal relationships.[2] Long before Talcott Parsons's coinage, Beddoes was well aware of the equivocations of the 'sick role';[3] it was a part which the patient could act to advantage, yet a device reciprocally giving society itself some leverage over the individual; not least, it was a cultural '*träger*' with a certain life of its own, which could victimize the minds and spirits, no less than penalize the bodies, of those it 'scripted'.

Beddoes was the finest anthropologist of cultural morbidity active in England between the death of Laurence Sterne and the emergence of Thomas Carlyle. And, like so many anthropologists, this medical missionary had dual citizenship, as rationalist and relativist, scientist and artist, outsider and insider. There was Beddoes the Enlightenment radical, doctor, inquirer, philanthropist, reformer – the man who, to adapt a phrase of his friend, Dr Erasmus Darwin, saw it as his mission to ride into battle against a fever. This Beddoes was frustrated by the follies and fatalism, the wilful blindness of people, privileged and poor alike, when assailed by sickness and suffering. This Beddoes wanted to slash through ignorance and error, to educate, advise, activate, harangue and heal. If, after around 1795, improvement could no longer be achieved on the national political stage, then the medical microcosm looked the most promising theatre for action.

But doubling this frustrated Beddoes, brusque, bloodied but unbowed, there was another, the Beddoes intrigued by sickness as fetish, as the object of ritual and intricate belief-systems, as an orchestrator of conversation and social intercourse, as the hermeneutic key to habits; sickness, in other words, as cult – an emotionally-entangled language of life which, however irrational, however contributory to tribulation, nevertheless articulated powerful moods and emotions, and radiated constant streams of meaning. As man, as *philosophe*, as physician, Beddoes despaired at the absurd health-lore practices of those poor people who knew no better, and raged at the grotesquely self-indulgent, self-pitying, health antics of rich and self-regarding folks who certainly should have known better. But, rather as Christian missionaries meticulously recorded the most obscene nuances of the pagan ceremonials they abominated, Beddoes became so enwrapped in all those fictions and fantasies, those affectations, silly clichés and stock repartee that took the terror out of disease and death by at least enabling them to be spoken, that he recorded this outlandish oral culture in remarkable detail, with the ear of a fine doorstep sociological investigator, a sympathetic novelist, and a satirical caricaturist rolled into one; and what he heard he tried to interpret.

I don't believe Beddoes the medical anthropologist wanted to go native; there is no warrant for suggesting that the doctor wished to climb into the sickbed with his patients. What may be said, however, is that he possessed sufficient empathy and insight to enable him to perceive certain symmetries and mutualities. If, *qua* doctor, he was to stand apart from (rather than be part of) a sickness culture which he deplored, not least because, by routinization, it unnecessarily protracted pain and suffering, he recognized that the medical profession at large was complicit in the perpetuation of that rigmarole. Doctors made people sick. Beddoes saw that was true, both thanks to their gross ineptitude, malpractice, and unsafe therapeutics, but also because it was the medical profession that 'trained' people to be conventional patients. And he could also, occasionally at least, hold the mirror up to himself, and acknowledge his own role in abuses he damned in others. Not least, the ironist in him appreciated the iatrogenic dangers of peddling still more print to eradicate the evils of a print-soaked culture.

Young man Beddoes had a fine feel for the times in which he lived. It was the century after Newton, the age of Enlightenment and politeness, of opulence, of the chemical revolution and the French Revolution. Everything was new, brilliant, in a whirl. Beddoes was a prophet of, and commentator upon, modernity; its problems and paradoxes perplexed him. He was a man less interested in timeless truths than in capturing what William Hazlitt soon would call the 'spirit of the age', and seeing the interconnections of the contemporaneous: illness, oppression, and the perversions of language; health, hope, happiness. In the flux of things, sickness somatized the complaints of the times, but sickness itself had to be expressed in idioms rooted in history, class, and culture. Hence, switching his attention from the histories of the sick to fundamental questions of power, professions, and politics, and then swinging back to the bedside stories, Beddoes constantly found himself arrested by the tricks of words, metaphors, and meanings, fibs and fictions. In the following chapters, I quote Beddoes at inordinate length, and linger over his prose, his forms of speech, his rhetorical strategies; and I do this because he himself heard that performance, and presentation mattered no less than content. More than any other doctor of his times – more than John Hunter, Edward Jenner, Thomas Percival, or others of equal eminence – it is Beddoes who allows us to hear, in however distorted a manner, illness and wellness on the airwaves. People talked themselves sick; Beddoes wanted to talk them well.

Those are some of the core issues this book will address. It will do so against a background agenda of questions concerning the meanings of sickness and the role of medicine in the long march to modernity. Close scrutiny of Beddoes's opinions, his eavesdropping on the dicta of the doctors, and his pugnacious confutations of received truths, will, I hope, afford evidence for the evaluation of these wider questions. In that rapidly industrializing society of which, as a Shropshire lad, Beddoes was very much an integral part – how did commentators assess the affinities between society, sickness and progress? Was it widely believed that the quantum of illness was growing or withering away? To what were disease outbreaks attributed? Did people expect that medicine was on the brink of revolution, rather like natural science in the age of Newton? And, if disease diminished, would doctors disappear with it? Or, if modern society might entail more and more trying forms of sickness, would the role of the physician be *enlarged*? What would the physician of the future do? In the nineteenth century the idea gained ground – take, for instance, Samuel Butler's *Erewhon* – that personal vices and society's evils were really forms of sickness, individual, social, political psychopathologies, needing treatment from statesmen-physicians: today we are said to live in the 'therapeutic state'.[4] In some respects, there is nothing new in such medicalizations of social life. Plato, of course, had likened the statesman to the physician; the image of the 'body politic', its 'constitution' perhaps corrupt and in need of the knife, was age-old; and it was not unusual for physicians to give their writings titles such as *Medicus Politicus*.[5] So what was distinctive about the 'medical politics' which Enlightenment apologists like Beddoes formulated and bequeathed to the future?

Beddoes was not a systematic thinker. He did not pass his career as a professor of medicine, delivering formal student lecture courses, nor compose medico-legal treatises in the manner of Johann Peter Frank.[6] He was a frantically busy man, engaged in myriad causes. Unlike Auguste Comte, no stately succession of writings followed from a youthful blueprint; many of Beddoes's writings were occasional pieces, impulsive or indignant responses to some particular crisis. Yet he was assuredly a thinker of great breadth of learning and culture. Few Englishmen of his time read more voraciously in so many modern languages. He was *au fait* with poetry, politics and philosophy, as well as science and medicine: he it was who reviewed *Wilhelm Meister* for the *Monthly Review*. His circle of companions ranged from Erasmus Darwin and James Watt to Samuel Taylor Coleridge and Humphry Davy. Though barely mentioned in standard histories of the *Aufklärung*, he is, was, in every important respect, a central late-Enlightenment figure, an inveterate battler against ignorance, obscurantism, priestcraft, and oppression, both autocratic and aristocratic; lifelong he vested his faith in the powers of reason, science, and education to improve the human condition. In 1789, he welcomed the cause of *liberté, égalité*, and *fraternité*, and, unlike such friends as Coleridge, he never backslid from his commitments, though he was not so blinkered as not to notice that the heady ideals of 1789 had become stained by blood, extremism, and events. Attached emotionally and ideologically to liberal values – to the people against the privileged, to science and *sapere aude*, Beddoes was nevertheless sufficiently alert as a social spectator, sufficiently responsive to the undercurrents of his times, sufficiently astute, one might say, as a doctor attuned to the precariousness of health and the double-dealings of disease, to be capable of appreciating the equivocal nature of the physician's role in society.

The early part of this book gives a thumbnail sketch of Beddoes's life against the eighteenth-century medical background. The lengthier chapters that follow do not then systematically examine the influences upon, or the year-by-year development of, Beddoes's views about illness, the community, and the doctor. Rather they selectively highlight certain core themes, ones that haunted Beddoes, and which we might see as indicative of the age. Could medicine be expected to march forward like physics or chemistry? This question, examined in Chapter Four, troubled Beddoes. The idealist in him sought experimental medicine, on the model of the natural sciences; the realist recognized that, whereas the physical sciences proceeded in the laboratory, medicine had to operate in the cottage, crescent, or the country house, and accommodate the fads and frailties of human subjects – patients, practitioners, politicians. Hence Beddoes's medical writings came round to addressing not disease in the abstract, but the peculiar forms of sickness in society, the limitations thereby imposed upon medicine, and strategies of damage limitation.

I proceed, from Chapter Five to Chapter Seven, to examine Beddoes's confrontations with the Enlightened classes, the propertied and the polite, and his belief that the commercial civilization driven by the triumphant market economy, the acquisitive ethos, and the fashionable ambience of the *beau monde*, were collectively breeding sickness even as they abridged many traditional evils. Alongside progress, there were new pathologies; civilization bred diseases and discontents.

And, as Beddoes saw it, not the least of the concomitant evils was that the medical profession itself had succumbed to participating in the palaver of polite sickness. Physic had thereby became part of the disease, rather than the cure. As I suggest in Chapter Eight, as a reformer Beddoes looked to the reform of the medical profession no less than of élite prejudice. Glaring paradoxes lurk in the politics of 'physician, heal thyself', no less than in the *aperçu* that a little learning can be a pathological thing.

Beddoes was a 'friend of the people', and he invested great effort in exposing the social, economic and political roots of ill-health, and in devising means to eradicate them. Here again, as Chapter Nine suggests, we run up against a paradox. If, combating Pitt or 'alarm', Beddoes was a spirited democrat, when confronting tuberculosis amongst the masses, his medical prescriptions and practices seem to have been more élitist and autocratic.

Thus core dilemmas are disclosed. What place was the doctor to occupy in society? Was he to be a private practitioner or a public functionary? Was his standing to be guaranteed by corporate professional authority, by the authority of science, or the plaudits of the people? Or was the physician to be an honest outsider, a prophet of pathology unhonoured in his own country?

I am not suggesting Beddoes solved any of these problems. I do believe he raised them, chewed them over, and perhaps possessed an unusually articulate grasp of the potential sociopathology of modernity and of the equivocal roles open to the physician and, more broadly, the intelligentsia, within a liberal, capitalist order. The following chapters use Beddoes's writings to ventilate a topic all too often ignored by historians of medicine: the making of the job description of the physician in modern society.

A few further points are worth mentioning. I do not want to make exaggerated claims for Beddoes, least of all concerning his 'influence', which was probably slight. Alive, he was too much of a loner, too much a curmudgeonly exponent of 'a plague on both your houses', to be an effective campaigner; dead, too many radical skeletons were rattling around in the cupboard – the revolutionary pamphleteer, the experimentalist drunk on laughing-gas – to permit him to be an eligible figurehead, even for progressives. I have, rather, distinguished Beddoes for several reasons. He was articulate and up-front, indeed, to the historian often gratifyingly opinionated. He was sensitive to the importance of form as well as content. In an age of Enlightenment pervaded by print culture, by newspapers, opinion, and ideology, the pen was perhaps as mighty as the sword, but, he recognized, the pen needed to be deployed with no less precision and flexibility than the rapier or the scalpel. Responding to what Jürgen Habermas, Raymond Williams and Terry Eagleton, in their various ways, have characterized as the emergent public sphere,[7] Beddoes, unlike most doctors, was path-breaking as a *writer*. Not least, he was creditably self-aware. He could see himself as part of the problem: he knew that sickness, at least psychologically speaking, was often iatrogenic, he diagnosed the diseases of print.

He was not alone: other medical writers possessed similar insights. As I discuss below, Beddoes's friend, Erasmus Darwin, was notable for his liberal-progressive vision of the doctor as crusader for social improvement. James Makittrick Adair was one of several medical essayists who transvalued physic into pantomime, and sickness into a satire upon the times. On the Continent, Tissot explored the diseases of civilization[8] while Cabanis was insisting that medicine was the key to a science of society.[9]

It would be highly desirable to have in-depth studies of the opinions and campaigns of other British medico-social reformers, for instance, John Coakley Lettsom, John Ferriar, or John Haygarth.[10] In their absence, however, I have felt obliged to bring Beddoes's views into prominence, when they might better be understood contextualized against the opinions of a wider cadre of the profession. Here and there, however, I have felt able to introduce comparisons and contrasts between Beddoes and his contemporaries – with William Buchan and James Parkinson as political radicals as well as medical reformers, or Thomas Trotter as a parallel morbid anatomist of the ills of modernity.

Before Beddoes can be fully understood, it would also be desirable to have a minute socio-topography of the Bristol intellectual community and its politics in the years of the doctor's residence there, the world of Southey and Coleridge, Davy and King. Studies by Michael Neve, Trevor Levere, Mark Harrison, and Mary Fissell have taken us far in that direction,[11] while Jan Golinski's superb new analysis of the shifting socio-cultural meanings of chemistry in Enlightenment England have further illuminated Beddoes's enterprise and provided its contextualization.[12] I see Golinski's reading of what chemistry meant to Beddoes as entirely in accord with my view of Beddoes's medical mission.

Third, and perhaps most basic to Beddoes, we badly need a comprehensive analysis of the politics of the English medical profession in the Revolutionary period. The work of Ivan Waddington established broad guidelines; John Pickstone and others have contributed valuable regional studies; and Irvine Loudon has given us an exemplary account of the reformist surge attending the emergence of the general practitioner.[13] But ignorance still shrouds the social, political and, above all, professional commitments and aspirations of the vast bulk of Beddoes's peers.

This is partly because the history of the English intelligentsia, in the transition from Enlightenment to Romanticism, still remains to be written. Historians of political thought have given us meticulous accounts of Burke and Paine, of Bentham and the rise of Utilitarianism. Literary historians, above all Raymond Williams and John Barrell, have heightened our awareness of contemporary perceptions of culture and society, the country and the city, community and alienation, provincialism and patriotism.[14] But we are still far from fully understanding the place and self-perception of intellectuals, such as Beddoes, in respect to the opportunities and threats posed by industrialization, by the growth of a commercial, consumer society, by wealth, luxury and their discontents.[15] What follows is some small contribution to these goals.

And so to Beddoes!

Notes

Throughout this book short titles are given in the Notes, keyed to full titles in the Bibliography. For the sake of clarity, however, works by Beddoes, on their first citation in each chapter, are given their long title together with date of publication.

1. Dorothy A. Stansfield, *Thomas Beddoes*; F.F. Cartwright, *The English Pioneers of Anaesthesia (Beddoes, Davy and Hickman)*; T.H. Levere, 'Dr Thomas Beddoes and the Establishment of his Pneumatic Institution'; *idem*, 'Thomas Beddoes, The Interaction of Pneumatic and Preventative Medicine with Chemistry'; *idem*, 'Dr Thomas Beddoes at Oxford, Radical Politics in 1788–93, and the Fate of the Regius Chair in Chemistry'; *idem*, 'Dr Thomas Beddoes (1760-1808): Science and Medicine in Politics and Society'.

2. For scholarship which discusses these dimensions, see H. Brody, *Stories of Sickness*; A. Kleinman, *Patients and Healers in the Context of Culture*; *idem*, *Social Origins of Distress and Disease*; *idem* and B. Good (eds), *Culture and Depression*; *idem*, *The Illness Narratives: Suffering, Healing and the Human Condition*; B.S. Turner, *The Body and Society*; *idem*, *Medical Power and Social Knowledge*; Roy Porter and Dorothy Porter, *In Sickness and in Health*.

3. Talcott Parsons, *The Social System*.

4. See the conceptualizations of Jacques Donzelot, *The Policing of Families*; Françoise and Robert Castel and Anne Lovell, *The Psychiatric Society*.

5. A good survey is needed of changing concepts of the status, social place, and function, of the doctor, building on P. Lain Entralgo, *Doctor and Patient*.

6. J.P. Frank, *A System of Complete Medical Police*; George Rosen, *A History of Public Health*; *idem*, *From Medical Police to Social Medicine*; R.A. Kondratas, 'Joseph Frank (1771–1842) and the Development of Clinical Medicine'.

7. For discussion of the intellectual's place, see Raymond Williams, *Culture and Society*; *idem*, *Keywords*; *idem*, *The Long Revolution*; *idem*, *The Country and the City*; Terry Eagleton, *The Function of Criticism*; Jürgen Habermas, *Knowledge and Human Interests*.

8. A. Emch-Deriaz, 'Towards a Social Conception of Health in the Second Half of the Eighteenth Century: Tissot (1728–1797)'; L.J. Jordanova, 'The Popularisation of Medicine: Tissot on Onanism'.

9. M. Staum, *Cabanis*.

10. Though see A. Marcovich, 'Concerning the Continuity between the Image of Society and the Image of the Human Body: An Examination of the Work of the English Physician J.C. Lettsom (1746–1815)'; Francis M. Lobo, 'John Haygarth, Smallpox and Religious Dissent in Eighteenth Century England'; R. Kilpatrick, '"Living in the Light": Dispensaries, Philanthropy and Medical Reform in Late-Eighteenth Century London'; Christopher Booth, *Doctors in Science and Society*; R.D. Thornton, *James Currie, The Entire Stranger and Robert Burns*.

11. M.R. Neve, 'Natural Philosophy, Medicine and the Culture of Science in Provincial England'; T.H. Levere, 'Dr Thomas Beddoes (1760–1808): Science and Medicine in Politics and Society'; Mary E. Fissell, *The Physic of Charity: Health and Welfare in the West Country, 1690–1810*; Mark Harrison, *Crowds and History: Mass Phenomena in English Towns, 1790-1835*.

12. Jan Golinski, *Science as Public Culture*.

13. I.S.L. Loudon, *Medical Care and the General Practitioner 1750–1850*.

14. John Barrell, *The Idea of Landscape and the Sense of Place*; *idem*, *The Dark Side of the Landscape*; *idem*, *English Literature in History, 1730–80*.

15. For background, see J.G.A. Pocock, *Virtue, Commerce and History*; John Sekora, *Luxury*; Linda Colley, 'The Apotheosis of George III'; *idem*, 'Whose Nation? Class and National Consciousness in England, 1750–1830'; Gerald Newman, *The Rise of English Nationalism*.

2
Life

> 'You are a philosopher', said the lady, 'And a lover of liberty. You are the author of a treatise called 'Philosophical Gas; or a Project for a General Illumination of the Human Mind'.
>
> (Peacock, *Nightmare Abbey*)

We are all children of our times. But if ever there was a person whose life appears the epitome of the currents and crises of his age, surely Thomas Beddoes was he.

Beddoes was born into a prosperous tradesman's family from Shifnal in Shropshire in 1760, the year of George III's accession.[1] He was, in other words, pretty much an exact contemporary of Pitt the Younger, Mary Wollstonecraft, Horatio Nelson, Emma Hamilton, and all the Williams: Cobbett, Godwin, Blake and Wilberforce. He was the junior by some years of those illustrious men of science, technology and letters who moulded his intellectual milieu: Matthew Boulton, James Watt, Erasmus Darwin, Joseph Priestley, Richard Lovell Edgeworth (who became his father-in-law), and all the other lights of the Lunar Society of Birmingham; and of Jeremy Bentham, Tom Paine and Edmund Burke; and he was somewhat senior to the geniuses of Romanticism – Wordsworth, Coleridge, Southey, Shelley, Byron, Hazlitt, and so forth.[2] Beddoes, as is evident, lived on a stage of intellectual, artistic and scientific incandescence, not surprisingly perhaps, as socio-economic and political cataclysms were changing the very face of the world.

Beddoes's father was a tanner, one of the droves of master craftsmen making up the middling ranks of that thriving heartland of early industrialization. The West Midlands character was recognized to be practical, thrusting, business-like and efficient.[3] All his life, Beddoes displayed such attributes. He aimed to rise by his own energies and industry. He believed that such was his birthright, and he had no truck with obstacles in his way: incompetence, tradition, privilege. As an orator he was fond of contrasting the energy of 'individuals' with the inertia of 'institutions'. At heart he was a tenacious liberal individualist, a typical bourgeois radical who dreamed of a society with room at the top.[4] Every step in his career tells a story not just about himself, but about the emergent society he helped to shape.

He was given a solid schooling by his ambitious father. Having proved highly intelligent, and blessed with an exceptionally retentive memory, he proceeded in 1776 – that extraordinary year! – to his local university, Oxford. Unlike Gibbon, Beddoes made the best of the opportunities afforded by that somnolent institution, securing for himself a comprehensive grounding in all the major European languages that later enabled him to excel as a cosmopolitan polymath.

Stimulated surely by his own roots in Midlands manufacturing, and by his father's trade, Beddoes somewhat unusually cultivated scientific interests as an undergraduate. He clearly decided at least to train and qualify, if not to practise, as a medical man, and sensibly chose, having obtained his B.A. in 1781, to quit Oxford, whose medical school was comatose,[5] and to move to Britain's premier centre for practical medical education, London. Beddoes became a pupil of John Sheldon, who succeeded the great William Hunter as proprietor of the unrivalled Great Windmill Street Anatomy School. While studying in London, he made the acquaintance of numerous leading men of science, particularly in such practical fields as chemistry. Beddoes always remained convinced of London's superiority in medical education. But he never settled in the metropolis, probably recognizing he lacked the grace and favour to shine on the London medical circuit, and perhaps later displayed the provincial's ambiguities towards gilded metropolitan fineries.

After London, Beddoes went on, in 1784, to complete his medical education in Edinburgh. This was a natural choice. For fifty years, Edinburgh had been offering the most systematic academic medical education in Britain.[6] By the time Beddoes arrived, the medical school was past its prime: the great Cullen was ageing, Alexander Monro II's teaching as anatomy professor had settled into a rut, and in any case Beddoes, accustomed to personal attention in London, felt too senior and accomplished to bear with good grace the round of rather elementary student lectures on offer. Though deploring the windy controversies raging throughout the faculty, he was somewhat attracted towards the 'young Turk' Brunonian movement, with its radical simplifications of medical science. By far his best experience in Scotland was the forging of a lasting friendship with Joseph Black. The professor became Beddoes's hero, combining, as he did, medical interests with international eminence as an innovator in chemistry, and commitment to the supreme importance of experimentation.

Oxford, London, Edinburgh: Beddoes availed himself of the best his nation had to offer in science and medicine, while not prematurely committing himself to a career. What next? He returned to Oxford in 1786, taking his M.D., and throwing himself into scientific research. The Oxford chemistry laboratory afforded him an ideal milieu for experimentation; no one hindered the solitary labours of the self-motivating young man, while there were just enough supportive colleagues distributed around the colleges to preclude isolation. And, though lacking a post on the establishment or a stipend, he soon launched into lecturing, assuming in 1788 the honorific title of 'Chemical Reader', and gaining a reputation as the reviver of university interest in the science. Around these years, his ebullient, Romantic enjoyment of Nature found outlet in geological expeditions in the 'Plutonist' terrain of the Welsh borderlands, and some of Beddoes's earliest papers offered valuable support for the Huttonian theory of the earth.[7]

Ever energetic, he widened his horizons by beginning to publish. Using his versatile linguistic skills, he brought out, during the 1780s, translations and editions of eminent Continental naturalists and experimentalists: Spallanzani, Scheele, and Bergman.[8] His scientific circle grew; warm friendships developed with members of the Lunar Society like Erasmus Darwin,[9] James Keir, and William Withering, with the Ketley iron-master, William Reynolds, and, slightly later, with James Watt. And in a bold move, Beddoes took a summer trip to France in 1787, visiting Guyton de Morveau in Dijon, and thereby signalling and cementing at first hand his enthusiastic espousal of the new French chemistry.

The eve of the French Revolution found Beddoes, approaching thirty, at the peak of his potential. He could hardly have given himself a better training for launching into a distinguished scientific career. He was already an internationalist and an experimenter; he had made contact, friends even, with the most productive and forward-looking men in the field. He had taken full advantage of the extraordinary openness of late-Enlightenment culture. Though a tanner's son, he perhaps had a career blossoming for him at august Oxford, as for a while the prospects seemed good for the founding of a chair of chemistry, for which he would be an obvious candidate. And his lectures were popular, to a degree that may belie the conventional image of Georgian Oxford as being at best indifferent to science. Yet residence in Oxford in no way had precluded him from the warmest contacts with Midlands industrialists, with Dissenting natural philosophers, and with Scottish literati. Everything was possible, nothing out of reach. To be young Beddoes was very heaven.

And then the French Revolution itself seemed to double his blessings. Nothing could better have captured his own outlooks or aspirations than the aims of the *citoyens* of 1789 and their great symbolic act of storming the Bastille. Down with tyranny, oppression, priestcraft! The age was dawning of liberty, opportunity, the rights of man, and government by the people. The French were at last gaining what had long been the birthright of the English; and in turn their courage would further promote at home the cause of progress – political, intellectual, and personal. Up to 1789, Beddoes appears to have been a political animal mainly implicitly, through what he did and represented; there had been no need to formulate a creed on paper. But his correspondence in the years from 1789 shows he rapidly became politicized: incendiary phrases leap from the pages of letters to his friend, Davies Giddy, with almost innocent abandon; on 14 July 1791, we find him sporting a tricolor, and singing revolutionary songs.[10] The cause of liberty and of destroying despots (or at least cheering their destruction from the touchline) was intoxicatingly simple and simply intoxicating.

This moment of infinite promise and possibility could not last. By 1791 the anti-revolutionary groundswell in Britain was growing menacing, particularly, of course, in Beddoes's *alma mater*, and he was finding that being honest Tom Beddoes – impulsively uttering radical opinions, passionately vindicating just causes, snatching up his pen to rebut reactionary nonsense – now won enemies as well as admirers.[11] Above all, the

Birmingham Riots of July 1791, in which loyalist Church and King mobs fired the library and laboratory of Joseph Priestley while the authorities looked on, or even egged them on, must have struck home. For in many respects Beddoes was a younger, and even more radical, version of Priestley. If Beddoes was not rendered anxious for his personal safety – one suspects that the 'little fat democrat' never felt physically afraid – he was at least made to recognize that opinion was rapidly polarizing, and forcing his hand. By 1792, he had made plenty of foes in the colleges, and can hardly have been finding his own position comfortable. And, though he presumably did not know this, the Home Office was having him watched.

He took some time out to take stock, going to stay with his friend, the iron-master, William Reynolds, and writing to compose his thoughts. He penned his epic poem, *Alexander's Expedition down the Hydaspes and the Indus to the Indian Ocean* (1792), supposedly to prove that it was possible to imitate the verse of Erasmus Darwin.[12] At around the same time, and showing his concern for popular welfare, there appeared his *The History of Isaac Jenkins, and of the Sickness of Sarah his Wife, and Their Three Children* (1792), an improving tract warning working people of the evils of drunkenness.[13] And he also set his thoughts about popular education down on paper, in *Extract of a Letter on Early Instruction, Particularly that of the Poor* (1792), passionate in its advocacy of 'direct methods' of instruction.[14]

In some ways, these literary and practical writings were a sidestep, a digression from politics. Yet Beddoes was never an emollient man, and even these became vehicles for the political rage now seething in his breast. *Alexander's Expedition* was an expression of vehement denunciation of imperialism and militarism, while his educational writings accused traditional schooling of serving as the tool of ecclesiastical obscurantism, in the best radical *philosophe* tradition dubbing religion a man-made monstrosity. *Isaac Jenkins* resonated with a sneering antipathy towards squires and parsons which echoes Paine and reminds one that Beddoes was Cobbett's contemporary.

Events came to a head. Before any action was taken to oust him, in 1793 Beddoes left Oxford on his own initiative, choosing to migrate some fifty miles south-west to Bristol, where he set up in practice in the fashionable new suburb of Clifton, rather touchingly in Hope Square. Perhaps he would have taken some such action anyway. His thoughts must have been turning to settling and marrying: a step that would have been out of the question given the insecurities of chemistry in monastic Oxford. In less than a year after installing himself in Clifton, he had, in fact, wed Anna, the daughter of his good friend, Edgeworth.[15] Only medical practice offered sure prospects of reliable remuneration. And Bristol was an attractive choice, a commercial centre that was beginning to support a fine artistic and literary culture.[16] Not least, Beddoes found himself in one of the nation's hotbeds of intellectual radicalism. He had for some time shared the radical opinions of the liberal intelligentsia: Price, Priestley, Horne Tooke, Thelwall, and so forth. He now came into direct contact with local activists. The years 1794 to 1797 saw Beddoes passionately involved in political campaigning, journalism, and pamphleteering with Thomas Poole, Joseph Cottle, the publisher, and above all with Robert Southey and Samuel Taylor Coleridge, then at the height of their radical phase, while enjoying the company of a circle of good friends, including the Edgeworths, Tom Wedgwood and other members of the Wedgwood clan, Gregory Watt and James Watt the younger – several of whom he was also treating for tuberculosis.[17]

It was the best of times, it was the worst of times. For, from the latter part of 1792, Beddoes become uneasy about the progress of the Revolution itself. In letters to his old Pembroke College chum, Davies Giddy, he had deplored the Terror, denouncing the 'infernal Club of Jacobins' as a gang of bloodthirsty fanatics whose self-important rhetorical rant had blown the Revolution off-course. Increasingly, his creed became radicalism with its heels dug in – defending the integrity of supporters of the Revolution and the rights of man, for if he could no longer applaud the Parisian politics of the guillotine, what was beyond doubt was that English *enemies* of the Revolution were his enemies. And he was increasingly, explicitly, and passionately hostile to government policy at home, with its clamp-downs on political associations and its arrests of radicals, which culminated in the suspension of Habeas Corpus in 1793 and the two Acts (the 'Gagging Acts') of 1795, restricting freedom of speech and assembly.

Quitting Oxford allowed Beddoes to voice his opinions for the first time. In a flurry of pamphlets, some reasoned and canny – *Where would be the Harm of a Speedy Peace?* (1795) – others exploding in righteous anger on behalf of the oppressed populace and in hatred of Pitt, and positively sinister in their tone – *Alternatives Compared: or, What Shall the Rich Do to be Safe?* (1797) – Beddoes won his spurs as a political activist.[18]

The early Bristol years saw Beddoes at his most politicized. Of course, these were terrible times: the outbreak of Anglo-French war, Pitt's campaign to silence opposition at home, rising inflation and taxation that ruined the domestic economy of the poor, provoked riots, and intensified class hatreds.[19] For a few years, Beddoes was at the very heart of democratic resistance in one of the most radical cities in the nation, actively and fruitfully collaborating with easily the most dazzling young thinker of the day, Coleridge, who was from 1796 editor of an anti-Pitt and pro-peace fortnightly, *The Watchman*.[20]

Thereafter the stuffing went out of radical protest, partly because what had first seemed a reactionary war to crush the rights of man was patently turning into a struggle of national survival against Napoleonic imperialism. Erstwhile 'friends of liberty' jumped ship and changed sides: first Southey and then Coleridge began their long slide into the High Tory 'Church and State' embrace. Beddoes himself grew politically quieter, and perhaps demoralized, but I see no sign that his anti-Establishment opinions ever moderated: till the very end of his life he was still referring to 'us plebeians' in a particularly bolshie manner. Rather, while remaining what Dr Johnson would have called 'a good hater', he internalized his disappointment, and learned to live those dark days with a sense of failure and bitterness.

In any case, Beddoes had other fish to fry. Around 1790, he had dreamed that a new age was dawning, not just in politics, but in natural philosophy. Exhilarating breakthroughs in gas chemistry, above all, the discovery of oxygen, would not merely transform science but would produce astounding medical advances. After his removal to Bristol, these dreams centred upon setting up a new medico-scientific site, the Pneumatic Institute, combining a laboratory and clinical services, to experiment upon the potential of gases for curing respiratory and other diseases. Through the 1790s, Beddoes nursed these plans. With extraordinary energy, he continued experimentation, above all with the cooperation of James Watt, whom he persuaded to design apparatus for his experiments and to provide funds (Watt proved an easy touch, as he himself had a tubercular son and daughter). In works such as *Observations on the*

Nature and Cure of Calculus, Sea Scurvy, Consumption, Catarrh, and Fever (1793) and *Considerations on the Medicinal Use of Factitious Airs* (1794), Beddoes broadcast his researches into a range of diseases, showing unusual capacity to combine clinical experience, physiological expertise, an experimental itch, a boldness, not to say rashness, in embracing new speculations, and an enviable familiarity with the current literature in all major languages.[21] He tirelessly publicized his plans, drummed up support, and solicited funding.

Collecting money proved a problem, but eventually, thanks to the generosity above all of Thomas Wedgwood, the Pneumatic Institute opened in 1799. It gave the opportunity to intensify Beddoes's gas researches; daring experiments with nitrous oxide (laughing-gas) were conducted by Beddoes's dazzling teenage protégé, Humphry Davy. But it did not prove, in any direct sense, a medical success: no clinical benefits followed, money ran short, the philosophic revellers, drunk on air, were ridiculed in the Tory press, and in 1801, perhaps worried for his reputation, Davy moved to London. Retrenchment, reorganization and rationalization were needed; by 1802, the Institute had been revamped into the Preventive Institution, with a scaled-down scientific programme but a renewed commitment to safeguarding the health of the poor through education and out-patient facilities.[22] Yet, once again, Beddoes's hopes were hardly realized.

The 1800s proved wretched. Politically, reaction was the order of the day. The struggle against Napoleon, if not exactly popular, was widely accepted as inevitable. Radical outrage was upstaged, dispersed. Beddoes's crusades for science, and for the people, had come to little. His marriage slipped into crisis. One senses a man growing bewildered, embittered even, busy as ever but having lost his former bee-line sense of direction. Perhaps, however, it was these disappointments which led him to reflect most fruitfully upon the human comedy, that strange mix of self-importance and suffering typical of the posher patients he attended every day. Certainly his most substantial writings of the new century – the remarkable *Hygëia: or Essays Moral and Medical, on the Causes Affecting the Personal State of our Middling and Affluent Classes*, which first came out in eleven monthly instalments in 1802 and 1803, and the literary experiment, the *Manual of Health: or, the Invalid Conducted Safely Through the Seasons* (1806) – engage with the foibles of his fellow men with a depth, if also with a despair, hitherto absent.[23] Ostensibly health manuals to be read by the educated classes, these works may be read as a hybrid of medical autobiography and soap opera, a death's jest book, in which Beddoes spelt out, almost free-associatingly, his final reflections upon the phenomenology and sociology of sickness in the modern commercial and industrial order, interspersed with a salmagundi of observations upon man, society, language, and literature, written in a style by turns experimental, facetious, self-indulgent, and anything but typical of standard health-education manuals. Medicine seems to have been leading the doctor into a new manner of writing.

If Beddoes kept diaries and other intimate musings, they have not survived (his widow, Anna, and the biographer she commissioned, J.E. Stock, apparently destroyed most of his papers). The inner man is somewhat elusive; he was perhaps that kind of personality who could express his innermost urges only through public activity, professional devices and literary displacements.

Beddoes died on Christmas Eve, 1808, aged just forty-eight, having suffered a steady deterioration in health. His death was little noticed. Although he died prematurely, he had outlived his moment. His radical, liberal faith in the marriage of science and revolutionary principles had long been overtaken by events. The mantle of chemistry had passed to the courtly Humphry Davy, now stunning the *noblesse d'orée* with his experiments not at the Pneumatic Institute but at the Royal Institution in fashionable Mayfair.[24] Poetry had moved to the Lakes. Enlightenment populism had given way to Romantic idealism. In Bristol, a new respectable intelligentsia was grouping, soon to embrace a culture of liberal Anglicanism and Peelite politics.[25] And, finally, in medicine, it was business as before.

It is to the state of the medical art that we now turn.

Notes

1. Practically all the following biographical information may be found in Dorothy A. Stansfield, *Thomas Beddoes*; much was first made public by Beddoes's first biographer, J.E. Stock, in his *Memoirs of the Life of Thomas Beddoes MD*. These standard sources will not be cited further.

2. Some introduction to the world of the late eighteenth-century intelligentsia may be found in Robert E. Schofield, *The Lunar Society of Birmingham*; Marilyn Butler, *Romantics, Rebels and Reactionaries;* Elie

Halévy, *The Growth of Philosophical Radicalism*; C.B. Cone, *The English Jacobins*; Gary Kelly, *The English Jacobin Novel, 1780–1805*; Raymond Williams, *Culture and Society*.

3. John Money, *Experience and Identity: Birmingham and the West Midlands 1760–1800*; B. Trinder, *The Industrial History of Shropshire*; A.E. Musson and E. Robinson, *Science and Technology in the Industrial Revolution*; Robert E. Schofield, *The Lunar Society of Birmingham*.

4. For an introduction to such political and social values, see Albert Goodwin, *The Friends of Liberty*; E.P. Thompson, *The Making of the English Working Class*.

5. C. Webster, 'The Medical Faculty and the Physic Garden'.

6. C.J. Lawrence, 'Medicine as Culture'.

7. Roy Porter, *The Making of Geology*, 141, 144, 175.

8. Thomas Beddoes (ed.), L. Spallanzani, *Dissertations Relative to the Natural History of Animals and Vegetables* (1789).

9. Thomas Beddoes's relations with Erasmus Darwin merit more study. Desmond King-Hele has entitled his latest biography of Darwin, *Doctor of Revolution*. The epithet seems more applicable to Thomas Beddoes.

10. This correspondence is unpublished, and is located in the Cornwall Record Office in Truro. For Giddy see A.C. Todd, *Beyond the Blaze*.

11. Beddoes was always headstrong and irascible. As early as 1787, he ventured to print a fierce attack upon the mismanagement of the Bodleian Library: *A Memorial Concerning the State of the Bodleian Library, and the Conduct of the Principal Librarian*. The point is that, before the 1790s, Beddoes could indulge his wrath without penalty to himself. Things changed.

12. Thomas Beddoes, *Alexander's Expedition down the Hydaspes and the Indus to the Indian Ocean* (1792).

13. Thomas Beddoes, *The History of Isaac Jenkins, and of the Sickness of Sarah his Wife, and Their Three Children* (1792).

14. Thomas Beddoes, *Extract of a Letter on Early Instruction, Particularly that of the Poor* (1792).

15. D. Clarke, *The Ingenious Mr Edgeworth*.

16. M.R. Neve, 'Natural Philosophy, Medicine and the Culture of Science in Provincial England'; F. Greenacre, *The Bristol School of Artists: Francis Danby and Painting in Bristol 1810–1840*.

17. Richard Holmes, *Coleridge: Early Visions*.

18. Thomas Beddoes, *Where would be the Harm of a Speedy Peace?* (1795); *idem*, *An Essay on the Public Merits of Mr Pitt* (1796); *idem*, *A Letter to the Right Hon William Pitt, on the Means of Relieving the Present Scarcity, and Preventing the Diseases that Arise from Meagre Food* (1796); *idem*, *Alternatives Compared: or, What Shall the Rich Do to be Safe?* (1797); *idem*, *A Word in Defence of the Bill of Rights against Gagging Bills* (1795).

19. Richard Holmes, *Coleridge: Early Visions*; J. Cottle, *Reminiscences of Samuel Taylor Coleridge and Robert Southey*.

20. Mark Harrison, *Crowds and History: Mass Phenomena in English Towns, 1790–1835*.

21. Dorothy A. Stansfield and Ronald G. Stansfield, 'Dr Thomas Beddoes and James Watt: Preparatory Work 1794–96 for the Bristol Pneumatic Institute'; W.D.A. Smith, *Under the Influence: A History of Nitrous Oxide and Oxygen Anaesthesia.*

22. Thomas Beddoes, *Rules of the Medical Institution, for the Benefit of the Sick and Drooping Poor* (1804).

23. Thomas Beddoes, *Hygëia: or Essays Moral and Medical, on the Causes Affecting the Personal State of our Middling and Affluent Classes* (1802–3); *idem, Manual of Health: or, the Invalid Conducted Safely Through the Seasons* (1806).

24. M.R. Neve, 'The Young Humphry Davy: or John Tonkin's Lament'.

25. M.R. Neve, 'Natural Philosophy, Medicine and the Culture of Science in Provincial England'.

3

The eighteenth-century medical milieu

> The learned doctor, who had studied with peculiar care the symptoms, diagnostics, prognostics, sedatives, lenitives, and sanatives of hypochondriasis, had arrived at the sagacious conclusion, that the most effectual method of curing an imaginary disease was to give the patient a real one.
>
> (Peacock, *Melincourt*)

Thomas Beddoes saw the time of Boyle, Newton, and the founding of the Royal Society, and, in medicine, of Sydenham, as ushering in a new era, the age of modern science. In this chapter, I shall scan features of the world of eighteenth-century science and medicine that constituted significant background to Beddoes's endeavours. How did he relate to the science and medicine of the previous century?

There has been little agreement amongst historians of medicine as to how to assess the state of medicine in the eighteenth century. They have been in no doubt that the nineteenth century saw a profound medical revolution in the biomedical sciences, thanks to Bichat, von Baer, Schwann, Ludwig, Bernard, Pasteur, and others – in short, with the rise of pathological anatomy, histology, cell biology, the advent of bacteriology and the germ theory of disease.[1] Charles Rosenberg has argued that there was a 'therapeutic revolution' in the nineteenth century,[2] and Bruno Latour has re-emphasized, albeit from the viewpoint of a new 'anthropological' perspective, the well-established concept that Pasteur was of cardinal importance in bringing together biology and medicine in the 'laboratory'.[3]

But before then? Today's historians of *science* are in no doubt that the seventeenth century – the age of Bacon, Galileo, Descartes, Boyle, Hooke, Newton, and so forth – saw a profound 'scientific revolution'. But did it also witness any significant transformation in *medicine*? Standard post-war histories of the rise of modern science – by Herbert Butterfield, A.R. Hall, C.C. Gillispie, and so forth – discern (if we except the solitary figure of Harvey) no 'medical revolution' to match the 'scientific revolution'.[4] One Harvey, in any case, does not make a summer.[5] And the synoptic histories of medicine canonical in the first half of the twentieth century typically dismissed the era from the time of Harvey through to around 1800 as a wasteland of speculative theorizing and arid rationalism; 'the lost half-century in English medicine' is the label used by William Lefanu to depict the post-1700 era.[6] Thus medicine apparently got left behind.

A revisionist historiography is, however, emerging. A recent volume of essays takes as its subject *The Medical Revolution of the Seventeenth Century*; a transformation, its editors argue, stimulated in part by the wider ferment of science itself.[7] The claim embodied in this title is certainly not unproblematic, but it is becoming more widely accepted amongst today's historians that, at least from the mid-seventeenth century, medical theory became confluent with the rapids of the scientific revolution.[8]

And rightly. For there is abundant evidence to show that leading medical thinkers in the early decades of the eighteenth century aimed to assimilate and capitalize upon the paradigms of science rendered so prestigious by Bacon, Descartes, the Royal Society, the Académie Royale des Sciences, and, above all, by Newton – aimed, in short, to bring themselves within the force field of modern natural philosophy.[9] Medical luminaries drew on the triumphs of the 'new philosophy' and the rhetoric of what Peter Gay has called 'the party of humanity'[10] to create progressive profiles for medicine itself. Alongside the mythic histories of the battles for political liberty, toleration and free thought forged by the *philosophes*, medical authors dramatized former struggles of reason against superstition, open-mindedness against dogmatism, experience against blinkered book-learning, to illustrate the adage that, in medicine too, truth was great and would prevail.[11] If the noble advances of the Hippocratics (supposedly the founding fathers of philosophical medicine) had been stifled throughout the Middle Ages by bigoted reverence for blind authority, the advent of printing, the genius of Leonardo, and the daring of Vesalius had re-kindled the investigative spirit.[12] And for many Enlightenment chroniclers of medical progress, Harvey was the ideal icon: his connections with Padua, his impeccable experimentalism – all bespoke the happy marriage of medicine and science, enshrined above all in the emblem of the heart as a pump, perfect proof that knowledge advanced when medicine and mechanical philosophy pulled together. Harvey's links with the Court told further exemplary tales of the place of patronage in the advancement of learning.[13]

Eighteenth-century medical propagandists harped on standard Enlightenment chords – the glories of Greece, revived by the Renaissance, the importance in later times of freedom, patronage, and public support – to evoke a medical past that rationalized the present and guaranteed future glories. These themes became very familiar indeed. In its article, 'Medicine', *Chambers' Cyclopaedia* traced the birth of medicine with Hippocrates and its corruption with the idolators of Galen:[14]

> At length, however, they [Galen's errors] were purged out and exploded by two different means; principally indeed by the restoration of the pure discipline of Hippocrates in France; and then also by the experiments and discoveries of chymists and anatomists; till at length the immortal Harvey overturning, by his demonstrations, the whole theory of the antients, laid a new and certain basis of the science. Since his time, Medicine is become free from the tyranny of any sect, and is improved by sure discoveries in anatomy, chymistry, physics, botany, mechanics &c. See MECHANICAL.

In short, concluded the historical part of this article, 'it appears, that the art originally consisted in the faithful collecting of observations; and that a long time after, they began to enquire and dispute, and form theories; the first part has ever continued the same; but the latter always mutable. See HYPOTHESES &c.'[15] The interpretative key evidently lay in the cross-referencing!

Above all, Enlightenment historiography named for medicine a noble mission. In North America, physicians such as

Benjamin Rush, Philadelphan signatory to the Declaration of Independence, and in France, the visionary Condorcet,[16] represented the improvement of health as essential to human emancipation – from fear, from want, from suffering. If, heretofore, the medical profession had, alas, all too often, taken a leaf out of the Church's book, pursuing a closed shop and cynically keeping the people in the dark, this 'dark age' was about to end: physic would be laid open to the people, health and humanity would march forward together.[17]

There were numerous different ways in which eighteenth-century medical thinkers expected to render their study truly scientific – or, in contemporary idiom, 'philosophical'. Observation and experiment became the watchwords of many. Baglivi, Mandeville and other early eighteenth-century polemicists advocated the bedside over the library, and experience over *a priori* rationalism, while nevertheless being careful to elevate 'philosophical' empiricism above the 'vulgar' empiricism of 'empirics', or quacks.[18]

Modern medicine tried to define a straight and narrow path between blind empiricism on the one hand and vain rationalism on the other. The jargon of traditional rational medicine, and such supposed entities as 'animal spirits' or 'black bile', was, of course, an easy target: were they not the relics of scholasticism, mere words, much bruited, never seen by the anatomist?[19] Mandeville made merry with Thomas Willis's rather similar attempts to explicate the internal workings of the body by means of mechanico-chemical analogies with stoves, stills, and circuitries of pipes and wires – what were these but the fancies of an idle brain?[20] Yet critics of rationalism themselves adopted a broadly mechanical approach to the animal economy, concentrating upon the gross anatomy of the major organs, and explaining health and disease in terms of the motions, pressures, and velocities of the fluids. Baglivi valued a mathematical approach, arguing in his *De Praxi Medica* (Lyon 1699), that 'the human body in its structure, and equally in the effects depending on this structure, operates by number, weight, and measure', and that herein lay the essence of science, for 'it operates thus by the wish of God, the highest Creator of all things, who, so that the framework of the human body should be accommodated more suitably to the capacity of the mind, seems to have sketched the most ordered series of proportions in the human body by the pen of Mathematics alone'.[21]

Amongst iatro-mechanists such as Archibald Pitcairn, the Scot who became Professor at Leiden and did much to put the Dutch university upon the medical map, sickness was resolved into hydraulic problems, health apparently depending upon the unobstructed passage of life-sustaining fluids throughout the physical system. The belief of late seventeenth-century iatro-chemists, -mathematicians and -mechanists that the human being could be represented as a machine which broke down when sick was inceasingly dismissed as crude and simplistic: doctors were not mere plumbers. All the same, Boerhaave's mechanical conceptualization of the body proved easily the most influential medical schema of the first half of the eighteenth century.[22]

It was, of course, superseded after around 1750; but the shifting of the accent from the vascular system to the nervous system (irritability, sensibility, excitability, reflex action) – in the work of Albrecht von Haller in Göttingen,[23] William Cullen,[24] John Brown (whose writings Beddoes edited),[25] and others in Scotland, and amongst the Montpellier 'material vitalists'[26] – indicates that the next generation was no less committed to the conviction that understanding the organic economy was a matter of the systematic investigation of corporeal fibres, tissues, vessels, and membranes. The pioneering by Morgagni of the theory and practice of morbid anatomy – the conviction that *post-mortem* dissections would reveal the lesions that were the seats of disease – followed naturally from the confidence in structural/functional correlations created by the mechanical outlook.[27]

Medicine was never monolithic. In Halle, Stahl repudiated the materialist reductionism implied in mechanistic theorizings, espousing an 'animism' that postulated a super-added non-mechanical soul ('anima'), acting purposively on various planes of consciousness, as the *sine qua non* of living beings.[28] The Stahlian view saw diseased conditions less as structural/functional breakdowns than as the attempt of the transcendent 'soul' to counter threats to its well-being from morbific matter. In stressing the limits of mechanism, Stahl was not alone; his doubts were echoed by Boissier de Sauvages's insistence that life required a central organizing principle.[29] And in their different ways, Bordeu in Montpellier,[30] Robert Whytt in Edinburgh,[31] and John Hunter in London,[32] equally denied the sufficiency of statics, hydraulics and mechanics for explaining animation and what may anachronistically be called homœstasis, postulating instead some form of vital force, and/or structured nervous organization that transcended the merely mechanistic.

Only a very few radical polemicists, of whom the mid-century French physician, La Mettrie, is of course, the most notorious, truly sought to reduce *l'homme* to *une machine.*[33] Even so, it is clear that eighteenth-century biomedical theory had substantially taken on board the terms and tenets posited and popularized by the new Newtonian natural philosophy. To some degree this shows the weathercock of intellectual fashion at work. But weightier matters were at stake. Confronted by the more bizarre, irrational manifestations of human behaviour – coma, convulsions, malformations, delirium, obsessions and the like – traditional opinion had commonly looked beyond, seeking explanation in Divine will or demoniacal possession, in astrological influences, or in imagination. Medical mechanists, by contrast, insisted that such phenomena could and should be comprehensively accounted for in terms of the internal organs and local operations of the body itself. The mechanistic programme thus promised to enlarge medicine's exclusive explanatory authority.[34]

Medicine sought in other ways to subject the mysteries of the organism to rational inquiry. Doctors participated in the wider quantifying quest. Seventeenth-century scientific metaphysics claimed that the real was what could be measured.[35] And, as has recently been emphasized by Ian Hacking, Lorraine Daston, Theodore Porter and others, the extension of the empire of science was furthered by the systematic reduction to intelligibility of the marvellous, the mysterious and the miraculous through fact-collection and -processing, through *l'esprit géometrique*, through application of the 'law of large numbers', and through the routine digestion of data in tables, algebraic formulae, equations, and ratios.[36] What could be enumerated could be formulated as natural laws, even if they might only be laws of probability. The empire of chance – so-called 'acts of God' – could thereby be tamed.

Falling sick had traditionally signified the arbitrariness of existence, or rather the essentially supernatural meaning of things. When mortal affliction struck ('out of the blue'), eyes had looked upwards.[37] From the mid-seventeenth century, physicians strove to extend their control over frail mortal existence, by plotting and investigating biomedical regularities. From the balancing chair of Sanctorius to the haemostatic experiments of Stephen Hales, the operations of the individual body were weighed, measured, and numbered. Collection of vital statistics led to life-tables and the calculation of differential life expectations, essential for assurance, annuities, and other actuarial computations. Bills of Mortality were increasingly published, upon which morbidity profiles could be based, and tracked against season, environment, and other variables. As Ulrich Tröhler has demonstrated, epidemic mortality ('mortality crises') became the object of investigation by army, navy and civilian doctors, especially after 1750, in the expectation that if periodicities in outbreaks of epidemic disorders such as smallpox, putrid and gaol fevers could be established, those infections might be predicted, controlled, and even prevented.[38] It is no accident that it was James Jurin, Secretary of the Royal Society as well as a prominent physician, who stated the superior benefits of smallpox inoculation in numerical terms.[39] By the close of the eighteenth century, birth and death, once those great mysterious ministers of Providence, had been reduced to a formula in the larger Malthusian ecobiology.[40]

The statistical worldview tended towards secularization:[41] a human destiny was implied whose key was not, it seemed, the decrees of Calvinist soteriology but the balance of possibilities. Numerical laws, even probabilistic laws, also entail a certain determinism: trends do not tarry for personal free-will. Attention to the masses as well as the individual thus beckoned medicine away from the bedside to the wider panorama of life chances in the context of the animal economy and the human comedy.[42]

Another initiative lay in classification. Ray, Tournefort, and, most systematically, Linnaeus, sought to enhance the power and glory of natural history by establishing a rational, coherent and organized inventory of creation, a '*systema naturae*', be it 'natural' or 'artificial'. It was obviously attractive for medicine to follow suit. In France, Boissier de Sauvages in his *Nouvelles classes des maladies* (1731), and in Scotland, William Cullen, devised particularly influential taxonomies.[43]

The rationales of such schemes partly lay in pedagogic needs: nosological charts of discrete diseases presented from the podium were easily assimilated by students, and readily applied on call. But, more significantly, and in line with Thomas

Sydenham's suggestion of a 'natural history of disease',[44] such taxonomies reinforced a growing conviction (itself marked in the shift from humoral fluidism to structural/functional solidism) that diseases truly were distinct entities, possibly localizable, possessing an ontological status perhaps analogous to chemical elements. Even more ambitiously, in his *Zoonomia*, Thomas Beddoes's friend, Erasmus Darwin, advanced a disease taxonomy – supposedly not just heuristic but natural, because grounded in physiology – predicated upon the organization of the nervous system: diseases were to be pigeon-holed as disorders of irritability, sensation, volition and association, according to the tier of the psychophysiological hierarchy they affected.[45]

No consensus clinched the objective truth or usefulness of such disease grids. Cullen's variegated disease-distribution map was challenged by John Brown's counter-insistence upon the unitary nature of disease; and Beddoes himself was deeply sceptical about the utility of medical taxonomies. Yet Brunonian medicine drew no less, in its own way, upon contemporary scientific idiom. Brown devised a disease barometer, calibrated upon a single arithmetic scale, running from zero (asthenic disorders: the *ultima thule* of under-stimulus) to 80 degrees (lethal over-stimulus), in which the mid-point represented a healthy equilibrium. The image of a single axis thus translated illness into an objective, quantifiable, tangible entity, and, in turn, made for a therapeutics that boiled down entirely into a matter of dosage size.[46]

Thus medical authors attempted to set their discipline upon a more scientific footing. The advances of the 'new philosophy' afforded many attractions. But scientific medicine was also a highly contentious shibboleth, a pawn in intra-professional rivalries, an ideological shuttlecock. After all, the relations between medical reality and medical philosophy were exceptionally problematic – large claims might be being staked for medicine's potential, to compensate for the fact that its actual state seemed the very reverse: an intellectual backwater, a sordid scandal. 'Scientific medicine' might, thus, be less a proud boast than a dream, even a wish-fulfilment. For what vexed many practitioners was that, in truth, medicine never had caught up with chemistry, or experimental physics, or even botany: high time it did.

Taking the long and broad view, we may see that – even if medicine did not achieve some sort of Newtonian 'paradigm revolution' in the eighteenth century, even if it lacked a towering genius, an icon, rather as, perhaps, Pasteur or Koch could serve for a later age – real, if somewhat unspectacular, advances occurred in medical theory and practice in eighteenth-century Britain. Some of these features may briefly be mentioned here. Anatomical and physiological expertise advanced, thanks for instance to the researches of the Hunter brothers, above all on the nervous system and the lymphatic system.[47] There were genuine improvements in operative surgery, in fields such as lithotomy and gunshot wounds; in obstetrics (to some small degree, thanks to the use of forceps); and in pharmaceutics (more widespread use of opiates as pain-killers, the popularization of digitalis for heart and dropsical conditions).[48]

Medical education undoubtedly progressed, with the founding and flourishing of the eminent Edinburgh medical school and the growing use of the London hospitals as sites for lecturing and clinical instruction.[49] Eminent teachers such as William Hunter set up private academies and anatomy schools.[50] The spread of medical information was expedited by the invention of medical journalism,[51] and the founding of groups such as the Medical Society of London.[52] Not least, medical services became more widely available. Due in part to growing affluence, the number of well-trained, competent medical practitioners operating in market-towns and country-villages steadily rose: this was the age when the 'general practitioner' became an established feature of the English landscape.[53] During the course of the century, charitable hospitals for the deserving poor were established, for the first time, in practically all major cities, as were more specialist institutions, such as lunatic asylums.[54] Dispensaries offering outpatient services often supplemented such facilities.[55] There was an extension of medical provision under the Poor Law.[56]

And in each instance, multiplier effects followed. More extensive medical provision encouraged higher degrees of competence and greater specialization. Better trained, more alert doctors led to more intelligent attempts to survey epidemiological patterns and to suggest preventive and remedial measures against sickness. There were campaigns for smallpox inoculation, hygiene, ventilation, and cleanliness, in civil society and in the armed forces.[57]

The list could be extended almost indefinitely. In ways often minor in themselves, but cumulatively significant, the medical enterprise (so we can see, with the benefit of hindsight) was becoming an integral feature of a modernizing, literate, society whose expectations were rising; and many features of Beddoes's career bear this out.[58]

It did not necessarily appear that way at the time. As has been amply documented in recent studies of Georgian public responses to medicine and the views of actual sufferers,[59] the medical scene could easily seem, on the contrary, a shambles or a scandal. Few major inroads had been made into the empire of Disease and Death.[60] With the exception of smallpox, the mortal diseases of 1700 remained at least as mortal in 1800.[61] Many of them – e.g., tuberculosis – had grown alarmingly more widespread.[62] There were more doctors in circulation, but was that an improvement? For of those, it was widely believed that many were unskilful, and that patients were more seriously jeopardized by the doctor's ministrations than by the disease. Many people thought of hospitals themselves as gateways to death. Commentators were outraged at the apparent epidemic of quackery;[63] regular doctors often complained about the continuation – spread, indeed – of ignorant self-medicating practices. Satirists, cartoonists and commentators widely portrayed medicos as pompous asses, seeking to hide their ignorance behind a veil of hard names in dead tongues, rapaciously exploiting the helplessness of the sick.[64] The internal wars amongst medicos – rivalries between physicians and surgeons, between Oxbridge-trained collegians and more plebeian practitioners with Scottish degrees – brought the profession into further disrepute.[65] Eighteenth-century literature teems with medical caricature: e.g., Dr Slop in *Tristram Shandy*.[66] It is hard to think of a single example of the physician as hero, or even as humane, in the fiction of the age.

In short, everybody could see that medicine was hardly making much real progress towards the goal of rendering life safe and healthy, and there was a widespread perception that a malaise infected the medical profession itself. Indeed, medicine lacked any eligible professional presence. The London colleges dwindled into insignificance and offered no leadership; Parliament took no interest in organizing medical provision or in central control of public health; and so, for better or worse, medicine in effect became a service supplied by individual practitioners, on an *ad hoc* basis, in the open market.[67]

This situation had virtues and vices. As perhaps compared with France, there were few official, formal, bureaucratic impediments to innovations in medical practice.[68] Competition and freedom had their merits. But there was little safeguarding of the public against medical incompetence or malpractice, and, operating in the market, practitioners had every incentive to milk the customer for all he was worth.

More high-minded and public-spirited (and one may say, more marginal) practitioners viewed this situation with distaste, alarm even. Many distinguished practitioners, particularly in the second half of the century – men such as John Haygarth, James Currie, and John Coakley Lettsom – developed a medical consciousness that went beyond the calls of improving private practice, and began to take the wider view of the health requirements of an industrializing society and the role that organized medicine should play within it.[69] It was against this background that Thomas Beddoes developed his own views of the place of medicine, past, present and future.

Notes

1. See standard surveys, such as Fielding H. Garrison, *An Introduction to the History of Medicine.*

2. C. Rosenberg, 'The Therapeutic Revolution'.

3. Bruno Latour, *The Pasteurization of France.*

4. Herbert Butterfield, *The Origins of Modern Science, 1300–1800*; A.R. Hall, *The Scientific Revolution, 1500–1800*; C.C. Gillispie, *The Edge of Objectivity*; Stephen Mason, *A History of the Sciences*; E.J. Dijksterhuis, *The Mechanisation of the World Picture.* It is highly indicative that I. Bernard Cohen, *Revolution in Science* has virtually no discussion of medicine.

5. In any case, Harvey is today often interpreted less as a modern than as a latter-day Aristotelian. See Andrew Cunningham, 'William Harvey'.

6. Fielding H. Garrison, *An Introduction to the History of Medicine,* who on p.303 speaks of the eighteenth century as the 'age of theories and systems' with a 'mania for sterile, dry-as-dust classifications of everything in nature'. By contrast the next chapter is headed, 'The Nineteenth Century: The Beginnings of Organized Advancement of Science'. See also Charles Singer, *A Short History of Medicine*; A. Castiglioni, *History of Medicine*; W.R. LeFanu, 'The Lost Half Century in English Medicine, 1700–1750'. For the best modern corrective, see W.F. Bynum, 'Health, Disease and Medical Care'.

7. Roger French and Andrew Wear (eds), *The Medical Revolution of the Seventeenth Century.*

8. See for instance Anita Guerrini, 'Isaac Newton, George Cheyne and the *Principia Medicinae*'; *idem*, 'James Keill, George Cheyne, and Newtonian Physiology, 1690–1740'; Lester S. King, *The Medical World of the Eighteenth Century*; *idem*, *The Road to Medical Enlightenment, 1650–1695*; *idem*, *The Philosophy of Medicine*; T. Brown, 'Descartes, Dualism and Psychosomatic Medicine'.

9. For the role of the Royal Society, see Roy Porter, 'The Early Royal Society and the Spread of Medical Knowledge'. For the interplay of medicine with general natural philosophy, see R.E. Schofield, *Mechanism and Materialism*. Good evidence of the Newton-worship is the number of medical writers who aped the form of the *Principia*. Boissier de Sauvages thus set out his *Dissertatio Medica de Motuum Vitalium Causa* using axioms, corollaries, lemmas, propositions and scholia, and discussing medical problems in the idiom of causes and effects, velocity, power, forces, etc. See the excellent discussion in Julian Martin, 'Sauvages's Nosology: Medical Enlightenment in Montpellier'.

10. Peter Gay, *The Party of Humanity*.

11. We lack a full account of the usable histories of medicine created by medics. For a helpful introduction for this period, see Julian Martin, 'Explaining John Freind's *History of Physick*'; and R.N. Schwab, 'The History of Medicine in Diderot's *Encyclopédie*'; *idem*, 'The Chevalier de Jaucourt, Physician and Encyclopaedist'.

12. For an assessment of Boerhaave's use of history, see Andrew Cunningham, 'Medicine to Calm the Mind'. For discussion of William Hunter's celebration of Renaissance breakthroughs, see Roy Porter, 'William Hunter: a Surgeon and a Gentleman'.

13. Robert G. Frank, *Harvey and the Oxford Physiologists*. Today we can, in a more rounded manner, see Harvey as no less an 'ancient' than a 'modern'. See Andrew Cunningham, 'William Harvey'; Andrew Wear (ed.), *William Harvey: The Circulation of the Blood and Other Writings*.

14. E. Chambers, *Cyclopaedia*, vol. 2, unpaginated, article 'MEDICINE'.

15. E. Chambers, *Cyclopaedia*, vol. 2, unpaginated, article 'MEDICINE'.

16. K. Baker, *Condorcet: From Natural Philosophy to Social Mathematics*.

17. C.J. Lawrence, 'William Buchan: Medicine Laid Open'.

18. G. Baglivi, *De Praxi Medica*; B. Mandeville, *A Treatise of the Hypochondriack and Hysterick Diseases*.

19. See V. Grosvenor Myer, 'Tristram and the Animal Spirits'.

20. K. Dewhurst, *Thomas Willis as a Physician*; Roy Porter, '"Expressing Yourself Ill": The Language of Sickness in Georgian England'.

21. G. Baglivi, *De Praxi Medica*, 29, quoted in Julian Martin, 'Sauvages's Nosology', 115. Excellent on Baglivi is S. Moravia, 'From *Homme Machine* to *Homme Sensible*'; see also H.L. Coulter, *Divided Legacy*, vol. ii, 215–20.

22. G.A. Lindeboom, *Hermann Boerhaave*, and Lester S. King, *The Medical World of the Eighteenth Century*, chs 2 and 3, offer a good conspectus on Boerhaave.

23. Karl M. Figlio, 'Theories of Perception and the Physiology of the Mind in the Late Eighteenth Century'.

24. C.J. Lawrence, 'The Nervous System and Society in the Scottish Enlightenment'; *idem*, 'Medicine as Culture'; W.F. Bynum, 'Cullen and the Study of Fevers in Britain 1760–1820'.

25. C.J. Lawrence, 'Cullen, Brown and the Poverty of Essentialism'; W.F. Bynum and Roy Porter (eds), *Brunonianism in Britain and Europe.*

26. François Duchesneau, 'Vitalism in Late Eighteenth-Century Physiology: the Cases of Bordeu, Blumenbach and John Hunter'.

27. Saul Jarcho (trans. and ed.), *The Clinical Consultations of Giambattista Morgagni*; Lester S. King, *The Medical World of the Eighteenth Century*, ch.9.

28. Johanna Geyer-Kordesch, 'Passions and the Ghost in the Machine'; *idem*, 'The Cultural Habits of Illness'; *idem*, 'Georg Ernst Stahl's Radical Pietist Medicine and its Influence in the German Enlightenment'. Another anti-mechanist view, which by its very existence demonstrates the power and prevalence of mechanism, may be found in Berkeley. See Marina Benjamin, 'Medicine, Morality and the Politics of Berkeley's Tar-water'.

29. Roger French, 'Sickness and the Soul'; Julian Martin, 'Sauvages's Nosology'.

30. Elizabeth Haigh, 'Vitalism, the Soul and Sensibility'; *idem*, 'The Vital Principle of Paul Joseph Barthez'; Karl M. Figlio, 'Theories of Perception and the Physiology of the Mind in the Late Eighteenth Century'; Theodore Brown, 'From Mechanism to Vitalism in Eighteenth Century English Physiology'.

31. R. French, *Robert Whytt, the Soul and Medicine.*

32. S.J. Cross, 'John Hunter, the Animal Economy, and Late Eighteenth Century Physiological Discourse'; June Goodfield-Toulmin, 'Some Aspects of English Physiology, 1780–1840'.

33. Ann Thomson, *Materialism and Society in the Mid-Eighteenth Century.* Ch.2 offers an excellent account of La Mettrie's medical outlook; see also Kathleen Wellman, 'Medicine as a Key to Defining Enlightenment Issues: The Case of Julien Offray de la Mettrie'.

34. For discussion of medicine and marvels, see K. Park and L. Daston, 'Unnatural Conceptions: The Study of Monsters in Sixteenth-Century France and England'; Simon Schaffer, 'Natural Philosophy'; Roy Porter, 'Monsters and Madmen in Eighteenth-Century France'.

35. E.A. Burtt, *The Metaphysical Foundations of Modern Science.*

36. And, one might add, through the technology that allowed measuring: see Simon Schaffer, 'Measuring Virtue: Eudiometry, Enlightenment and Pneumatic Medicine'; see more generally Ian Hacking, *The Taming of Chance*; Gerd Gigerenzer, Zeno Swijtink, Theodore Porter, Lorraine Daston, John Beatty, and Lorenz Kruger, *The Empire of Chance*; Tore Frängsmyr, J.L. Heilbron and Robin E. Rider (eds), *The Quantifying Spirit in the Eighteenth Century.*

37. Andrew Wear, 'Puritan Perceptions of Illness in Seventeenth-Century England'; *idem*, 'Historical and Cultural Aspects of Pain'; *idem*, 'Interfaces: Perceptions of Health and Illness in Early Modern England'; P. Curry, *Prophecy and Power. Astrology in Early*

Modern England; A.D. Farr, 'Medical Developments and Religious Belief'; Roy Porter, 'Medicine and the Decline of Magic'; *idem*, 'Medicine and Religion in Eighteenth-Century England: A Case of Conflict?'. For the medical view from the eighteenth century, see J. Haygarth, *Of the Imagination, as a Cause and as a Cure of Disorders of the Body*.

38. For Hales, see D.G.C. Allan and R.E. Schofield, *Stephen Hales*; Ulrich Tröhler, 'Quantification in British Medicine and Surgery 1750–1830'. See also P.C. Cohen, *A Calculating People*.

39. G. Miller, *The Adoption of Inoculation for Smallpox in England and France*.

40. Catherine Gallagher, 'The Body Versus the Social Body in the Works of Thomas Malthus and Henry Mayhew'.

41. The case for the eighteenth-century secularization of medicine is forcibly made in the Introduction to Andrew Cunningham and Roger French (eds), *The Medical Enlightenment of the Eighteenth Century*, which emphasizes the shifts from soul to psyche, to psychology, pneumatology, and the replacement of the priest by the physician. Compare M. Bloch, *The Royal Touch*.

42. James C. Riley, *Sickness, Recovery and Death*.

43. Knud Faber, *Nosography*; Lester S. King, *The Medical World of the Eighteenth Century*, ch.7; Julian Martin, 'Sauvages's Nosology'; Roger French, 'Sickness and the Soul'.

44. K. Dewhurst, *Dr Thomas Sydenham 1624–1689;* Andrew Cunningham, 'Thomas Sydenham'; O. Temkin, 'The Scientific Approach to Disease; Specific Entity and Individual Sickness'.

45. Roy Porter, 'Erasmus Darwin: Doctor of Evolution?'.

46. W.F. Bynum and Roy Porter (eds), *Brunonianism in Britain and Europe*.

47. W.F. Bynum and Roy Porter (eds), *William Hunter and the Eighteenth-Century Medical World*.

48. Edward Shorter, 'The Management of Normal Deliveries and the Generation of William Hunter'; J.K. Aronson, *An Account of the Foxglove and its Medicinal Uses, 1785–1985*.

49. Roy Porter, 'Medical Education in England Before the Teaching Hospital: Some Recent Revisions'; C. Lawrence, 'Medicine as Culture'; S. Lawrence, 'Science and Medicine at the London Hospitals'; *idem*, 'Entrepreneurs and Private Enterprise'.

50. W.F. Bynum and Roy Porter (eds), *William Hunter and the Eighteenth-Century Medical World*; Anne Darlington, 'The Royal Academy and its Anatomical Teachings'.

51. Roy Porter, 'Medical Journals to 1800'.

52. Thomas Hunt (ed.), *The Medical Society of London 1773–1973*.

53. I.S.L. Loudon, 'The Origins of the General Practitioner'; *idem*, 'The Nature of Provincial Medical Practice in Eighteenth-Century England'; *idem*, *Medical Care and the General Practitioner 1750–1850*.

54. Roy Porter, 'The Gift Relation: Philanthropy and Provincial Hospitals in Eighteenth-Century England'; J. Woodward, *To Do The Sick No Harm*.

55. I.S.L. Loudon, 'The Origins and Growth of the Dispensary Movement in England'.

56. E.G. Thomas, 'The Old Poor Law and Medicine'; J. Lane, 'The Provincial Practitioner and his Services to the Poor 1750–1800'.

57. U. Tröhler, 'Quantification in British Medicine and Surgery 1750–1830'.

58. This is well stated in Christopher Booth, *Doctors in Science and Society*, 202–14, 'The Development of Medical Journals in Britain'.

59. L.M. Beier, *Sufferers and Healers*; Dorothy Porter and Roy Porter, *Patient's Progress*; Roy Porter and Dorothy Porter, *In Sickness and in Health.*

60. M.J. Dobson, 'Population, Disease and Mortality in Southeast England, 1600–1800'; *idem*, 'A Chronology of Epidemic Disease and Mortality in Southeast England, 1601–1800'; G.M. Howe, *Man, Environment and Disease in Britain.*

61. J.R. Smith, *The Speckled Monster.*

62. For discussion, see below, ch.6.

63. Roy Porter, *Health for Sale.*

64. G.S. Rousseau, *Tobias Smollett*; Kate Arnold-Forster and Nigel Tallis, *The Bruising Apothecary: Images of Pharmacy and Medicine in Caricature.*

65. I. Waddington, 'The Struggle to Reform the Royal College of Physicians, 1767–1771'.

66. L. Sterne, *The Life and Opinions of Tristram Shandy.*

67. A point emphasized in Dorothy Porter and Roy Porter, *Patient's Progress.*

68. M. Ramsey, *Professional and Popular Medicine in France, 1770–1830.*

69. Christopher Booth, *Doctors in Science and Society*, 202–14; J.J. Abraham, *Lettsom.*

4

The advancement of scientific medicine

Found a philanthropic college of anti-contagionists, where all the members shall be inoculated with the virus of all known diseases. Try the experiment on a grand scale.
(Peacock, *Crochet Castle*)

Unlike most medical practitioners, Thomas Beddoes was, first and probably foremost, a natural philosopher, or as we would say today, a scientist. Had not the unpopularity of his radicalism driven him from Oxford University in 1793, he would probably have devoted his career to research and teaching in chemistry and cognate sciences such as mineralogy, albeit with medical applications in mind. It was to earn a living and support a family that he gave himself to medical practice in Bristol. The signs are that he did not find daily practice gratifying; it was clearly the Pneumatic Institute (founded 1799), and, later, the Preventive Institution (1802) that kept his enthusiasms aflame.

Beddoes was thus at heart a scientist. His ideal for medicine was to create a science of sickness. He never wavered in that unalloyed faith in science, in the scientific method, and in the benefits of the application of science to society, which he shared with such other late-Enlightenment *philosophes* as Condorcet, and, nearer home, those cronies and co-workers associated with the West Midlands Lunar Society.[1]

Inspired by his Enlightenment convictions,[2] Beddoes painted human history as a broadly progressive diorama. As naturalists and philosophers, he held the Ancients in no special esteem, being – and here he was the typical *philosophe* – apt to chide Plato for his 'mystic passages'.[3] The Christian Middle Ages appeared far worse; a slough of dogma, bigotry, and superstition (the ultimate vestige of monasticism, he believed, was the English public school).[4] Beddoes had no religious sensibility – he could, indeed, be rabidly anti-clerical, seizing every opportunity for lambasting ecclesiastical establishments and disparaging theology.

Modern times were more enlightened. Beddoes unreservedly celebrated the scientific breakthroughs of the age of Boyle, Newton, and the early Royal Society. Indeed, early in his career he republished the pioneer writings on airs and respiration of the mid-seventeenth-century Oxford natural philosopher, John Mayow, an act of homage that simultaneously staked out a pedigree for himself.[5] Mayow, Beddoes noted in his 'Introduction', 'not only discovered several elastic fluids, and the essential properties of the most active of them all', but also 'aspired to change the whole face of medicine and physiology, by the application of his wonderful discoveries to the appearances of animal nature'.[6] One might surmise that the editor was chiselling his own epitaph.

Beddoes commonly referred to his century as remarkable for philosophy, improvement and hope. He applauded the astounding advances in chemistry associated with Lavoisier, Guyton, Fourcroy, and the French School. He idolized Joseph Black.[7] And, especially in his early years, he was fervent about the shape of things to come in scientific medicine. Convinced of the applicability of pneumatics to the cure of such afflictions as consumption, he prophesied in 1793 that 'from chemistry, which is daily unfolding the profoundest secrets of nature, we can hope for a safe and efficacious remedy for one of the most frequent painful and hopeless of diseases'.[8] To the youthful Beddoes, science's future seemed dazzling. In his *Chemical Experiments and Opinions* (1790), he forecast that 'however remote medicine may at present be from such perfection', there was no reason to doubt that,[9]

> by taking advantage of various and continual accessions as they accrue to science, the same power will be acquired over living, as is at present exercised over some inanimate bodies, and that not only the cure and prevention of diseases, but the art of protracting the fairest season of life and rendering health more vigorous will one day half realise half the dream of Alchemy.

Chemistry held the key to the medical millennium.[10] 'In a future letter', he announced to Erasmus Darwin in a public epistle in 1793,[11]

> I hope to present you with a catalogue of diseases in which I have effected a cure. The power of the various elastic fluids, and of a diet and medicines calculated according to the theory, which prescribes a particular mixture of airs in any given case, will I hope soon be determined. There are many diseases in which neither patients nor practitioners have much reason to be satisfied with the state of medicine; and multitudes will, no doubt, concur with me in endeavouring to put it upon a better footing. Many circumstances indeed seem to indicate that a great revolution in this art is at hand. We owe to pneumatic chemistry the command of the elements which compose animal substances. . . . And if you do not, as I am almost sure you do not, think it absurd to suppose the organization of man equally susceptible of improvement from culture with that of various animals and vegetables, you will agree with me in entertaining hopes not only of a beneficial change in the practice of medicine, but in the constitution of human nature itself.

Beddoes's expectations for the perfectibility of science, and especially its potential for revolutionizing human life, were thus, as can be seen, underpinned by a dynamic philosophy of human nature and a psychology of learning. Far from being flawed by original sin, man was a malleable creature of infinite possibility. Human attributes were not fixed, mind was not bounded by innate ideas. Explicit in his embracing of Locke, Hartley and the British school of philosophical empiricism and physiological psychology, Beddoes set no limits upon the human capacity to respond to the stimulus of sense experience, and to progress through dynamic interaction with the environment, natural and social.[12] He was, in fact, a standard-bearer for the anti-authoritarian theory of education, pioneered by Locke, extended by Rousseau, and re-anglicized by his father-in-law, Richard Edgeworth, and his colleague, Thomas Day.[13] According to these progressives, true education and knowledge, indeed truth itself, could not be received *ex cathedra* from teachers or books.[14] It must develop from first-hand experience of the outside world, gained through the medium of the senses, and above all by doing. Knowledge was interactive. Convinced that Nature's truths were capable of discovery through the five senses, Beddoes regarded education as necessarily, in the widest sense, experimental. Experimentalism in science and medicine was thus congruent with, and guaranteed by, the elementary laws of learning and mental development. Small wonder, then, that sciences like chemistry were leaping ahead. Precisely because they hinged upon experimentation, they were epitomes of the paths to progress trodden by the human race itself – instances of ontogeny recapitulating phylogeny.

But if chemistry's triumphs glowingly attested man's ameliorative capacity, all in the garden was not rosy. In practical medicine, expectations had outrun achievements. Indeed, surveying attitudes to health held amongst even well-educated and articulate lay people, a gloomy Beddoes put a standard Enlightenment topos to a new use:[15]

> So much is there to unlearn on the present subject, that to reduce the mind to that *blank* state in which, according to Locke, it originally exists, would be no mean advantage to four out of five among those, who may take up these essays.

Thus, in stark contrast to his balance-sheet for chemistry, Beddoes despaired of the actual state of clinical medicine. It seemed barely to be progressing at all. Why was this? The explanation lay, in Beddoes's eyes, in the particular social relations stifling medicine. Clinical medicine ought to be – like chemistry – a rational practice. History-taking, diagnosis, prognosis, therapeutics – all should proceed according to the best scientific knowledge and techniques known to the open-minded clinician. Actuality was quite the opposite. Practical medicine had been perverted by the cash nexus in Britain's booming commercial economy, private practice rendered irrational by the prejudices of rich patients and of greedy, servile doctors alike.[16]

In genteel society, rank commanded authority and money talked. The spread of polite learning and accomplishments – indeed, the Enlightenment agenda of the diffusion of knowledge – ironically increased the confidence of the better sort in their own taste, opinions and skill. Under such circumstances,

Beddoes complained, patients from the *beau monde* demanded deference from doctors, interfering with proper practice.[17] In truth, such members of polite society were the very worst judges of their own ailments: fickle, dogmatic, rash:[18]

> in questions of medicine, the most obstinate belief is usually coupled with the most profound ignorance. What we hear uttered with oracular confidence, in sick apartments and at convivial meetings, over wine and round the tea-table, when it is considered as idle speculation, can only provoke a smile. But if it be regarded as, one day, destined to decide the fate of infants and of invalids, it must excite pity and horror.

Thus, on the one side of the clinical encounter was the misinformed, but influential sufferer. On the other was the doctor. Despite its patina of liberality and learning, Beddoes believed the British medical profession had sold its soul to trade. Physicians jostled to get on, get rich, and get reputations. Hence they toadied shamelessly to their patrons' prejudices, needlessly multiplying visits, persisting with therapies patently worthless, and, above all, prescribing mountains of medicaments – a device lucrative to themselves and their apothecaries. In fact, so disgracefully had they reduced the calling of physic to the profitable business of prescribing, that 'the Materia Medica . . . is now regarded as little else than a collection of stimuli, [and] medicine is become an art of administering drams'.[19] Some were furthermore involved in such exorbitant practices as the spa racket, to be discussed in a later chapter.[20] In general, Beddoes concluded, practitioners prostituted their art, to maximize gain and ingratiate themselves with the high and mighty. Mammon had seduced Aesculapius.

So while chemistry was blazing its scientific trail, medicine had been reduced to a charade, a corpus of quackery not confined to bare-faced charlatans. Beddoes vilified quacks and their inanities. As an instance of the trash the laity would swallow whole from them, he recalled that the notorious Liverpool nostrum-monger, Samuel Solomon, on being asked one day, 'what was the cause of the late bilious flux at Liverpool? *Sir,* answered he, *I can attribute it to nothing but the prodigious quantity of flies this summer. Never were so many flies. All the meat was fly-blown!*'.[21] The horror was that such balderdash – the idea that meat exposed to flies could cause dysentery – might equally have come from the lips of some fashionable regular. Beddoes boldly advocated legislation against quack medicines.

But regular medicine also had to be changed. 'Is so salutary a revolution in medicine possible?' he asked: 'I do not know; but is it not worth while to enquire?'[22] What measures, then, might be taken to improve understanding of the laws of health and disease, and promote therapeutics? Beddoes, as we have seen, staked his faith on science. But science could be advanced only by proper methods in appropriate centres. Various potential channels for the regeneration of medical knowledge seemed to him less than promising.

There is no sign, for example, that Beddoes believed that the 'decline of medicine' problem could be solved by radical restructuring of the existing chartered medical corporations.[23] He never drew up blueprints for remodelling the medical profession, never even hinted that the Royal Colleges could spearhead the purification of the art. Nor did he assign responsibility for such tasks to the state. Though noting that the establishment of a parliamentary Board of Agriculture, in the absence of a corresponding Board of Health, betrayed bizarre priorities,[24] he never looked to the battery of state-centralized medical and scientific institutions in Paris as a paradigm for progress on the near side of the Channel.[25] Beddoes was a liberal, disposed to regard the state and its corporations more as obstacles than as aids to progress.

Nor did Beddoes look to academe as the nursery of medical advance. Throughout his writings, the university is treated as an organ, at most, of medical instruction, and never of medical research. And even in their instructional role, the universities as then constituted left much to be desired. Oxbridge had slumbered.[26] And for their part, the Scottish universities, though energetic, had become doctor-factories, spewing 'half-drilled medical recruits' prematurely off the pedagogic assembly-line.[27] Edinburgh graduates were not trained to think. Moreover, because there were too many students sharing too few cadavers, anatomical skills remained imperfect – the very field of competence upon which clinical progress must depend, for it was, judged Beddoes, 'the grammar of universal medicine'. The result?[28]

> The pupils of most schools, for want of being thoroughly grounded in it, are turned loose upon the sick, not only with scanty and confused notions, but with very inadequate power of acquiring others. Hence, in many emergencies, they must act at random, and will call a disorder incurable when, to successful treatment, there was merely wanting a better introduction into the penetralia of animal nature.

Given the cardinal importance of anatomy (paired with 'universal experience', it comprised the 'two eyes of medical men'),[29] Beddoes believed, surely extrapolating from personal experience, the best prospects for its improvement lay in the metropolis, because of its wealth of hospitals, private anatomy schools – and corpses! 'London is the spot in Great Britain, and probably in the whole world, where medicine may be taught as well as cultivated to most advantage'.[30] After all, the Hunter brothers had done more for the subject than all the Edinburgh professors put together – as Beddoes knew, having studied under William Sheldon, William Hunter's successor.[31] All that was needed in the capital, he growled, was a pinch of public spirit, it being not 'easy to estimate the number of persons, whom our government has suffered to linger in misery, or to die in the flower of their days, simply from having so long neglected to found a compleat medical seminary there'.[32]

Neither state-funded institutions nor the universities would be the nodes of medical science. Nor, though this may *prima facie* sound surprising, would the hospitals. Beddoes had negative views about infirmaries. In general, he judged them unhealthy sites, breeding-grounds of disease.[33] They also, he believed, tended to be misgoverned by boards of Lords and Ladies Bountiful, besotted by their own conspicuous philanthropy, and served by idle honorary physicians and fractious surgeons.[34] 'To be a physician to an infirmary is often more a title than a function, and retained out of jealousy or pride.'[35] Nor were they patient-friendly. 'Charity' had degenerated into 'cabal'[36] and 'the most odious feelings seem sometimes to operate against the sufferers within their walls'.[37]

So had infirmaries advanced medical knowledge? 'I could name a variety of hospitals', Beddoes answered, 'which in a long course of years have furnished nothing or next to nothing to medical philosophy'.[38] He was keen to improve such institutions, advocating rotation of offices and the grassroots stimulus of greater 'public participation', to 'rouse the ingenious from their indolence, and deprive the incapable of that credit which the public ignorance suffers them to acquire, and which they abuse'.[39] But he never gave hospitals pride of place in his reform schemes. How far was he *au fait*, one wonders, with those developments in Paris, then just beginning to turn the hospital into the nerve-centre of a clinical science based upon the 'clinical gaze', pathological anatomy, and the *méthode numérique*?[40]

For promoting medical science, Beddoes seems to have favoured smaller, more informal gatherings. Fired perhaps by his sturdy, provincial plain-man's faith in self-help, and surely inspired by the example of the Lunar Society and the new Literary and Philosophical Societies, he looked to groupings of friends and peers. His preferred model for biomedical research was the Pneumatic Institute, which finally opened its doors in Clifton in 1799.[41]

As is well known, this body consisted of himself, the young Davy, who in effect became the chief researcher, and a handful of helpers, notably the Swiss-born doctor, John King, Robert Kinglake, the young Peter Mark Roget, and friends like Coleridge. The aim was to pursue laboratory research, testing developments by means of clinical trials upon poor patients. Funding came through voluntary donations from well-wishers (Joseph Banks conspicuously declined to make a contribution, excusing himself on the grounds that research into the curative properties of gases would prove to be all hot air.)[42] This informal structure, linked to energetic postal networking with fellow-workers elsewhere, appears to have appealed to Beddoes, being in tune with his vocal distrust of corporate bodies and faith in autonomy.[43] Funding was his headache. Noble lords such as the Duke of Bedford, who gave handsomely to agricultural improvement, should spare a thought, and some guineas, for health as well.[44] 'I do not for example see', Beddoes commented sardonically, 'why at some future period persons of fortune may not like to maintain as many animals for the prosecution of physiology, as they do at present for barking after hares, stags, and foxes'.[45]

Beddoes's researches through the 1790s, and the workings of the Pneumatic Institute itself, its successes and failures, are familiar enough thanks to lengthy accounts published by

Beddoes and Davy, and excellent recent historical analyses.[46] Beddoes the physician had special hopes for the curative properties of artificial airs, seeing respiration as a particularly direct form of therapeutic intervention, above all in cases of lung complaints. He recorded extensive self-experimentation, including a substantial record of 'an experiment upon myself' which consisted of putting himself on a course of oxygen for several months, 'to attempt to throw some light upon the nature of consumption'. 'I was rather fat, but during this process I fell away rapidly, my waistcoats becoming very much too large for me'.[47] His pulse quickened, he became hectic, he suffered nose-bleeds – in short, he developed the characteristic symptoms of consumption – so exactly that 'I am almost afraid lest they should be considered as imaginary or fictitious'.[48] Thanks to these experiments, he convinced himself, temporarily at least, that tuberculosis was caused by hyper-oxygenation. The increased incidence and severity of consumption was due, he rather implausibly suggested, to the fact that the moderns were breathing 'a purer air than their ancestors'.[49]

Beddoes believed the Institute's strength lay in the opportunities afforded for integrating laboratory experiments with clinical findings. It was necessary to know the sick, not just their diseases, or their corpses. One-to-one doctor-patient relationships were indispensable to medical advance. Throughout his writings he insisted upon the need for thorough medical histories. 'When I meet with invalids observant of themselves and disposed to communicate', he noted:[50]

> it has long been my custom to request a particular narrative, in writing of all the circumstances which they suppose to have any relation to their complaint. It is the only way, I believe, to get at the knowledge of the original causes of disorders when they lie any way remote.

Hence it would be at such sites as the Pneumatic Institute that medical research would thrive. Meantime, however, information routinely coming to light in other settings but scandalously neglected, could be put to far better use. Beddoes deplored the fact that the atomization of private medical practice discouraged data-pooling. Too little clinical material entered the public domain.

In life-and-death matters like clinical medicine, deliberate concealment was an abomination, and, for that reason, the arcana of quacks were insufferable. 'Secrecy, as you well know', Beddoes reminded Erasmus Darwin, 'and promises unrestrained by sense or shame, constitute the *essential character* of empiricism'.[51] It was easy, of course, he added – as so often, in his somewhat curmudgeonly way, not missing the opportunity for a barb against his brethren – for regulars to parade their virtue in this matter; and they 'should perhaps hesitate before they proclaim a man a monster for not making an unconditional surrender of a medical secret. Least of all, have we practitioners of medicine a right to act that any one more ingenious than ourselves should empty his brains into our pockets? Are *we*, forsooth, so disinterested with our pittance of skill?'[52] If an individual were to sink time and money into improving pharmaceuticals, equity demanded that his efforts, if proven successful after suitable trials, should receive public reward.

Little better than the deliberate secrecy of the charlatans, however, was the near-universal oblivion which overtook clinical case-experience. Mountains of valuable data were daily being inscribed in the minds, if not the notebooks, of doctors, and it was scandalous that most vanished without trace, rarely being systematically preserved for public consultation.[53] This 'waste of facts'[54] was shocking, for 'the grand expedient for rendering physiology popular and medicine certain, is to enlarge our stock of observations on animal nature'.[55]

Beddoes proposed two solutions. First, more energetic medical publication. He was himself a copious author, as well as being editor of *Contributions to Physical and Medical Knowledge* (1799), a compendium of medico-scientific papers written largely by his friends. Looking back, he saw it as no accident that the revival of medicine from around 1500 had followed hard on the heels of the invention of printing – the superiority of the Moderns over the Ancients was largely thanks to Gutenberg.[56]

Second, he urged more systematic collection and indexing of medical facts in convenient archives.[57] 'Why should not reports be transmitted at fixed periods from all the hospitals and medical charities in the kingdom to a central board? The regulation would prove beneficial beyond all calculation, both to patients within the house and to those out of doors'.[58] Other 'charitable establishments for the relief of the indigent sick' should also supply all possible medical information.[59] System was of the essence. 'The medical functionaries of hospitals should be required at fixed, perhaps monthly, periods to furnish an account of their respective departments, particularly noticing such phaenomena as should appear to them instructive or singular'.[60] Physicians at large should also be encouraged to submit information. A paid clerical staff should process the data, making it freely available to all – and opportunities for seminars should be afforded: the stimulus they could offer to comparison and criticism would sift good from meretricious practice. 'What would be the effect', Beddoes mused,[61]

> of register offices, not exactly for receiving votive tablets, like certain ancient temples, but in which attestations, both of the good and of the evil, that appears to be done by practitioners of medicine, should be deposited? We can never come at the just balance between regular and irregular practice, without having the accounts on both sides.

Without systematic data-storage and -retrieval, medicine would never flourish as a progressive science.[62] 'To lose a single fact may be to lose many lives. Yet ten thousand, perhaps, are lost for one that is preserved; and all for want of a system among our theatres of disease, combined with the establishment of a national bank of medical wealth, where each individual practitioner may deposit his gains of knowledge, and draw out, in return, the stock, accumulated by all his brethren'.[63]

Two new types of medical institution were proposed specifically to capitalize this 'national bank'. He advocated 'a species of dispensary, to which I have ventured to give the name of preventive medical institution'.[64] This would comprise a medical charity for the poor, obliged to harvest medical data as well as offering treatments. And, second, more energetic pathological investigation was needed. Morbid anatomy was clearly the highroad to medical progress,[65] for improvements in practical medicine were bound to be[66]

> owing to our advancing knowledge of the changes, wrought by disease. To the same are we chiefly to look for future improvements. Unless the practitioner be aware to what a disorder is tending, how can the patient expect preservative measures to be planted in the exact place between himself and danger?

Thanks to enlightened princely patronage, anatomy had taken root in Renaissance Italy. In the eighteenth century it blossomed in France. Britain, however, was in danger of lagging behind, on account of the foolish statutory and moral pressures restricting the legal supply of cadavers for dissection and leading to recourse to body-snatchers.[67] 'Is it not too absurd', he asked, 'that enquiry into the state of dead bodies should be carried on almost always in haste, and often by chance or stealth; and that mankind should absolutely not suffer an art, which concerns all alike, to acquire a juster title to their confidence?'[68] The solution? A new public forum for pathology. 'An institution for the minute examination of dead bodies and for inventing superior methods of examination might be so conducted in the metropolis as possibly to double the number of facts, useful to medicine, in twenty years'.[69]

The collection, systematization, and evaluation of data to be accomplished by his schemes would produce, Beddoes opined, an enormous boost in medical morale. It would militate against that isolation that made for complacent, conservative practice, and stimulate practitioners to pull their weight in a forward-looking community. Indeed, Beddoes suggested, one could divide up practitioners into two camps. There were the 'routine' medics, who scaled their practice down to the expectations, prejudices, and anxieties of their patients. These constituted the great majority of practitioners operating within genteel patronage networks and on the free market. By contrast, there were the vanguard of 'experimentalists', amongst whom Beddoes clearly counted himself.

As earlier emphasized, Beddoes vested great faith in laboratory experimentation, developing factitious airs and conducting vivisection to investigate physiological and pharmacological problems. Nor did he spare readers even of his popular books the gory details.[70] Did mercurial medicines cause tuberculosis? He tried out this hypothesis upon dogs, as he explained to readers of *Hygëia*:[71]

> I accordingly caused two puppies to be procured. Into the crural vein of each, at the age of about six weeks, running mercury was injected. The animals appeared not to suffer in the least for nine days. On the tenth one was killed and on examination of the lungs, tubercles were discovered in considerable number.

But for Beddoes, 'experimentalist' carried a far wider meaning. The epithet applied to any doctor promoting medicine as a progressive science, and eager to put new approaches to trial. Yet, in commending to the public the experimentalist as the model physician, Beddoes knew he was skating on thin ice. For one thing, by advocating 'experimentalism' he risked tarring himself with the brush of quackery, via the punning verbal association with 'empiricism'.[72] Relating to Erasmus Darwin his own atmospheric experiments, Beddoes confessed, 'of course, I must expect to be decried by some as a silly projector, and by others as a rapacious empiric'.[73]

In addition, Beddoes was sensitive to the fact that scientific innovation, particularly anything smacking of a speculative or hypothetical nature, or, above all, carrying a French connection, had fallen under public suspicion in the reactionary atmosphere of 'alarm' shrouding Britain from the early 1790s. He had personally become a target of lampoons in the *Anti-Jacobin Review* that hinted that his gas experiments were wild, hysterical, and orgiastic.[74] Worse still, reactionary opposition to medical experiments could speciously be clad in the attractive garb of 'humanitarianism'. 'The protective feeling of indignation against men supposed capable of sporting with life and suffering – and this alone – has set the public against experiments, as they are called, in physic'.[75] The experimental physician, Beddoes riposted, was often in reality more genuinely humane than the self-promoting philanthropist. 'The public forget that the experimentalist, from the way in which he takes up the consideration of a case, must enter into all the patient's sufferings; and probably therefore will feel for him without making a show, whereas it is ten to one but that the *routinier* makes a great show without feeling in the least'.[76]

Emotive issues – at a time when scientists were often accused of heartless cruelty to dumb animals, and hospitals were widely suspected of being experimental stations. 'Whenever the making of experiments in medicine is mentioned, people's feelings, I observe, always wax warm. This is right'.[77] But Beddoes believed he could win over the public through the testimony of history, by painting an epic canvas, in the philosophical manner, of the centuries-long struggle of the experimental against the dead hand of routine.[78] 'It would be a waste of words to speak generally of experimental philosophy. Every person of education knows what it is. Since the reign of James I experimenters have prodigiously thriven in this country . . . Boyle and Newton are names as familiar to every one as his A, B, C'; in medicine, their blessed spirit had been embodied in 'the immortal Sydenham'.[79] Beddoes invited reflection upon the special qualities of such 'experimentalists': 'they take the utmost pains to inform themselves of the previously discovered qualities of the objects to which they direct their attention. They apply their faculties coolly that they may not impose upon themselves, and report scrupulously that they may not impose upon others'.[80] In short, experimenters were 'in earnest to discover truth',[81] and the leading lights of modern medicine – 'Our Potts and Hunters' – had 'made all their improvements in defiance of routine'. Indeed, Beddoes insisted, it should be understood that 'the improvements in medicine which at this moment occupy the attention of civilized society are due to experimenting. There is the cow-pock inoculation, which had its way prepared before it by the small-pox inoculation – a practice boldly experimental. There is also affusion with cold water in fevers'.[82]

By contrast, the 'antagonists of research',[83] as Beddoes respectfully called them, were easy-going men, tailoring their practice not to truth but to demand: they were 'perfectly content with their acquisitions, provided the public be content with *them*'. Such men naturally 'spare no pains', Beddoes conceded – 'in adjusting their address and demeanour'. If experimentalists were medicine's front-line scientists, these traditionalists were its orators and thespians. 'They study a part, and rehearse to all intents and purposes as much as comedians. Their stage is the sick room. There they direct their speeches and gestures to the by-standers with as deep calculation and anxiety as the theatrical performers before a crowded audience'.[84] Bad enough if the routine doctor were just a posturing old ham. What truly damned him in Beddoes's eyes was that he made sure his patient went on 'paying and swallowing'.[85]

Mindless prejudice assumed that *routiniers* were less risky. Not so! 'If in the bills of mortality', countered Beddoes, 'there were a column for those that die of the doctor, fifty would be seen to die of his dulness for one who dies of his ingenuity'.[86] And fashion ensured that routine physic still held the citadel: 'it would be happy if there were three or four experimental doctors in repute at the west end of the town, and as many in the City' – unless, bantered Beddoes, one conceded that the routine doctor was himself rather experimental, albeit in his own way,[87] 'for example, as taking upon himself to ascertain how often a given right hand will ascend emptying phials into the stomach, and descend drawing single and double fees out of the pocket, without being wearied'.[88] 'Who but must shudder', he concluded, with an irony that became second nature, 'at the idea of the havoc that would ensue, if a tribe of Bergmans, Lavoisiers, Berthollets, and Cavendishes, were to break in among us under the guise of physician'.[89]

In short, Beddoes commended the medical experimentalist as the twin of the chemist or natural philosopher. Such medical luminaries 'may be said to enter the temple of nature with as pure a spirit of devotion as ever inspired religious votary'; they 'believe in cool dedication', 'they press forward as if they acquired new vigour at every advance. When one mode of investigation does not succeed, they lose no time in recruiting their thoughts and returning to the charge'.[90]

Thus Beddoes imagined the physician of the future as an experimental scientist, treating patients within a progressive investigative procedure. The sick would necessarily shed the interactive role they enjoyed in routine traditional practice. Yet they too in time would recognize the benefits: 'the better people are informed concerning medical practice, the less will they intermeddle', he opined, hopeful about the powers of knowledge, 'the less frequently also will they be the dupes of the crafty and inert part of the faculty, and the more readily will they cooperate with those, who, spare neither their faculties nor their credit in behalf of the sick'.[91]

This is not to imply, however, that Beddoes aimed to 'expropriate health', that is, entirely to exclude the lay public from the healing arts.[92] Rather, he wanted radically to alter the role of the sick in medical transactions. In scientific medicine, lay people ought to have no active part, because medicine must be the exclusive domain of the expert physician. Rather the public should be inducted into the science of *prevention*. Theirs, as subsequent chapters will show, was properly the field, not of medicine, but of health.[93]

Taking stock of the medical art, Beddoes faced the familiar progressive's paradox. Here was a branch of inquiry that should be leaping forward with its sister sciences: in reality stagnation prevailed. Why? Following the Baconian theory of the four idols, and drawing upon Enlightenment analyses of religion, Beddoes evoked convenient socio-psychologies of error.[94] For one thing, the talents of the human race had long been fixed upon higher things: 'an infinitely small portion of genius has hitherto been exerted in attempts to diminish the sum of our painful sensations; and the force of society has been exclusively at the disposal of Despots and Juntos, the great artificers of human evil'.[95] High time that political and military rivalry gave way to scientific, and swords were beaten into scalpels; 'there is no improvement in the condition of the World, for which we might not hope from the bloodless rivalship of nations'.[96]

But human understanding also had its own intrinsic obstacles. The primitive or untrained mind (Beddoes explained) is swayed by emotions and leaps to conclusions. A wound starts to bleed. Instinctual association of ideas makes a bystander take up a red object. The bleeding stops (in truth, quite independently), but the seeds are thereby sown for a crude theory of signatures; and, building on such imaginative flights, 'the doctrine of diseases gradually puts on a more scholastic form'.[97] Error is codified into theory, theory in turn into dogma; and overall, concluded Beddoes, 'it is wonderful with what avidity prejudices in physic as well as in religion are imbibed, and with what obstinacy they are retained by the untutored mind'. Indeed, he added, since such 'vulgar errors' arose from a universal psychology, his strictures applied equally to 'the peasant in the field and the philosopher in the closet'.[98] Thus edifices of error would ascend on the flimsiest of foundations, and only the stern criticism of facts would periodically detonate them; hence the need for central information bureaux, and for the ceaseless vigilance of scientific thinking.

Of course, the practice of physic needed mending too, so that plain truth regarding diagnoses and therapies would no longer be routinely subordinated to the whims of the paying patient and the sycophancy of the mercenary physician. The clinical encounter needed the candour of the laboratory experiment. And that, insisted Beddoes, ever the passionate didact, meant firing the rising generation with the love of truth. To which end, what better than to encourage every girl and boy to take up the most progressive science of all: chemistry?[99] Chemistry would not merely school the mind; it would serve as a prophylactic against disease itself. 'I should not be surprised', ventured the irrepressible *philosophe*, 'if, in a few years, it should become as common for persons to go about to instruct private families in chemistry, mechanics, in tangible geometry and various sorts of manufactures, as it now is in music and drawing. The lessons . . . would help to save many from falling into nervous indispositions'.[100]

Beddoes never wavered in his espousal of science and its methods. Physics and chemistry had been galvanized by their scientific revolutions; they were shooting ever forward. Medicine lagged; to remedy this, Beddoes outlined institutional changes to expedite medical research, and a reformation in doctors' attitudes – from routinism to experimentalism – to render clinical practice more scientific.

But Beddoes was well aware, as social observer and critic, that it was simplistic to attribute medicine's stagnation simply to the failure to adopt scientific principles, or to expect that such adoption would work instant revolution. Medical problems and medical progress were matters not solely of science but of society. It is to this issue that we turn.

Notes

1. See Jan Golinski, *Science as Public Culture: Chemistry in Enlightenment England.*

2. See Roy Porter, 'The Enlightenment in England'; *idem*, 'Was There a Medical Enlightenment in Eighteenth Century England?'.

3. Thomas Beddoes, *Hygëia: or Essays Moral and Medical, on the Causes Affecting the Personal State of our Middling and Affluent Classes*, 3 vols (1802–03), vol. 1, Essay iv, p.5 [future references to *Hygëia* will be given in the form 1 iv 5.]

4. Beddoes, *Hygëia*, 1 iv 7. Beddoes was a lifelong anti-cleric, inclined to characterize organized religion as a tool of mind control. See the opening pages of *Hygëia*, 1 iv 2; and Thomas Beddoes, *Extract of a Letter on Early Instruction, Particularly that of the Poor* (1792).

5. Thomas Beddoes (ed.), *Chemical Experiments and Opinions; Extracted from a Work Published in the Last Century* (1790); R. Frank, *Harvey and the Oxford Physiologists.*

6. Thomas Beddoes, *Observations on the Nature and Cure of Calculus, Sea Scurvy, Consumption, Catarrh, and Fever: Together with Conjectures upon Several Other Subjects of Physiology and Pathology* (1793), 42.

7. Stansfield, *Thomas Beddoes.*

8. Beddoes, *Observations on the Nature and Cure of Calculus*, 13.

9. T. Beddoes (ed.), *Chemical Experiments and Opinions*, 60. Beddoes quoted this in his *Letter to Erasmus Darwin*, M.D., *on a New Method of Treating Pulmonary Consumption and Some Other Diseases Hitherto Found Incurable*, 29.

10. Beddoes, *A Letter to Erasmus Darwin*, 58.

11. Beddoes, *A Letter to Erasmus Darwin*, 60. Beddoes appears to be familiar with Darwin's evolutionist leanings.

12. For the psychological background see J. Yolton, *John Locke and the Way of Ideas*; *idem*, *Thinking Matter*, Robert M. Young, 'Association of Ideas'; David Spadafora, *The Idea of Progress in Eighteeenth Century Britain*; Hiram Caton, *The Politics of Progress*.

13. D.A. Stansfield, 'Thomas Beddoes and Education'; D. Clarke, *The Ingenious Mr Edgeworth*; W.A. Campbell Stewart and W.A. McCann, *The Educational Innovators, 1750–1880*.

14. Beddoes, *Hygëia*, 1 i 37; *idem*, *Extract of a Letter on Early Instruction, Particularly that of the Poor*. Beddoes was an early advocate of rational toys.

15. Beddoes, *Hygëia*, 1 i 53.

16. For Beddoes on the shortcomings of regulars see below, ch.8.

17. For Beddoes's account of the evils of patient power see Roy Porter, 'Reforming the Patient in the Age of Reform: Thomas Beddoes and Medical Practice'; and, for wider analysis, N. Jewson, 'Medical Knowledge and the Patronage System in Eighteenth Century England'; *idem*, 'The Disappearance of the Sick Man from Medical Cosmology, 1770–1870'.

18. Beddoes, *Hygëia*, 1 i 45, 48.

19. Beddoes, *Observations on the Nature and Cure of Calculus*, viii.

20. See below, ch.7.

21. Beddoes, *Hygëia*, 1 i 50. For Beddoes's detestation of Solomon as the king of the quacks see Roy Porter, *Health for Sale*, 177–8; more generally, for hostility to quacks, see Irvine Loudon, '"The Vile Race of Quacks With Which This Country is Infested"'; R. Cooter (ed.), *Studies in the History of Alternative Medicine*.

22. Beddoes, *Observations on the Nature and Cure of Calculus*, viii.

23. For medical reform movements see I. Waddington, 'The Struggle to Reform the Royal College of Physicians, 1767–1771'; *idem*, 'General Practitioners and Consultants in Early Nineteenth Century England'; *idem*, *The Medical Profession in the Industrial Revolution*.

24. Thomas Beddoes, *Manual of Health: or, the Invalid Conducted Safely Through the Seasons* (1806), 420f.

25. M. Ramsey, *Professional and Popular Medicine in France*; D. Vess, *Medical Revolution in France*; Erwin H. Ackerknecht, *Medicine at the Paris Hospital, 1794–1848*; M. Foucault, *The Birth of the Clinic*.

26. C. Webster, 'The Medical Faculty and the Physic Garden'; John Gascoigne, *Cambridge in the Age of the Enlightenment*.

27. T. Beddoes, *A Letter to the Right Honourable Sir Joseph Banks . . . on the Causes and Removal of the Prevailing Discontents, Imperfections, and Abuses, in Medicine* (1808), 37. On Beddoes's attitudes to medical education in the universities, see Roy Porter, 'Plutus or Hygeia? Thomas Beddoes and Medical Ethics'.

28. Beddoes, *A Letter to the Right Honourable Sir Joseph Banks*, 60.

29. Beddoes, *A Letter to the Right Honourable Sir Joseph Banks*, 75.

30. Beddoes, *A Letter to the Right Honourable Sir Joseph Banks*, 77; S. Lawrence, 'Science and Medicine at the London Hospitals'; R.

Kilpatrick, '"Living in the Light": Dispensaries, Philanthropy and Medical Reform in Late-Eighteenth Century London'.

31. S.W.F. Holloway, 'Medical Education in England, 1830–1858'; on medicine in Edinburgh see C.J. Lawrence, 'Medicine as Culture'; and, more broadly, Roy Porter, 'Medical Education in England Before the Teaching Hospital'; W.F. Bynum and Roy Porter (eds), *William Hunter and the Eighteenth-Century Medical World*; S. Lawrence, 'Science and Medi- cine at the London Hospitals'; *idem*, 'Entrepreneurs and Private Enter- prise'; *idem*, 'Educating the Senses'; Anne C. Darlington, 'The Royal Academy and its Anatomical Teachings'.

32. Beddoes, *A Letter to the Right Honourable Sir Joseph Banks*, 79.

33. T. Beddoes, 'Considerations on Infirmaries', appendix 3 to J.E. Stock, *Memoirs of the Life of Thomas Beddoes*. For hospitals in Bristol, see M.E. Fissell, 'The Physic of Charity'.

34. T. Beddoes, *Contributions to Physical and Medical Knowledge* (1799), 11. For assessments of the validity of such a view see J. Woodward, *To Do The Sick No Harm*; Roy Porter, 'The Gift Relation'.

35. Beddoes, *Contributions*, 11.

36. Beddoes, *Contributions*, 25.

37. Beddoes, *A Letter to the Right Honourable Sir Joseph Banks*, 84.

38. Beddoes, *Contributions*, 13.

39. Beddoes, *Contributions*, 12. The same themes are to be found in Beddoes's *Suggestions Towards an Essential Improvement in the Medical and Surgical Departments of the Bristol Infirmary* (1798).

40. M. Foucault, *The Birth of the Clinic*; Erwin H. Ackerknecht, *Medicine at the Paris Hospital, 1794–1848.*

41. On the Pneumatic Institute, see F.F. Cartwright, 'The Association of Thomas Beddoes, M.D. with James Watt, F.R.S.'; *idem, The English Pioneers of Anaesthesia*; S. Forgan *et al.* (eds), *Science and the Sons of Genius*; L.S. Gottlieb, 'Thomas Beddoes M.D. and the Pneumatic Institution at Clifton 1798–1801'; J.E. Hodgson, 'James Sadler of Oxford, Aeronaut, Chemist, Engineer and Inventor'; T.H. Levere, 'Dr Thomas Beddoes and the Establishment of his Pneumatic Institution'; A.H. Miller, 'The Pneumatic Institution of Thomas Beddoes at Clifton'; M.R. Neve, 'The Young Humphry Davy: or John Tonkin's Lament', 1–3; *idem*, 'Natural Philosophy, Medicine and the Culture of Science in Provincial England'.

42. T.H. Levere, 'Dr Thomas Beddoes and the Establishment of his Pneumatic Institution'.

43. See M. Berman, '"Hegemony" and the Amateur Tradition in British Science'; D.M. Knight, 'Science and Professionalism in England, 1770–1830'.

44. Beddoes, *A Letter to the Right Honourable Sir Joseph Banks*, 122.

45. Beddoes, *A Letter to the Right Honourable Sir Joseph Banks*, 122.

46. F.F. Cartwright, 'The Association of Thomas Beddoes, M.D. with James Watt, F.R.S.'; T.H. Levere, 'Thomas Beddoes, The Interaction of Pneumatic and Preventative Medicine with Chemistry'; Dorothy A. Stansfield and Ronald G. Stansfield, 'Dr Thomas Beddoes and James Watt: Preparatory Work 1794–96 for the Bristol Pneumatic Institute'.

47. Beddoes, *A Letter to Erasmus Darwin*, 50–1.
48. Beddoes, *A Letter to Erasmus Darwin*, 54.
49. Beddoes, *A Letter to Erasmus Darwin*, 21.
50. Beddoes, *Hygëia*, 2 vii 9; see also A. Kleinman, *The Illness Narratives*; H. Brody, *Stories of Sickness*.
51. Beddoes, *A Letter to Erasmus Darwin*, 4.
52. Beddoes, *A Letter to the Right Honourable Sir Joseph Banks*, 92.
53. For an active contributor, Beddoes has curiously little to say about the role of medical journalism. See Roy Porter, 'Medical Journals to 1800'. In Beddoes's day, one solution to the problem of preserving and diffusing information was the medical society. See Thomas Hunt (ed.), *The Medical Society of London 1773–1973*.
54. Beddoes, *A Letter to the Right Honourable Sir Joseph Banks*, 85.
55. Beddoes, *Contributions*, 6.
56. Beddoes, *Contributions*, Introduction.
57. Beddoes, *A Letter to the Right Honourable Sir Joseph Banks*, 82.
58. Beddoes, *A Letter to the Right Honourable Sir Joseph Banks*, 83.
59. Beddoes, *Contributions*, 9.
60. Beddoes, *Contributions*, 9.
61. Beddoes, *A Letter to the Right Honourable Sir Joseph Banks*, 93.
62. Beddoes, *A Letter to the Right Honourable Sir Joseph Banks*, 83.
63. Beddoes, *A Letter to the Right Honourable Sir Joseph Banks*, 85.
64. Beddoes, *A Letter to the Right Honourable Sir Joseph Banks*, 86.
65. Thomas Beddoes, *Considerations on the Medicinal Use of Factitious Airs and on the Manner of Obtaining Them in Large Quantities*, Part I by Thomas Beddoes, Part II by James Watt, 2 parts (1794), 230.
66. Thomas Beddoes, *Researches Anatomical and Practical Concerning Fever, as Connected with Inflammation* (1807), 229.
67. Beddoes, *Researches Anatomical and Practical Concerning Fever*, 230. See also R. Richardson, *Death, Dissection and the Destitute*.
68 Beddoes, *Researches Anatomical and Practical Concerning Fever*, 230.
69. Beddoes, *Researches Anatomical and Practical Concerning Fever*, 231.
70. Beddoes, *Hygëia*, 2 vii 49.
71. Beddoes, *Hygëia*, 2 vii 49.
72. Beddoes, *A Letter to Erasmus Darwin*, 4; see Porter, *Health for Sale*, 187f.
73. Beddoes, *A Letter to Erasmus Darwin*, 4.
74. Seamus Deane, *The French Revolution and Enlightenment in England 1789–1832*; N. Garfinkle, 'Science and Religion in England, 1790–1800'.
75. T. Beddoes, *A Manual of Health*, 416.
76. Beddoes, *A Manual of Health*, 416.
77. Beddoes, *A Manual of Health*, 410.
78. Beddoes, *A Manual of Health*, 416.
79. Thomas Beddoes, *A Lecture Introductory to a Course of Popular Instruction on the Constitution and Management of the Human Body* (1797), 56.
80. Beddoes, *A Manual of Health*, 412.

81. Beddoes, *A Manual of Health*, 411.
82. Beddoes, *A Manual of Health*, 417.
83. Beddoes, *A Manual of Health*, 413.
84. Beddoes, *A Manual of Health*, 417.
85. Beddoes, *A Manual of Health*, 415.
86. Beddoes, *A Manual of Health*, 418.
87. Beddoes, *A Manual of Health*, 419.
88. Beddoes, *A Manual of Health*, 415.
89. Beddoes, *A Manual of Health*, 419.
90. Beddoes, *A Manual of Health*, 413.
91. Thomas Beddoes, *Observations on the Medical and Domestic Management of the Consumptive; on the Powers of Digitalis Purpurea; and on the Cure of Scrophula* (1801), 13.
92. The phrase comes from I. Illich, *Limits to Medicine.*
93. Roy Porter, 'Reforming the Patient. Thomas Beddoes and Medical Practice'.
94. For Enlightenment fears that Enlightenment might prove counter-productive, see Roy Porter, 'Civilization and Disease: Medical Ideology in the Enlightenment'.
95. Beddoes, *Observations on the Nature and Cure of Calculus*, iv.
96. Beddoes, *Observations on the Nature and Cure of Calculus*, iv.
97. Beddoes, *Hygëia*, 1 i 50.
98. Beddoes, *Hygëia*, 1 i 51.
99. Beddoes, *Hygëia*, 3 ix 108.
100. Beddoes, *Hygëia*, 3 ix 108.

5

The problem patient

> Opinion governs all mankind
> Like the blind leading of the blind.
> (Samuel Butler, *Miscellaneous Thoughts*)

In full-time medical practice from 1793 till his death fifteen years later, Beddoes acquired enlarged face-to-face experience with a broad band of sufferers. During those years, he produced a stream of works addressed to reforming medicine. Unlike some contemporaries who were primarily concerned with reorganizing the statutory basis of the professional superstructure, Beddoes principally sought to improve health care at the contact point of clinical relations, and, more broadly, to revitalize medicine as an engine of social improvement.

Beddoes's directives towards the poor, such as *The History of Isaac Jenkins, and of the Sickness of Sarah his Wife, and Their Three Children* (1792), are the staple admonitory pap of the times. Be thrifty, be frugal, be industrious, be regular, be clean, be hardy, be continent, be temperate, be satisfied, and, above all else, be sober, Beddoes instructed the labouring classes in a prose not wholly escaping Hannah More's egregiously patronizing anodynes.[1] Beddoes aimed to teach habits to the indigent that would strengthen their health, keep them in work, and minimize the need for doctoring. I shall further explore these somewhat stereotyped writings in Chapter Nine.

In sharp contrast, Beddoes wrote with zest, originality, and rare passion about health care amongst the polite and propertied in a series of expansive works, above all *Hygëia*,[2] published in eleven monthly instalments from 1802 to 1803 and running to some 1500 pages, and the *Manual of Health* (1807)[3]

– a terse five hundred pages – both targeted at the 'middle and more opulent classes'[4] (for they alone, Beddoes observed, had the 'necessary degree of intelligence').[5] His professed aim, in these works and elsewhere, was to expose defects in the daily practice of doctoring – the pragmatism of practitioners,[6] the cozenings of quacks,[7] and, above all, the vanities of the genteel classes themselves – in the hope that, suitably chastened, these 'intelligent' readers would mend their ways.

Improvement was in the air. The bracing breezes of freedom and criticism (so ran the familiar Enlightenment rhetoric that Beddoes himself broadcast)[8] were fanning the fires of science and practical knowledge. Should not these be yielding tangible health improvements, affording prospects of future sanative paradise? Far from it.

Beddoes's writings for the cultured layman painted sombre scenes of stagnation and sufferings. Traditional infections and fevers continued unabated, endangering even the privileged. Other fatal diseases were daily growing more rampant, above all, tuberculosis. And a host of chronic conditions, not lethal perhaps but nonetheless disfiguring, debilitating, or disabling, were also growing worse: gout, nervous maladies, scrophula, hysteria, hypochondria, chlorosis, and digestive disorders. Beddoes pointed the accusing finger at his readers: 'our chronic maladies are of our own creating'.[9]

Nor was there cause for complacency on the therapeutic front. Few successful cures had been discovered: Beddoes's own aspirations for oxygen as a panacea for lung conditions did not outlast the century. Worse, Beddoes believed that the medical profession itself had become almost terminally corrupted by the lure of lucre, and quackery was all the rage, hoodwinking even 'people who have enjoyed the most liberal education'.[10]

So why was progress proving pathological? Neither a reactionary nor a Rousseauvian, Beddoes did not believe in Original Sin, nor that the civilizing process entailed an inevitable decline and fall from some pristine natural state of health and happiness, holiness or wholeness. Hence the signs of deterioration in health and, perhaps, also in medicine, demanded explanation and rectification. The heart of the matter, Beddoes believed, lay in the triumph of commercialism and its associated *mores*, which had brought about a 'society in its complicated state'.[11]

Fundamental was the allure of affluence. 'In the social arrangements which have gradually formed themselves in Europe', he observed, 'WEALTH, the most general object of power, becomes the most general object of desire'.[12] Mercantile success was creating a restless, mobile, emulative, achiever society, new urban conveniences, domestic luxuries, greater freedom of life style ('in no country is there so large a proportion of inhabitants with such liberty of choice, as in Great Britain'),[13] and super-sophisticated manners – all accompanied by that enlarging of personal, intellectual and cultural horizons we call the Enlightenment.[14] Such developments, though broadly desirable in themselves, were, however, unsettling; and as Beddoes was anxious to show, they were, perhaps more alarmingly, further warping *attitudes* towards health, sapping abilities to cope with sickness, and sabotaging therapeutic relations between patients and practitioners.

Britain, Beddoes reflected in *Hygëia*, took pride in its liberty, its international commercial and imperial power, its riches. Yet 'Is all this solid benefit or empty boast?' This was no idle question. 'What revenue of health and comfort has our vast dominion over art and nature yielded?. . . . Has Britain wasted her vigour in the debauches of glory?' – indeed, was Britain poised to suffer, as widely prophesied by revolutionaries and reactionaries alike, an imminent 'millennium of misery'?[15]

The crux of the health problem, as Beddoes saw it, lay in the ascendancy of commodity capitalism. The manufacturing system was destroying the strength of workers, cooped up for long hours in cramped, polluted workshops, and exposed to noxious fumes, heat and dust. 'The encouragement of manufactures', he remarked, almost epigrammatically, in *Hygëia*, 'is the creation of a miserable and sickly population'.[16] But commerce was hardly less deleterious for the employing classes, all too often rendered permanently poorly by 'early confinement in compting-houses' in dark-roomed towns that 'abridged health'.[17] With his extensive West Midlands and Bristol experience, Beddoes particularly deprecated the growing habit amongst business men of 'sacrific[ing] their offspring to Moloch', by sending out their sons as merchants' clerks at far too tender an age: their fate? – to end up as stunted hypochondriacs with ruined stomachs.[18]

The bilious, however, got off lightly. For the fury of financial speculation, with its 'bubbles' and crashes, was liable to drive votaries of greed to distraction.[19] 'Go for instance to the scenes of trade at London or at Bristol', Beddoes urged the sceptical:[20]

> Among the faces that appear at high 'Change, mark those that bespeak the cares attendant upon wealth already accumulated; and those others, where an added air of wildness characterises the speculator, too much in haste to wait for the reward of regular industry, and burning to get rich by the lucky hit. Some of these men will grow mad enough to be watched at home or sent to a lunatic asylum, where they will be haunted by the fear of coming upon the parish.

But money madness destroyed the health not only of 'yuppie' speculators. What C.B. MacPherson has called the 'opportunity society'[21] created unease, anxiety, and restlessness for everyone consumed by getting and spending. Money was itself a devil. 'The universal facility of credit in this country', Beddoes alleged, was often disastrous for health, especially for 'those students who are in haste to ruin their constitution'.[22] Easy come, easy go: credit today, the Clink tomorrow.[23] '*All the world is melancholy, because all the world is in debt*' – this commonplace 'observation', Beddoes reflected, 'certainly, will not account for the whole of the melancholy among us. . . . But it will account for a great many of those unwelcome visitations, against which no gaiety of apparel is able to protect many a snowy bosom.'[24]

Less advanced societies, Beddoes suspected, might suffer worse from acute disorders; but urban affluence, with its 'over-fondness for the *good things* of life', was proving the seedbed for terrible new chronic malaises[25] that sealed 'the fate of those who consume [no less than] of those who manufacture various articles of luxury'.[26] Frankenstein-like, *homo economicus* had spawned monstrous desires and demands, above all 'a taste for more refined luxuries', with which he could not cope, psychologically or physiologically, for 'the appetite is found too strong for the mind, and for the body too'.[27]

Beddoes was thus distressed by the diseases of civilization produced by acquisitiveness. 'The English', he noted, 'are more remarkable than any other nation on the globe for the accumulation of *comforts*, and indeed unhappily we pique ourselves upon the distinction'.[28] Why 'unhappily'? While scouting the draconian solution – that the reader should 'discard his or her comforts all at once' – it was, nevertheless his duty, Beddoes insisted, to 'open a course of reflexion', thanks to which readers might 'satisfy themselves that the reliance they place on externals is vain'. They must ponder the seeming paradox that 'those who have most comforts about them, are commonly the most comfortless of all mortals',[29] for 'those who want nothing else very commonly want health'.[30]

Here lay the nub of the matter. This flourishing economic order blessed, or cursed, with multiplying wealth, and addicted to the pleasures of property and 'passive enjoyments'[31] proved, in many respects, damaging to equilibrium, both physical and mental. Fluent, like many an earlier medical moralist, in the idiom of civic humanism, Beddoes declared war on luxury.[32] But, unlike Dr George Cheyne a couple of generations previously, Beddoes did not feel the need to target his attacks against gross gluttony and habitual drunkenness.[33] For that gargantuan personal greed condemned by Cheyne had itself seemingly undergone its own civilizing process and grown less grotesque. Appetites had already become more refined – now the rage was for 'sauces as kill hunger by inches'![34] Yet, in the process, they had, in Beddoes's view, also thereby grown all the more insidious, because greed had camouflaged itself in the diplomatic fictions of politeness.

Listen to the buzz of background chat at dinner parties: '" – do let me send you some more of this mock turtle" – "another paté" – "Sir, some of the trifle", "a few slices of cucumber" – "I SHALL INSIST upon your trying this nice melon"'. Better to drop the genteel pretence, and to talk straight in bluff medical lingo about the health risks: '"shall I send you a fit of the cholic" – "do let me help you to a little bilious vomiting and purging" – "Ma'am, you cannot refuse a touch of inflammation in the bowels – It may come to a tight race between your intestines and your physician. But I hope it will stop before it gets quite to the undertaker and the sexton"'.[35]

Refinement was thus a false friend: 'every half hour, spent out of the carpeted, stuccoed, and stoved sitting room, will contribute towards the redemption of the constitution from oppressive languor and sickliness'.[36] Leisure attended and contributed to other evils – above all, paradoxically, the business of doing nothing, the vertiginous hurry of modern vacancy, growing ever more hectic and confused. '*Did you see the papers today? Have you read the new play – the new poem – the new pamphlet – the last novel?*' was all one heard nowadays, Beddoes complained. 'You cannot creditably frequent intelligent company, without being prepared to answer these questions, and the progeny that springs from them'. The consequence? 'You must needs hang your heavy head, and roll your bloodshot eyes over thousands of pages weekly. Of their contents at the week's end, you will know about as much as of a district, through which you have been whirled night and day in the mail-coach'. Sick headaches were the reward of this regime of 'quick desultory reading': 'What wonder then that we should hear complaints against the age as wanting energy of feeling and compass of mind?'.[37]

Fast living, idle business, and the itch for novelty – the two phrases on all smart-set lips were '*as soon as possible*' and '*as fast as possible!*'[38] – reinforced emulation and competition, the urge to scintillate in the eyes of the world, seeing and being seen. 'An universal interest must be taken in the condition of those about us, not less lively than the desire we see so prevalent of dazzling strangers by the splendour of an equipage or by the lights of the understanding'. People craved admiration, deplored Beddoes, wanting 'every thing about us – cloaths, tables, chairs, pictures, statues – all exquisite in their kind'; the only thing neglected in this sumptuous parade? – our health, and that of our offspring. One ought to be 'shocked at seeing, under the same roof, perfect representations of the human figure' – *viz*, paintings, ornaments, and statues – 'in contrast with the most wretched realities. . . . Parents, in short, must find and seek honour in the healthiness of their children'.[39]

This fetishism of objects was driven, of course, by that 'fawning, treacherous divinity', fashion.[40] 'The despotism of fancy' was the most degenerate, desolating despotism of all: 'what elicits . . . sparks of emulation from the eyes, and induces agitations that equally disturb the rest, of thousands of striplings and of damsels, panting for celebrity in Britain?' teased Beddoes – 'why, may be, a nosegay of artificial plumes, or a well-stiffened collar'.[41] Indeed, in the carnage of civilization, he noted, presumably glancing sidelong at Malthus's new theory of demographic checks, 'neither war nor pestilence [had] a larger share perhaps than the prevailing modes of female dress',[42] for modern taste made the sex primp and preen in diaphanous cottons, 'half naked, all evening, braving disease and death', falling sacrificial victims 'in countless numbers, at the altar of fashion'.[43]

Fashion was generally judged one of the evils of *modernity*.

Better, perhaps, to class it a vestige of savagery, a survival of the tribesman's adoration of gaudy beads. Whichever, as a blind, fetishistic force, this 'barbarous despotism of Fashion' tyrannized over commercial Britain no less than the Terror decimated revolutionary France:[44]

> Their requisitions are as imperious as those of ROBESPIERRE, and as tamely endured. A table of diseases and of deaths, directly and indirectly produced by these requisitions, with the manner of their production . . . might be inscribed; THE REVENGE OF THE SLAVES OF REFINEMENT UPON THEIR TASKMASTERS.

In fine, 'it seems impossible to live in the fret and fume of fashion without direct injury'.[45] Nor was it only in dress that fashion exercised its diabolical sway.

For the 'spoiled children of art' had now become addicted to a proliferation of artificial desires and phoney wants – in a word, 'a new world of objects'. Enter consumer man. Indeed, judged Beddoes, 'it is upon an endless variety of ephemeral appendages to himself, to his retinue, or his mansion, that the heart of him who means to figure in the beau monde, is eternally set'. Yet such 'passion' for novel acquisitions was sick – in fact, 'more tormenting' even than the miser's 'thirst' for gold. For our Timons could at least store up 'solid and durable treasure'; but all was weariness, fever, and fret in the 'mart of the mode' wherein 'every new pattern makes all the old purchases worthless' – the result being that 'what these have cost creates a sense of vexation more violent, than a large stake, lost at the gaming table'.[46]

Thus fashion whipped up storms of disappointment and exhaustion for the 'I want it now' generation.[47] People were chasing their tails. 'The multiplication of the roads to wealth unavoidably keeps pace with the multiplication of gratifications, and of those contrivances for displaying accomplishments, which wealth can command', explained Beddoes, 'for it is by profiting from the sale of these gratifications and these contrivances (that is, of the various luxuries of the table, of the toilet, of furniture, of equipage, of the fine arts) that more and more members of society grow rich'.[48] The outcome? More work, more worry, more waste, people running ever faster to stand still. Whereas 'savage life is uniform and dull', modern times had turned into a 'dance', a 'drama', an 'ever-moving picture'.[49] Yet this frenzy of fashion fast ceased to be fun. The man of mode laid waste his power and ended up jaded, suffering *ennui* and a 'want of relish'.[50] 'The cells and conventicles of gentility . . . harbour beings, upon whose wearisome uniformity the tumult of pleasure never breaks in'.[51] As a result, those addicted to 'ephemeral appendages' and the 'rage for parties', were condemned to spicing up their dreary days with such 'provocatives' as alcohol and narcotics, that merely 'render the succeeding listlessness more intolerable, and another forced orgasm more indispensable'.[52]

In short, modern *mœurs* were a health hazard, especially to the eighteenth-century forerunners of 'yuppies' and the idle rich. 'Wealth exempts from certain kinds of labour. But the wealthy stretch this privilege a great deal too far for their good. . . . If we reckon from the middle station upwards, it would, I believe, be more just to assert, that the unhealthiness of families is in the direct, than that it is in the inverse proportion, of their wealth'.[53] After all, demanded Beddoes, explaining his sanative inverse square law, 'does not gold bring with it its plagues?'[54] Those seduced by *la dolce vita* ended up 'visited by the GOUT, the DROPSY, the PALSY – by the BLUE DEVILS, and OTHER COLOURED DEVILS lodged in the system'.[55]

The quintessential vice of the times, was not, however, gross greed, gluttony, or mindless acquisitiveness. It was, in Beddoes's view, the craving of the 'haves' to distinguish themselves over and against the 'have nots', through ever more precious refinements of life style, conspicuous indices of genteel superiority.[56] Sensibility was the special escutcheon of success in this endeavour. Pursuit of refinement meant abandonment of, and contempt for, the full-blooded active habits of ordinary tradesmen and farmers. After all, was not rude health *rude*, the birthmark of the *hoi polloi*? Such snobbery, judged Beddoes, was the slippery slope to sickliness.[57]

That conspicuous opulence 'which enables a greater proportion of the British to lead a life of comfort . . . than of the people of any other country', inevitably sapped the constitution of those 'who in shrinking from every comfortless sensation that may be occasioned by the action of the elements, are obliged to lead for a great part of the year a dusky chamber life. The foot that has always rested upon a carpet will be chilled if it tread upon a marble floor. . . . at how much pains we have been to make ourselves too tender for the climate in which we live'.[58] Thus refinement was enfeebling, reducing resistance.

Delicacy, enervation ('relaxation' in the original sense of that term),[59] and nervous sickliness were thus the brood of cossetting and idleness – 'diseased sensibility is among the effects of long habituation to a high temperature in an atmosphere without motion'.[60] What particularly riled Beddoes, as he embroidered his black comedy of manners, was the fact that, being such patent proof of fortune, sickliness had become a status symbol. All manner of stuff and nonsense was being talked, he grumbled, about 'the advantages of a feeble constitution', amidst those self-same smart circles parroting the modish humbug of Rousseau's 'disparagement of art and science'.[61]

Thus, Beddoes complained, modern mamas *à la mode*, anxious to hook husbands for their daughters, invested vast effort in rendering them 'languid', lest one 'brought up with a sovereign regard to health, should not be delicate enough for the present demand'.[62] And the torture chamber *de rigueur* to render the daughters of the *nouveaux riches* Twiggy-like votaries of the Graces was the boarding school. Cold, damp, stingy with rations, and entirely without exercise facilities, the fashionable academy was guaranteed to make girls 'puny and drooping' and even terminally pretty – for the modern establishment 'has greatly contributed to multiply the genteel, linear consumptive make, now or lately so much in request'.[63] It was all good business for the 'sick trade': than proprietors of girls' schools 'medical men have few better patrons'.[64]

No surprise, then, that the medical miseries of modernity 'have been laid to social refinement as its genuine but monstrous offspring'.[65] Victims of vanity, gentlefolk cultivated an air of sensibility, but 'they find they have embraced sickliness instead of delicacy' – 'Alas for the abuse of terms', Beddoes riposted: 'do we not hear the diseased perpetually styled *delicate*? Heaven knows how many this one *catachresis*, for that is the name of the said figure of speech, may have led to become candidates for disease, or at the least seduced into self-neglect.'[66]

Top people had to be persuaded to 'practise for improvement in health'.[67] But putting a stop to their absurd affectations was, however, no easy matter. The problem lay in convincing 'the ghastly beauties of the court and city' – those for whom 'the ruddiness of the milk-maid has been a standing jest'[68] – that robustness wasn't incurably vulgar, even a 'curse'.[69] Direct means were doomed: health could not be sold to bright young things as natural or normal, still less as a duty. The answer lay, hinted the canny doctor, in fobbing it off as 'SOMEWHAT OF AN ACCOMPLISHMENT'.[70] Yet such a ruse could be but a beginning. 'The first great preservative of mental, as of bodily health, is active occupation'.[71] Unfortunately, affluence had rendered strenuous exertion frightfully uncouth in genteel circles: there was no Spectatorial or Chesterfieldian equivalent of the muscular Christianity popular in later generations.[72]

With its train of luxury, fashion, and refinement, commercial civilization thus hazarded the health of the affluent and aspirant. But equally deleterious was the *mental* culture gracing, or perhaps disgracing, Quality Steet: the Addisonian ambience of the Enlightenment. In smart circles, Beddoes chided, the *comme il faut* was to pass oneself off as tasteful, witty, brimful of news, opinions, and 'smart tripping chat' about faces and places, and all the latest. Boorish Squire Westerns were out, polite accomplishments in. So the better sort were now bingeing on booklets, rather as once they had on beefsteaks – and mental and moral indigestion were the inevitable *sequelae* of such 'cramming the head with dose after dose of heterogeneous ideas, before the first have had time to settle'.[73] Days better given over to the farm or the field were being wasted on the sofa, eyes glued to duodecimos. And what were folks the better for all this diet of instant opinions and *ersatz* stimulus? Beddoes took a very dim view of this addling of the élite's brains by light reading in the name of amusement, accomplishments and improvement: empty heads were being force-fed with trivial ideas.

Beddoes scouted the political hot-air literature of the time advanced by 'second-rate reformers'.[74] Worse by far, however, were those terrible innovations, novels, which 'render the sensibility still more diseased': 'I cordially assent to the opinion of almost all men of reflection', thundered the doctor, echoing Mrs Malaprop, that of all popular writing, 'NOVELS undoubtedly are the sort most injurious. . . . They increase indolence, the imaginary world indisposing those, who inhabit it in thought, to go abroad into the real'.[75] Here was yet another instance of fiction fostering head-in-the-clouds fantasizing: 'The common love-stories are justly regarded as abominable. They relax soul and body at once' – and, Beddoes implied, though in the most mealy-mouthed terms, they initiated teenagers into masturbation.[76]

More pernicious still, all this *belles lettristic* trash was seeping down to the young, for this was a new age of children, in which 'parents overlay their young in blind fondness'.[77] Foolish faith in genteel accomplishments had made schooling ever more bookish, and the specialist children's writer had taken up residence in Grub Street. However well-meaning such authors might be, the genre was inevitably ruinous to physical and mental health, because the young should be exercising their muscles, not their sensibilities. 'The juvenile library!', he fumed, 'with submission, I must consider it as little better than a repository of poisons. What acrimonies will it not engender in the habit! what obstructions in the body!'[78] Premature bookishness begat terrible maladies. 'The parent, when he brings a daughter or a son, "morbidly alive in every nerve", to the physician, should be candid enough to tell, how many dozens of Lilliputian volumes he devoured within a few years after he learned to read, and of how many hours' use of his limbs and sense he was daily defrauded in consequence'.[79] Ever faithful to the learn-by-doing pedagogics of his father-in-law, Beddoes insisted that education should be rendered 'less dependent upon books': otherwise the rising generation would grow up with enfeebled frames and crooked spirits.[80]

In all such ways, modern expectations, not least the march of mind, were increasing susceptibilities to sickness. Particularly disturbing was the fact that the misguided illusions of polite culture further promoted wrong-headed ideas specifically about maladies and medicine. If indiscriminate reading itself induced a certain nausea, people's noddles were also, in the process, being stuffed with simplistic, ill-digested medical maxims, culled from that very circulating-library reading. The better sort plumed themselves upon understanding their own health. Not so! 'Nothing is more fallacious than the common saying that every man of sense at forty knows what is good for his constitution'.[81]

The masses, naturally, swore by their bits and pieces of medical magic, saws, and sayings: they knew no better. But such prejudices, Beddoes insisted, were not unique to yokels. In truth, 'medical superstition is to be sought, not only in the peasant's hut, but in the city and in the palace; beside the toilette of the lady of first fashion, and in the cabinet of the philosopher – more or less disguised perhaps, but still the same in substance'. Innumerable 'vulgar errors' were bobbing about, buoyed up by the hot air of lay opinion.[82]

Moreover a 'trickle down' process was also at work, whereby, through books and gossip, professional medical arcana seeped into the public mind.[83] The trouble was that such ideas 'made their fortune in the world' only after being 'exploded' by science.[84] 'Opinions cast off, like threadbare apparel, by the faculty, go each in their turn to the public. *In the politest and best informed circles*, according to newspaper phraseology, no day probably passes without its victim to some antiquated hypothesis concerning the *purity of the blood, the acrimony of the juices, the transmigration of humours, the salubrity of the air of this or that spot*'.[85] Similarly with scrophula: just *everybody* knew that the proper thing to take was scurvy grass, convinced that this would 'attenuate the humours, purify the blood or clear the passages' – but *everybody* was wrong, for this was an obsolete recourse, resting, Beddoes assured his readers, 'upon a wrong principle'.[86]

Tea-table chit-chat was a Babel of 'erroneous domestic opinion'.[87] Some know-alls insisted it would be a mistake to let skin ulcers dry up, because, while running, they drained off peccant humours. No, others countered: dry up the offending swellings, and the trouble would go away. Both were wrong.[88] And who knows how many bizarre ideas had accreted around gout? Sufferers were, preposterously, pleased to get a bout of gout, convinced the disease protected them from more serious disorders. Totally absurd! Yet that was far from the only instance:[89]

> In questions of medicine, the most obstinate belief is usually coupled with the most profound ignorance. What we hear uttered with oracular confidence, in sick apartments and at convivial meetings, over wine and round the tea-table, when it is considered as idle speculation, can only provoke a smile. But if it be regarded as, one day, destined to decide the fate of infants and of invalids, it must excite pity and horror.

After all, Beddoes insisted, the hypochondria epidemic was proof of the power of all this insidious mental garbage. 'Some philosopher remarks, that a life would hardly suffice to enumerate the vain fantasies of mankind. No title in the list would, perhaps be more copious than that of suppositious and exaggerated diseases'.[90]

The smattering of medical pseudology picked up and passed on by the laity produced one specially unfortunate outcome. It gave the public the gall to pose as infallible oracles upon the merits of doctors themselves: patients thought they knew best. Eavesdrop upon a dialogue (Beddoes invited his readers) between a Spectator – such as himself – and a wiseacre patient, who has just rejected the services of a particular physician:[91]

> "But why?" you inquire, "has *he* any marked deficiency of common sense?"
> "Oh! As to common sense! I do not say that. But what is common sense! Is not something more wanted, where life itself is at stake?"
> "True. In that I perfectly agree. But he has had, I am told, the usual opportunities for becoming thoroughly acquainted with his profession. Did he shew any particular negligence of disposition at the time of his studies? Or has he been a dissipated man since? Have you heard anything to that effect?"
> "I cannot say I have. But this I know. For it came to me from one, who had it from a particular friend to the family. In my Lord Burroughdale's last illness, he certainly mistook a putrid for an inflammatory sore-throat; and had one ounce more of blood been taken, his lordship, I am confidently told, must have been rotten in his grave, by this time – Nay, the surgeon himself, it is whispered, hesitated about obeying the prescription for bleeding."
> "Such mistakes, sure enough, are far from pleasant."
> "Pleasant! what security have you against one as bad now? Such blunderers, really ought not – but I wonder how he ever got patients after my Lord's narrow escape".
> "Well, then, I thank you for your caution. And I believe I must call in Dr ———."
> "What, Dr ——." That notorious man of experiment, whom every body is crying out against! Did not he give iced water in a burning fever, though the whole world knows it is so hazardous to drink cold things, when hot? Nay, by carrying the prescription himself, my very next door neighbour discovered at the apothecary's, that he had ordered for his daughter arsenic, think of that! under

> a different name. Such a violent thing for such a poor puny creature as that girl! My God, and are human creatures then, not better than rats, that they are to be enticed to swallow poison in disguise!"
> "Suppose then I send to Dr F. Nothing like this can be alleged against him."
> "He! a mere Dr Slop. I'll answer for it, where something must be done without delay, you will as soon trust to your housekeeper's panada, as to Dr F.'s medicine."

'In this manner', concluded Beddoes, 'would a determined private practitioner traverse the whole list of graduates, English and Scotch. . . . His own recipe, he would still persevere in pressing as infallible'.[92]

'Private practitioner?' This, Beddoes glossed, was smart slang for a lay person who fancied his medical know-how. It was a scandalous semantic fraud – 'what a winning thing is a genteel name' – on a par with calling an assasin a 'private gentleman soldier'.[93] Such folk – and the worst of them were the women ('busy-bodies in petticoats', asided the rather misogynistic Beddoes, deploring 'the fatal authority of the sex in medicine')[94] – felt no compunction about offering medical advice, forming diagnoses, and 'prescribing to the prescriber'. Admixtures of 'self confidence and distrust of others',[95] 'these good people . . . have, strong upon them, the passion for snapping up verbal and written recipes for every current *name* of disease'. Some were 'public minded, and know no greater pleasure than in drawing from their magazine for the benefit of every acquaintance within reach of a call or a note';[96] others 'treasure up these stores for family use', taking pride in the charity that began at home: 'with what an air of satisfaction does one often hear it said; *we do such and such things within ourselves.* The phrase carries a happy union of œconomy, independence, security and mutual affection . . . what hedgehog, rolled up round, tight, and warm, in his skin, on a frosty morning, is more an object of envy than so close a family circle?'[97]

These self-styled 'private practitioners' commonly trafficked in remedies, 'circulating scraps of paper, marked with medical hieroglyphics, just as they circulate scandal, for want of other employment';[98] and many such parlour prescriptions acquired spurious sanctity from being passed down in manuscript, having been 'originally transcribed from obsolete works, published during that barbarous state of pharmacy, from which this art has been of late much reclaimed. Of course, above ninety-nine times in a hundred, practitioners of medicine have, in common use, improved formulas'. Yet further proof here that vernacular medicine was but a vestige of antiquated professional practice.[99]

This proliferation of 'drugs in hands not taught their use' was specially disgraceful.[100] 'Beware how you play the doctor's part', Beddoes warned his readers:[101] was not ignorant family dispensing the equivalent of being 'turned blindfold into a apothecary's shop and giv[ing] your child the first drug you may lay your hands upon'? Imagine the outrage, 'were a lady, educated and endowed as ladies usually are, to produce, from her pocket, a case of surgeon's instruments . . . nobody, I suppose, would submit to the hands of the operator'. For some fatuous reason, however, no one blanched at the thought of these Ladies Bountiful dishing out drugs by the dozen, 'the equally dangerous tools of the *physician*'.[102]

Drugging one's family, friends and familiars could lead to dire consequences. It had become the done thing to dose oneself with 'opiates in colds, whether as poppy syrup, or in the more fiery form of paregoric elixir, which is the base of many of our advertised cough drops. Whether disfigured, or prepared simply according to the college of physicians, the paregoric elixir has aggravated all the mischiefs which I have described as resulting from protracted colds'.[103] Not least, as Beddoes well knew from such acquaintances as Coleridge and Tom Wedgwood, the medicinal self-administration of opiates could be the slippery slope to addiction.[104]

Overall, these 'private practitioners' were guilty of a mischievous 'disposition to interfere . . . with the personal management of others'.[105] By contrast to sage regulars, they were at best like 'one rushing to the rescue in the dark'.[106] So why did they do it? Nothing but 'vanity' was 'the grand principle of this contraband trade' – such adepts having an itch 'for being admired on account of trifles'.[107]

Yet the fault did not entirely lie with the sick. For alongside the 'private practitioner', Beddoes also condemned the 'polite practitioner', for his eager and self-serving collusion in the medical pretensions of prestigious patients.[108] One gross mercenary imposition of this kind was the publication, by regulars no less than by quacks and hacks, of handbooks of kitchen medicine and 'Every Man His Own Physician' manuals. Many of these, in particular the evergreen *Domestic Medicine* (1769) by William Buchan, brazenly justified the enterprise of 'laying physic open' by trading on the Enlightenment idiom of freedom and popular rights.[109]

Beddoes, who, of course, in the political sphere, subscribed to ideals of popular education and empowerment, deemed them inapplicable to medicine. Consumers assumed a spurious medical expertise on the strength of ownership of such pestiferous volumes. They 'lay in a thick close-printed publication, purporting to be a family compendium of the practice of physic; then they place it, as shelf-companion to the bible, and hold it next in veneration to the sacred volume; the one being the fund from which they draw and dispense what is necessary to happiness in the life to come, the other in the present life'[110] – recall that Beddoes regarded religion as a phantom of the brain. 'Certain adventurers' – no names, no pack-drill, but Beddoes probably had Buchan in mind – had undoubtedly 'obtained a degree of public confidence by their endeavours to popularize the practice of medicine',[111] but, in truth, do-it-yourself domestic medicine was as nonsensical as teach-yourself shoemaking.[112] Medicine could not be picked up from the circulating library: 'one has infinitely less chance of becoming an adept in medical matters without regular study, than of becoming rich without regular industry'.[113]

Hallowed as treasuries of wisdom, such tomes were invested with unwarranted confidence: 'if there were safety in the multitude of books', Beddoes chaffed, 'parents would have little to apprehend for their progeny'.[114] In reality, however, the public mind was being stuffed with junk medical reading. 'I may, I believe', Beddoes commented, 'presume upon it as a pretty generally allowed fact, that in no line is there so large a proportion of bad hands as in that of book-making . . . none in which the wholesale vendors more frequently contrive to pass worthless articles upon the consumer'.[115] Almost by definition, no worthwhile work of domestic medicine existed – 'I doubt whether any physician of avowedly large experience . . . has ever undertaken to instruct the unprepared public, in the general knowledge and treatment of disorders'[116] – so what could a wretched book of home physic be but 'productive of disastrous consequences'?[117]

The *literati* and the *glitterati* thus made rods for their own backs. They pursued sickly life styles; they were infatuated with their own medical skills; and, by suborning their medical attendants, they sapped the salubrious powers of physic. Their error? They wanted it both ways. 'A child is ridiculed for thinking that he can eat his cake and have it. Are not grown people equally ridiculous, if they complain of ailments at the time they are doing every thing in their power to bring them on? – There can be no hope of avoiding them, unless we be filled by a *sentiment* of the value of health, at least as lively as that which animates us to the pursuit of any other temporal blessing . . . . Whoever', concluded Beddoes, one hopes with a blush, 'can inspire the public with this sentiment will do more good than the discoverer of twenty specific remedies'. Things had to change.[118]

For one thing, the public needed to learn never to mess with medicine. Every churchyard was a *memento mori* showing the 'fatal effects, arising from domestic errors'.[119] Keep off! Beddoes warned, for[120]

> Persons out of the profession incur too great a risk, and I wish they could be made to feel more responsibility, when they meddle with the administration of medicines. If they think it too much to call in a physician on every *slight* occasion, they may change this opinion in some degree, if they consider that they must be very imperfect judges concerning occasions, and that a physician, acting with success on seeming slight occasions, will render his unavailing assiduities in emergencies less frequently required. So that there will be a certain œconomy of the person, and a probable one of the purse.

But Beddoes had positive recommendations too. Rousseau may have judged the 'state of nature' the 'sole preventive for the diseases of society', but his was a wayward, wilful pessimism. There was no future in fatalism. True, curative medicine had far to go, 'the imperfection of the healing art being an incontestable fact, to which not only every bill of mortality, but every assemblage of grave-stones bears witness'.[121] But there could be no going back: 'to accelerate the progress of civilization is probably our only practical and only effectual plan'. No time for nostalgia or hand-wringing, for it.[122]

> may, at least, be worth while to consider, whether the exertion of intellect cannot repair mischiefs, which it must be allowed to have incidentally produced, and whether that havoc of health and life, with which our civilization is justly upbraided, may not be the effect of the barbarism which it still retains in its composition.

Thus progress must solve its own problems. Wisdom would not come spontaneously – 'it must, no doubt, be taught', indeed, esteemed, so that eventually 'consciousness of health, thus contemplated, will become just as much a source of pleasure as consciousness of virtue'.[123]

To secure such improvements, researchers must advance medical science, and clinicians deploy it. So what role was left for the public? Their lot lay not with 'remedying' disorders but with 'preventing' them – for 'prevention is better than cure'.[124] Assigned thus to 'preservation', not 'restoration',[125] the people thereby had an active, prophylactic, role in health, acquainting themselves with the 'diseases of society',[126] and acting to anticipate them. Yet prevention, though a 'great and precious . . . art', was 'neglected'.[127] Hence Beddoes needed to cajole his readers to pursue 'habitual well-being'.[128] Eclipsed by the morbid glamour of medicine, the meaning of health – that 'first of blessings'[129] – had wellnigh been forgotten, to say nothing of its value. Beddoes sketched another scene from clinical life:[130]

> "What is good against the head-ache, Doctor?" "Health, Madam." "Well, if you feel no interest about an old woman like me – Marianne there, you perceive, has been hacking all the afternoon. Do tell her of some little thing, that is good against a cough." "Health, Madam." "But are you resolved not to give a more satisfactory answer? In that case, I shall take the liberty of guessing why." "Poh! Mrs W. —", cried a grave person in spectacles, from behind a full hand of cards – "you should know that it is the trick of these gentlemen NEVER TO SPEAK PLAIN, as some great man says. And if they will not in a tete-a-tete, can you expect it before company?" "I am not conscious of having uttered any enigma. I am sorry for the young lady. But I must still answer – health, Sir, health, Madam".

'The lady', Beddoes concluded, 'it will appear from the preceding little fragment, belongs to the corps, from which I am ambitious to enlist recruits'.[131]

Thus the laity should not trespass upon the practitioner's healing vocation; its task was safeguarding its health. In this, doctors could help. For, while anatomizing the abuses of high society, Beddoes also sought to instruct readers in the laws of hygiene. Indispensable was increased attention to the body, its operations and hazards. Indifference and prudery had to cease.[132] 'The exterior of the human body', Beddoes reflected, 'is frequently contemplated with the highest delight and but seldom, in its healthy state, with disgust'. By contrast, there was too little 'familiarity with the internal parts', and unfortunately, thanks to common customs, 'it requires an exemption to overcome the repugnance which arises on observing them attentively for the first time'. (The stomach, confessed the tubby physician, 'in man and in animals resembling man is far from recommending itself by any elegance of appearance'.)[133]

To this end, Beddoes proposed courses of anatomical and physiological lectures for the public, women included, and also, more daringly, open clinical lectures, involving demonstrations upon volunteer 'indigent sufferers'.[134] Anticipating opposition, he explained:[135]

> I do not see why popular CLINICAL lectures should not be joined to popular anatomical lectures . . . . It must be their aim to make fully sensible the mischiefs arising from systematic irregularity; from injudicious management after exposure to the inclemencies of the weather, and from the other innumerable ordinary errors of individual conduct. They must explain the origin and conduct, much more minutely than the treatment of diseases. They may be conveniently undertaken wherever there exists an infirmary.

Such demonstrations would help secure the happiness of posterity 'in the most effectual manner'.[136] Protests would flood in, but how stupid of society to teach the 'anatomy and physiology of external prosperity', while ignoring the welfare of people's very bodies, for 'the very same reason that makes it advantageous to be able, at the shortest warning, to call before us a summary of our *pecuniary* circumstances, applies with at least equal force to our *personal* circumstances'.[137]

Of course, objections would, as ever, be raised to instruction. Touting the highly radical suggestions of setting up 'in every one of our considerable towns, lectures for a *mixed* audience, on select subjects of ANATOMY', Beddoes predicted such a proposal would be deemed un-English, impious and immodest; and[138]

> innumerable mothers, though accustomed to consider themselves but as instruments for promoting the well-being of their offspring, will feel an unconquerable repugnance against paying any sort of attention to our internal conformation, even though the means of instruction be placed ever so conveniently within their reach. That we are *fearfully* and *wonderfully made* they will piously believe, but every particular proof of this proposition they will consider as lying beyond their province.

How absurd that those itching to meddle with medicines should disdain truly to corroborate health![139]

In short, the public needed knowledge of the 'laws of their own existence' and the 'science of the human structure and functions'.[140] Thereby 'physiology will come to be considered as the domestic science *par excellence*'.[141] His writings were a step in that salutary direction, since they contained not a syllable about home-dosing or -surgery, being entirely devoted to 'applying physiological knowledge to domestic use'.[142]

Beddoes deplored the blindspots of the *glitterati* who neglected their health, but loved playing the doctor. They enthusiastically patronized Humane Societies for resuscitating the drowned – it was all a vicarious thrill; but they hardly gave a thought, or a penny, to the infinitely larger numbers of routine tuberculosis victims – 100,000 a year, he guessed.[143] Lumbered with 'legislators equally unacquainted with the subject of national health',[144] Beddoes aimed to launch a drive for 'education, in the enlarged, proper sense of that term', whose first goal would be to dispel error:[145]

> The author is certainly accumstomed to see invalids, for whom it would be happy if their whole mass of ideas –

> provided those were included that relate to the means of their recovery – could be abolished. No physician but must have found disorders less difficult to manage than patients, and both disorders and patients together, less difficult than the friends of patients.

Having thus wiped clean the slate, the health educator could at last reconstruct the patient, by laying bare the social and personal sources of sickness, and by giving instruction, not in physic, but in health. Still, it would be a Herculean task. If, at the dawn of the French Revolution, Beddoes trumpeted the imminent millennium in curative medicine, by the 1800s, when tackling health education, his tone had grown sombre, sardonic, self-mocking even. Thanks to his own and his colleagues' writings, he noted, children were beginning to enjoy a more wholesome diet: 'and so happy a change is probably an indication that strong public and private remonstrances from medical men, if they be continued half a century, will have a real influence on the condition of their fellow creatures'.[146] The millennium was thus postponed, but not cancelled.

In such self-deflating irony lies the heart of the matter. Beddoes hoped that, as a doctor, educator, writer, and *philosophe-médecin,* he could promote solutions to ill-health. He was also sufficiently self-aware that he and his ilk might be part of the problem. After all, his own profession had to shoulder responsibility for the perversions of medical practice, for it was practitioners who had condoned whatever nonsense the laity wanted to believe (illness was business), and who were profiteering from such obscene temples to Mammon as watering-places.[147] After all, the spirit of the Enlightenment – as expounded by Buchan and his followers – was for putting medicine in lay hands. After all, Beddoes was himself a compulsive writer of tomes targeted at the public. If authorship were counter-productive, if being hooked on books were a health risk, could Beddoes himself – writing books against bookishness, in a manner compounding the paradoxes of Burton and Sterne – escape censure? ('Will this be good for your worship's eyes?') Beddoes was not unaware of the ironies of his own stance.[148]

In the end, the cause of health hinged upon education. Would it work? Was it even a consistent, credible option? Everyone wanted to teach, no one to learn. 'There is a foible, even more common among the instructors of little people, than among us authors, who pretend to instruct the large public. Both take much greater pleasure in giving than in following good advice. Both would rather find faults in others than amend their own'.[149] Wasn't dishing out yet more opinions to the opinionated self-evidently self-defeating?

Beddoes devoted no fewer than a couple of hundred pages of that work of 'moral materia medica', *Hygëia*, to savaging public schools for boys (which prized 'emulation [and] confinement',[150] neither a very estimable quality) and boarding schools for girls. The negation of paedeia, such establishments ruined morals and health in one fell swoop. All the same, he never wavered from his Locke- and Hartley-derived vision of mankind as essentially educable. And that meant *all* folks – even the lower orders, and not excluding domestics ('It is by no means so impracticable as many would fain make us believe, to eradicate . . . prejudices from the minds of female attendants'.) All minds were much of a muchness – 'there is much less disparity in the power of apprehension of different ranks, than the superior members of society are willing to flatter themselves'.[151] What was crucial was the right method of teaching – 'it can very seldom be done by threats or by commands'; what maids needed were not orders, but explanations – and these could be given 'without derogation from authority'.[152] Thus, there were grounds for hope, and certainly scope for improvement.

This chapter, it goes without saying, has not been claiming that we hear, in Thomas Beddoes's sometimes almost Chekhovian texts, the authentic tones of *fin de siècle* high society, drawling out its own vulgar errors. Beddoes, it is true, may be credited with paying attention to his patients, and with having a good ear. Illness was verbalized as well as somatized, and good physicians, he believed, must first be good listeners – though it was a much-neglected skill: 'physicians have been at little pains to record the history of patients'.[153]

Even so, the voice of the sick as recorded at the Beddoesian medical cocktail party is obviously a construct, a fiction, a moral fable deftly crafted to suit his strategies. As a medical meritocrat, he needed to forge myths of lay meddlesomeness – all those ghastly petticoat doctresses! – as a foil to his new model future of unchallenged, altruistic, professional authority. Yet as a populist and radical, Beddoes was eager, while excoriating aristocratic decadence, not to silence the people but to reform them, turning them from would-be Aesculapians into devotees of Hygeia.

Notes

1. Beddoes detested Hannah More, in his correspondence with Davies Giddy calling her 'hypocritical' and a 'bigot'. Yet he had no doubt that it was the job of the educated to instruct the poor, and was paid the rather ambiguous compliment of being asked, by Miss More's supporters, for permission to reprint his tract against drunkenness, *The History of Isaac Jenkins, and of the Sickness of Sarah his Wife, and Their Three Children* (1792). This book was reissued by do-gooders many times in the nineteenth century.

2. Beddoes, *Hygëia: or Essays Moral and Medical, on the Causes Affecting the Personal State of our Middling and Affluent Classes* (1802–3).

3. Beddoes, *Manual of Health: or, the Invalid Conducted Safely Through the Seasons* (1806).

4. Beddoes, *Hygëia*, vol. 1, Essay i, p.8. [future references will appear in the form 1 i 8].

5. Beddoes, *Hygëia*, 1 i 9.

6. For Beddoes on the shortcomings of regulars see below, ch.8.

7. For Beddoes on quacks see Roy Porter, *Health for Sale*, 199–202.

8. For a characterization of the Enlightenment in England see Roy Porter, 'The Enlightenment in England'; *idem*, 'Was There a Medical Enlightenment in Eighteenth Century England?'; Seamus Deane, *The French Revolution and Enlightenment in England 1789–1832*.

9. Beddoes, *Hygëia*, 2 vii 98.

10. Beddoes, *Hygëia*, 1 i 46; T. Beddoes, *A Letter to the Right Honourable Sir Joseph Banks* (1808), 108, 97, 100; Roy Porter, 'Plutus or Hygeia?'

11. Beddoes, *Hygëia*, 1 i 9. For eighteenth-century views of the perverting effects of commerce see J.G.A. Pocock, *Virtue, Commerce and History*; John Sekora, *Luxury*. For contemporary perceptions of the relations between the march of civilization and growing threats to health see Roy Porter, 'Commerce and Disease in Eighteenth Century England'. For today's sociological debate, see also D. Miller, *Material Culture and Mass Consumption*.

12. Beddoes, *Hygëia*, 1 ii 52.

13. Beddoes, *Hygëia*, 1 iii 11.

14. For these views, see Roy Porter and Mikuláš Teich (eds), *The Enlightenment in National Context*; John Brewer and Roy Porter (eds), *Consumption and the World of Goods*; Carole Shammas, *The Pre-Industrial Consumer in England and America*; Mihaly Csikszentmihalyi and Eugene Rochberg-Halton, *The Meaning of Things*. See Beddoes, *Hygëia*, 1 iii 81: 'British consumers are supplied not only by British producers but the labourers of almost every other country administer to the sensuality or to the indolence of our richer classes'.

15. Beddoes, *Hygëia*, 1 iii 6 and 10. On rival prophecies in the 1790s, see Seamus Deane, *The French Revolution and Enlightenment in England*; C.B. Cone, *The English Jacobins*; Iain McCalman, *Radical Underworld*.

16. Beddoes, *Hygëia*, 1 iii 84. See also Thomas Beddoes, *A New Method of Treating Pulmonary Consumption* (1794); and Roy Porter, 'Consumption: Disease of the Consumer Society?'.

17. Beddoes, *A Manual of Health*, 143, 135.

18. Beddoes, *Hygëia*, 2 viii 91. Bristolians were proverbially money-grubbing: see M. Neve, 'Natural Philosophy, Medicine and the Culture of Science in Provincial England'; J. Barry, 'The Cultural Life of Bristol, 1640–1775'. On the general effects of urbanization, see Peter Borsay, *The English Urban Renaissance*; *idem* (ed.), *The Eighteenth Century Town. A Reader in English Urban History 1688–1820.*

19. Beddoes, *Hygëia*, 3 x 77.

20. Beddoes, *Hygëia*, 3 x 77.

21. This felicitious phrase is in C.B. Macpherson, *The Political Theory of Possessive Individualism.*

22. Beddoes, *Hygëia*, 1 iv 29. On credit see John Brewer, 'Commercialization and Politics'; Julian Hoppit, 'The Use and Abuse of Credit in Eighteenth-Century England'.

23. Beddoes, *Hygëia*, 1 ii 71.

24. Beddoes, *Hygëia*, 1 ii 72.

25. Beddoes, *Hygëia*, 1 ii 52.

26. Beddoes, *Hygëia*, 1 ii 58 and 60.

27. Beddoes, *Hygëia*, 1 ii 57 and 58.

28. Beddoes, *Hygëia*, 3 ix 207. Such views had earlier been expounded by George Cheyne. See the 'Introduction' by Roy Porter to G. Cheyne, *The English Malady.*

29. Beddoes, *Hygëia*, 3 ix 207.

30. Beddoes, *A Manual of Health*, 33.

31. Beddoes, *A Manual of Health*, 131.

32. See Sekora, *Luxury*.

33. On the differences between Cheyne's and Beddoes's critiques see below, ch.6.

34. Beddoes, *Hygëia*, 1 ii 64; see also Roy Porter, '"Expressing Yourself Ill"'.

35. Beddoes, *Manual*, 307. For polite fibs, see Roy Porter, '"Expressing Yourself Ill"'; S. Mennell, *All Manners of Food.*

36. Beddoes, *Hygëia*, 2 v 60.

37. Beddoes, *Hygëia*, 3 ix 163. '*Hypocrite auteur, mon semblable, mon frère*', one is tempted to respond.

38. Beddoes, *Hygëia*, 1 ii 65.

39. Beddoes, *Hygëia*, 2 vii 99. For the eighteenth-century child as consumer object and status symbol, see Linda Pollock, *Forgotten Children*; *idem, A Lasting Relationship*; J.H. Plumb, 'The New World of Children in Eighteenth-Century England'.

40. Beddoes, *Hygëia*, 1 ii 62. Compare the views of the contemporary Bath physician, J.M. Adair, *Essays on Fashionable Diseases*:

'fashion, like its companion Luxury, may be considered as one of those excrescences which are attached to national improvement' (p.1); 'As societies advance in civilization, the active mind of man, not contented with the means of satisfying our natural wants, is anxiously employed in creating artificial wants, and inventing the means of their gratification' (p.2); 'the empire of fashion has now become universal; it is not confined to the decorations of our persons, or the embellishment of our houses and equipages; but extends to our politics, morals, religion, and even in some degree to our sciences. Men and women of fashion are supereminently distinguished from those of no fashion, or whom, no-body knows' (p.2). For general discussion of changing tastes, see A. Forty, *Objects of Desire.*

41. Beddoes, *Hygëia,* 1 ii 81 and 71.
42. Beddoes, *Hygëia,* 1 iii 75 and 1 ii 71.
43. Beddoes, *Hygëia,* 1 iii 74.
44. Beddoes, *Hygëia,* 1 ii 73, 75–76.
45. Beddoes, *Hygëia,* 1 ii 70.
46. Beddoes, *Manual,* 163; *Hygëia,* 1 ii 70. For discussion of consumption and the meaning of things see N. McKendrick, John Brewer and J.H. Plumb, *The Birth of a Consumer Society*; John Brewer and Roy Porter (eds), *Consumption and the World of Goods*; Lorna Weatherill, *Consumer Behaviour and Material Culture, 1660–1760*; *idem,* 'Consumer Behaviour and Social Status in England'; *idem,* 'A Possession of One's Own'; A.O. Hirschman, *The Passions and the Interests.*
47. Beddoes, *Hygëia,* 1 ii 52.
48. Beddoes, *Hygëia,* 1 ii 53.
49. Beddoes, *Hygëia,* 1 ii 53 and 54. This acceleration of life is well conveyed by F.D. Klingender, *Art and the Industrial Revolution*; H. Jennings, *Pandaemonium.*
50. Beddoes, *Hygëia,* 1 ii 62.
51. Beddoes, *Hygëia,* 1 ii 62.
52. Beddoes, *Hygëia,* 1 ii 70. 'Orgasm' here does not have a narrowly sexual meaning. See also 1 ii 65; 1 ii 62, and for the wider problem of alcohol and addiction, the 'Introduction' by Roy Porter to Thomas Trotter, *An Essay, Medical, Philosophical and Chemical, on Drunkenness*; and Thomas Trotter, *A View of the Nervous Temperament,* 105.
53. Beddoes, *Hygëia,* 1 ii 54.
54. Beddoes, *Hygëia,* 1 ii 57.
55. Beddoes, *Hygëia,* 1 ii 57.
56. On the separation of élite and popular culture see Pierre Bourdieu, *Distinction*; J.M. Golby and A.W. Purdue, *The Civilization of the Crowd*; Peter Burke, *Popular Culture in Early Modern Europe.*
57. Janet Todd, *Sensibility.*
58. Beddoes, *A Manual of Health,* 132.
59. Roy Porter, '"Expressing Yourself Ill": The Language of Sickness in Georgian England'.
60. Beddoes, *A Manual of Health,* 134.
61. Beddoes, *A Manual of Health,* 3.
62. Beddoes, *Hygëia,* 1 iii 62.

63. Beddoes, *A Manual of Health*, 214, 233.
64. Beddoes, *Hygëia*, 1 iii 12.
65. Beddoes, *Hygëia*, 1 i 87.
66. Beddoes, *Hygëia*, 1 iii 63; *A Manual of Health*, 17.
67. Beddoes, *A Manual of Health*, 21.
68. Beddoes, *A Manual of Health*, 14.
69. Beddoes, *A Manual of Health*, 7.
70. Beddoes, *A Manual of Health*, 7.
71. Beddoes, *Hygëia*, 3 x 79.
72. B. Haley, *The Healthy Body and Victorian Culture.*
73. Beddoes, *Hygëia*, 1 iii 32.
74. Beddoes, *Hygëia*, 1 iii 78. I do not believe that the fiery radicalism that Beddoes espoused in the 1790s ever diminished. His expectations of rapid and imminent political improvement did not, however, last beyond about 1793.
75. Beddoes, *Hygëia*, 1 iii 77.
76. Beddoes, *Hygëia*, 1 iii 78. On masturbation see see P.-G. Boucé, 'Les Jeux Interdits de l'Imaginaire': E.H. Hare, 'Masturbatory Insanity'; R.H. MacDonald, 'The Frightful Consequences of Onanism'; J. Stengers and A. Van Neck, *Histoire d'une Grande Peur: La Masturbation*; L.J. Jordanova, 'The Popularisation of Medicine: Tissot on Onanism'.
77. Beddoes, *A Manual of Health*, 38; Linda Pollock, *Forgotten Children*; J.H. Plumb, 'The New World of Children in Eighteenth-Century England'.
78. Beddoes, *Hygëia* 3 ix 166.
79. Beddoes, *Hygëia*, 3 ix 167. On Edgeworth see W.A.C. Stewart and W.P. McCann, *The Educational Innovators, 1750–1880.*
80. Beddoes, *Hygëia*, 3 ix 169. D. Clarke, *The Ingenious Mr Edgeworth.*
81. Beddoes, *Hygëia*, 2 viii 54.
82. Beddoes, *Hygëia*, 2 vi 64.
83. See N. McKendrick, John Brewer and J.H. Plumb, *The Birth of a Consumer Society*; John Brewer and Roy Porter (eds), *Consumption and the World of Goods.*
84. Beddoes, *Hygëia*, 1 i 51 and 52.
85. Beddoes, *Hygëia*, 1 i 52. For lengthier discussion see Roy Porter, 'The People's Health in Georgian England'; and Dorothy Porter and Roy Porter, *Patient's Progress*, ch.11.
86. Beddoes, *Hygëia*, 2 vi 66.
87. Beddoes, *Hygëia*, 2 vi 64.
88. Beddoes, *Hygëia*, 2 vi 72.
89. Beddoes, *Hygëia*, 1 i 45; 1 i 48. For lay opinion see Dorothy Porter and Roy Porter, *Patient's Progress*, ch.3.
90. Beddoes, *Hygëia*, 1 i 58; on hypochondria see E. Fischer-Homberger, 'Hypochondriasis of the Eighteenth Century – Neurosis of the Present Century'; S. Baur, *Hypochondria.*
91. Beddoes, *Hygëia*, 1 ii 23.
92. Beddoes, *Hygëia*, 1 ii 25.
93. Beddoes, *Hygëia*, 1 ii 20. *Cf.* J.M. Adair, *Essays on Fashionable Diseases*, 73, with its condemnation of 'the empiricism of lady and gentleman doctors'.

94. T. Beddoes, *A Letter to the Right Honourable Sir Joseph Banks*, 113.

95. Beddoes, *Hygëia*, 1 ii 22; *idem*, *Rules*, 133.

96. Beddoes, *Hygëia*, 1 ii 16.

97. Beddoes, *Hygëia*, 1 ii 17; see also Dorothy Porter and Roy Porter, *Patient's Progress*, ch.3.

98. Beddoes, *Hygëia*, 1 ii 29.

99. Beddoes, *Hygëia*, 1 ii 29.

100. Beddoes, *Hygëia*, 1 ii 22.

101. Beddoes, *Hygëia*, 2 vii 94.

102. Beddoes, *Hygëia*, 1 ii 40 and 38.

103. Beddoes, *A Manual of Health*, 197.

104. Roy Porter and Dorothy Porter, *In Sickness and in Health*, ch.11; V. Berridge and G. Edwards, *Opium and the People*; N. Fruman, *Coleridge, the Damaged Archangel*.

105. Beddoes, *Hygëia*, 1 ii 40.

106. Beddoes, *Hygëia*, 1 ii 46.

107. Beddoes, *Hygëia*, 1 ii 27.

108. Beddoes, *A Manual of Health*, 358; for further discussion, see Roy Porter, 'Plutus or Hygeia? Thomas Beddoes and Medical Ethics'.

109. Roy Porter, 'The Patient in Eighteenth Century England'; *idem*, 'The People's Health in Georgian England'; Paul Slack, 'Medical Practitioners and Treasures of Poor Men'; Ginnie Smith, 'Prescribing the Rules of Health: Self-Help and Advice in the Late Eighteenth-Century England'.

110. Beddoes, *Hygëia*, 1 ii 18.

111. Beddoes, *Hygëia*, 1 ii 33.

112. Beddoes, *Hygëia*, 1 ii 19; C.J. Lawrence, 'William Buchan: Medicine Laid Open'; C. Rosenberg, 'Medical Text and Medical Context'.

113. Beddoes, *Hygëia*, 1 ii 15. For Beddoes's extremely demanding notion of a proper medical education, see below ch.8.

114. Beddoes, *Hygëia*, 2 v 6.

115. Beddoes, *Hygëia*, 1 ii 18.

116. Beddoes, *Hygëia*, 1 ii 31.

117. Beddoes, *Hygëia*, 1 ii 19.

118. Beddoes, *Hygëia*, 1 iv 97.

119. Beddoes, *Hygëia*, 3 xi 92.

120. Beddoes, *A Manual of Health*, 193.

121. Beddoes, *Hygëia*, 1 ii 33.

122. Beddoes, *Hygëia*, 1 i 89.

123. Beddoes, *Hygëia*, 1 i 84.

124. Beddoes, *Manual*, 200.

125. Beddoes, *A Manual of Health*, 32.

126. Beddoes, *Hygëia*, 1 i 88.

127. Beddoes, *Hygëia*, 3 xi 86.

128. Beddoes, *Hygëia*, 1 i 16.

129. Beddoes, *Hygëia*, 1 i 16.

130. Beddoes, *Hygëia*, 1 ii 14 and 15. Beddoes's emphasis upon the positive importance of health squares well with the discussion in Michel Foucault, *The History of Sexuality: Introduction*, except, of course,

that Beddoes claimed that the bourgeoisie neglected their health whereas Foucault's argument is that they seriously cultivated it.

131. Beddoes, *Hygëia*, 1 ii 15.

132. Beddoes, *Hygëia*, 2 viii 6.

133. Beddoes, *Hygëia*, 2 viii 7; see Roy Porter, 'Bodies of Thought: Thoughts about the Body in Eighteenth Century England'; Hillel Schwartz, *Never Satisfied.*

134. Beddoes, *Hygëia*, 2 vi 92.

135. Beddoes, *Hygëia*, 2 vi 91.

136. Beddoes, *Hygëia*, 2 vi 91.

137. Beddoes, *Hygëia*, 1 i 29.

138. Beddoes, *Hygëia*, 1 i 37 and 39.

139. Beddoes, *Hygëia*, 1 i 40. Beddoes gave such lectures, which were apparently a success.

140. Beddoes, *Hygëia*, 1 i 34; 36.

141. Beddoes, *Hygëia*, 2 vi 48.

142. Beddoes, *Hygëia*, 1 i 54.

143. Beddoes, *Hygëia*, 3 xi 3.

144. Beddoes, *Hygëia*, 1 ii 81.

145. Beddoes, *Hygëia*, 1 i 53.

146. Beddoes, *Hygëia*, 1 iii 28.

147. See below ch.7.

148. L. Sterne, *The Life and Opinions of Tristram Shandy*, 265. See also Roy Porter, 'Against the Spleen'.

149. Beddoes, *Hygëia*, 1 iii 15.

150. Beddoes, *Hygëia*, 1 iii 59.

151. Beddoes, *Hygëia*, 2 v 16.

152. Beddoes, *Hygëia*, 2 v 16. For the psychological background see J. Yolton, *John Locke and the Way of Ideas*; *idem*, *Thinking Matter*; Robert M. Young, 'Association of Ideas'.

153. Beddoes, *Hygëia*, 2 viii 127; H. Brody, *Stories of Sickness*; A. Kleinman, *The Illness Narratives.*

6

Enlightenment and pathology

How can we be cheerful when our nerves are shattered?

(Peacock, *Nightmare Abbey*)

Beddoes conjured up, I have been arguing, a theatre of health in which the life styles of the giddy and the gay were undermining well-being. Patient patronage was exacerbating the problem, by neutralizing the powers of medicine. I wish now to show that Beddoes's critique of the health threats of enlightened living in commercial society expressed a widely shared medical diagnosis of the pitfalls of progress. I shall examine two themes in particular; first, 'nervousness', with its associated notion of addiction; and then the problematization of 'consumption'.

In a major discussion in his 'The Enlightenment as Medicine and as Cure', developed in his *The Enlightenment. An Interpretation*, Volume 2, Chapter 1, 'The Recovery of Nerve', Peter Gay painted a sunny picture of medical progress.[1] At the dawn of the Enlightenment, according to Gay, humoralism was still hegemonic, and medical practice hidebound.[2] But things were changing. Inspired by Bacon, Descartes, Locke, and, above all, Newton, medicine began to swim in the scientific mainstream. 'By the time of Locke. . . . Medicine, it seemed, was transforming itself from a medieval mystery . . . into a thoroughly philosophical science', through the abandoning of tradition, authority and rationalism, the pioneering of observation, and the embracing of cognitive pluralism.[3] Boerhaave was particularly significant. In time, 'all this stress on experience, on clinical study and experimentation, revolutionized medicine'.[4]

Medical progress boosted Enlightenment optimism. If 'the most powerful agent in the recovery of nerve was obviously the scientific revolution',[5] medical improvements also played a key part, for in many fields, the 'results were impressive'.[6] With the success of smallpox inoculation, 'the recovery of nerve was visible on men's very faces'.[7] Indeed, 'for observant men in the eighteenth century, *philosophes* as well as others, the most tangible cause for confidence lay in medicine', 'the most highly visible and the most heartening index of general improvement'.[8]

Philosophes, of course, made merry with physicians' follies. Yet medical advances were 'the object of their admiration'.[9] Not surprisingly, therefore, they liked to cast themselves as doctors to society. The *ancien régime* was sick: mentally (the diseases of poverty, hunger, violence), and psychologically (ignorance and folly, superstition and enthusiasm). *Philosophes*-physicians were needed to diagnose social pathology and prescribe reformed regimens. 'If the philosophes were missionaries, they were medical missionaries'.[10]

To our eyes, Gay's late-'60s account of eighteenth-century medical progress looks uncritically euphoric. Research and rethinking have queried whether Boerhaavian 'scientific medicine' truly advanced understanding of disease or paid clinical dividends (Rosenberg has postponed the 'therapeutic revolution' to the nineteenth century, Shorter and others to the twentieth).[11] Gay's suggestion that medicine contributed to the population explosion would no longer be accepted by demographers, who stress not a falling death rate but a rising birth rate, attributing this to earlier marriage.[12]

Even so, today's medical historians would not be unsympathetic to Gay's more general case that Enlightenment ideologies shaped attitudes and practice towards illness and even, perhaps, contributed towards healthy living. Religious and secular philanthropy extended the range of medical facilities through the founding of hospitals, dispensaries, lying-in charities, poor-law services, etc. McKeown's damnation of eighteenth-century hospitals as 'gateways to death' – a view which, oddly, still haunts Gay's account – is now discounted; and if the Enlightenment infirmary wrought no miracle cures, it probably, as Risse has suggested, did some small-scale good.[13] Enlightenment outlooks also filtered down into other areas of health, including childbirth, child-rearing,[14] and deathbeds.[15]

How far, however, can we accept Gay's main reading, his

linkage of the *philosophes'* optimism ('recovery of nerve') with their medical confidence? Regarding the past as a sea of suffering, many *Aufklärer* looked to medicine as one of many promising technologies of hope to build a better future. Was it not the job of medical science and practice to turn sick populations healthy?

Mankind had slowly progressed (so ran Enlightenment speculative 'conjectural histories') through a series of socio-economic stages rising from hunting, through pastoralism and feudalism, to commercial capitalism. In this process, the growing division of labour had multiplied wealth. Gains in political liberty had created free markets which liberated human energies. Intellectual and religious toleration sped the advancement of knowledge, science, and technology, for 'the relief of man's estate', as Francis Bacon put it. Progress, apologists proclaimed, was realising man's right to happiness. Must it not also be ameliorating health? After all, the environment was being tamed and famine conquered, anatomy and physiology were beneficiaries of the 'new philosophy', the Old World and the New were yielding wonder drugs such as opium and 'Peruvian bark' (quinine), and smallpox inoculation was spreading.[16]

Many *philosophes* conjured up noble visions of medical progress, none more eloquently than Condorcet, whose *Esquisse* (1794) forecast that scientific medicine in a rational society would conquer disease and even death itself.[17] These prophecies echoed in Britain. 'Who shall undertake', Thomas Beddoes himself wondered, 'to tell the fortune of the coming generations?', before proclaiming, in his *Letter to Erasmus Darwin* (1793), that 'a great revolution in this art is at hand', thanks to the imminent great leap forward in pneumatic chemistry.[18]

Beddoes's contemporary, William Buchan, was similarly convinced that the business of Enlightenment was to improve *salus populi* through 'the progress of knowledge'. The right to health was fundamental to all the other rights of man. Ignorance, he announced, echoing Benjamin Rush,[19] was the root of sickness:[20]

> While men are kept in the dark, and told that they are not to use their own understanding, in matters that concern their health, they will be the dupes of designing knaves.

Enlightened peoples, by contrast, would treasure their health and value good medicine. In any case, Buchan stressed, in many maladies, intelligent self-help was sufficient: bed-rest, wholesome diet, attention to the non-naturals, hygiene, cleanliness, and not least, trust in the healing powers of Nature. Even with sexually transmitted diseases, 'in nineteen out of twenty cases, where this disease occurs, the patient may be his own physician'.[21]

Thus *philosophes* and doctors widely foretold a brighter medical future. Yet a darker vision was also looming:[22] might the progress of civilization be leading not to the promised land of salubrity but to the sickbed? Might the march of medicine not be rectifying, but exacerbating, this situation? To toy with Gay's terms, Enlightenment, far from offering 'medicine' and 'cure' was, many feared, itself the 'disease', or at least one of its co-factors.

Anybody could see, for one thing, that disease had neither been vanquished nor had withered away. Many statesmen and commentators believed the great nations were actually becoming depeopled – a sure sign of both biomedical and socio-moral crisis. And the English were winning notoriety for a range of nervous, hysterical and mental disorders, ensuring the island's reputation as a suicide black-spot.[23]

Peace, prosperity, politeness, and the advancement of knowledge should surely have led to betterment. It was thus a puzzle if wealth were seemingly at odds with health. So what *were* the relations between disease and commercial society?

The solution, theorized by *philosophes* and physicians alike, was that civilization might itself be the provocation of sickness. In primeval times, it was claimed, needs had been few, exercise plentiful, food plain and wholesome. Necessity made men hardy, and hardiness inured them to pain. 'True health and vigour of body', argued Beddoes's contemporary, the Scottish physician, Thomas Trotter, 'are the inheritance of the untutored savage'.[24] Disease, by contrast, was the child of 'excess' or 'debauch'.

Thus the civilising process itself begat deleterious life-styles. Luxury, thundered critics, corrupted private morals, public virtue, and, not least, physical stamina. The cancer seemed to be spreading. In the 1730s, George Cheyne gauged that a third of all disorders were nervous.[25] Seventy years later, Thomas Trotter guessed they constituted 'two thirds of the whole, with which civilized society is afflicted'.[26] For disease, ominously like fashion, obeyed the 'top down' effect: 'we shall find', warned

Trotter, that nervous ailments are no longer confined to the better ranks in life, but rapidly extending to the poorer classes'.[27]

It is worth examining in greater depth the meta-history of health formulated by George Cheyne, the Scottish physician whose impeccable Enlightenment credentials included espousal of the iatro-mechanistic doctrines of the Leiden-Edinburgh school and adulatory popularization of Newtonian natural philosophy.[28] Cheyne was convinced that as England rose to riches, the people's health was sinking, succumbing to that clutch of chronic, constitutional conditions he dubbed 'The English Malady'.[29]

Why so? 'If we suppose, as we must, that Mankind at first, were Healthy, and Sound', explained the pious Scotsman, it followed that 'none but Men themselves' could have initiated this plague of disorders.[30] Cheyne span a primitivist tale: 'when Mankind was simple, plain, honest and frugal, there were few or no diseases. Temperance, Exercise, Hunting, Labour, and Industry kept the Juices Sweet and the Solids brac'd.'[31] As early as the Ancients, however, the rot had set in. Conventional wisdom had praised the Greeks for inventing medicine. But had they not been *driven* to it by the proliferation of sickness provoked by their softened, sedentary, urban existence?[32]

> The antient *Greeks*, while they lived in their Simplicity and Virtue were Healthy, Strong and Valiant: But afterwards, in Proportion as they advanced in Learning, and the Knowledge of the Sciences, and distinguished themselves from other Nations by their Politeness and Refinement, they sunk into *Effeminacy*, *Luxury*, and *Diseases*, and began to study *Physick*, to remedy those Evils which their Luxury and Laziness had brought upon them.

Thus Enlightenment – the *first* Enlightenment – had proved the cradle of sickness. Thereafter, it was downhill all the way. Prosperous England suffered in particular for,[33]

> Since our Wealth has increas'd, and our Navigation has been extended, we have ransack'd all the Parts of the *Globe* to bring together its whole Stock of Materials for *Riot*, *Luxury*, and to provoke *Excess*.

Many facets of England's mercantile and social success were conspiring to exacerbate the menace:[34]

> *The* Moisture *of our* Air, *the Variableness of our* Weather, *(from our Situation amidst the* Ocean) *the* Rankness *and* Fertility *of our Soil, the* Richness *and* Heaviness *of our Food, the* Wealth *and* Abundance *of the Inhabitants (from their universal Trade) the* Inactivity *and* Sedentary *Occupations of the better Sort (amongst whom this* Evil *mostly rages) and the Humour of living in great, populous and consequently unhealthy Towns, have brought forth a* Class *and* Set *of Distempers, with atrocious and frightful* Symptoms, *scarce known to our Ancestors, and never rising to such fatal* Heights, *nor afflicting such* Numbers *in any other known Nation.*

The more 'luxurious, rich and wanton' the nation grew, the more distempers mushroomed.[35] Sophisticated living in high society carried high health risks, especially thanks to the elaboration of cuisines culled from all corners of the globe, involving dishes, salted, smoked, and highly-seasoned, all washed down with distilled liquors and ardent spirits.[36]

Alongside his chronicle of disease, Cheyne also proposed a differential sociology. Agricultural labourers were the 'here and now' analogues of savages, being 'No Thinkers' but physically robust: '*Fools, weak* or *stupid* Persons, *heavy* and *dull Souls*, are seldom much troubled with Vapours or Lowness of Spirits'.[37] By contrast to these happy morons, top people routinely sacrificed their physique and fitness to the calls of business, leisure, pleasure, and fashion. The intelligentsia was particularly vulnerable, for:[38]

> Since this present Age has made Efforts to go beyond former Times, in all the Arts of *Ingenuity, Invention, Study, Learning,* and all the contemplative and sedentary Professions (I speak only here of our own Nation, our own Times, and of the better Sort, whose chief Employments and Studies these are) the Organs of these Faculties being thereby worn and spoil'd, must affect and deaden the whole *System,* and lay a Foundation for the Diseases of Lowness and Weakness.

Doubtless with his own 'case' in mind – his *bon viveur* habits at one point swelled him up to thirty-two stone – Cheyne noted that '*Great Wits* are generally great *Epicures*, at least, Men of *Taste*'.[39] If creativity needed the stimuli of the bottle and the table, no wonder the nerves became damaged, or even deranged.

Sickness, Cheyne believed, was ravaging the superfine consciousnesses of those fine spirits blessed with exquisite feelings and racing minds. Such volatile souls were trapped in a vicious circle. When business and success bred '*Anxiety* and *Concern*', they fled to diversions in dissipation – resorting to '*Assemblies*, Musick Meetings, Plays, Cards, and *Dice*', or drowning their sorrows, but such dissipations inevitably carried heightened health risks.[40] In short, the irony (or Providential Justice) was that top people were doomed to suffer for their talents.[41]

Cheyne's conceptualization of the 'English Malady' as an élite disorder at once constitutionally crippling yet highly eligible as a badge of success has been widely analysed;[42] a few facets are, however, worth underlining here. First, Cheyne was emphatic that such sicknesses were sociogenic. 'These monstrous and extreme *Tortures*, are entirely the Growth of our own Madness and Folly, and the Product of our own wretched Inventions'.[43] Second, espousal of such a tenet did not make him a primitivist ranter, or a Rousseauvian *avant la lettre*. Critics of his recommended light diet – he urged lean meat, less meat, and even vegetarianism – were misrepresenting him, he insisted, in accusing him of being '*at Bottom a mere* Leveller, and for destroying Order, Ranks *and* Property'.[44] For – my third point – Cheyne was not for rejecting the good life but refining it. He wanted to sublimate the corporeal grossness of modern opulence into more elevated and aetherial consumption patterns. To achieve such a lightness of being, he formulated a new sociology (élite living savoured as an aesthetic experience), a new psychology (heightened sensibility, indeed, delicacy of *taste*) and predicated them upon a new physiology, which replaced Galenic humoralism with the iatro-mechanical idiom of the nerves[45] as the key to 'the Human *Machin*'.[46] For health, contended *The English Malady*, depended not upon exploded humoral equipoise but upon nervous tone. Being so delicate, nerves were readily clogged and obstructed. In particular, acidities produced irritations encouraging ulcerations, inflammations, and other impediments. Weakened ('relaxed') nerves would finally induce diarrhoeas, rheums, dropsy, diabetes, scrophula, and other chronic malaises.

Fine physical health, it followed, depended upon keeping these vital nerves springy and tonic. All the more so as the *beau monde* 'have a great Degree of Sensibility; are quick Thinkers, feel Pleasure or Pain the most readily, and are of most lively Imagination'.[47] Psycho-physiology thus supported the 'common Division of Mankind into *Quick Thinkers, Slow Thinkers* and *No Thinkers*'; 'Persons of slender and weak Nerves are generally of the first Class: the Activity, Mobility and Delicacy of their intellectual Organs make them so'. Indeed, nervous affliction[48]

> *never happens or can happen, to any but those of the liveliest and quickest natural Parts, whose Faculties are the brightest and most spiritual, and whose Genius is most keen and penetrating, and primarily where there is the most delicate Sensation and Pain.*

Such highly-strung people (as we would put it, still deploying the same idioms), living on their nerves, were particularly prone to debility.

Cheyne's moral tale of the health hazards of modernization evidently struck chords with his contemporaries. Robert Campbell, social commentator and author of *The London Tradesman*, applied it to the enigma of the rise of the medical profession. 'In the first Ages of the World' – yet another just-so story – 'Mankind subsisted without this Species of Men'. How so? It was because 'their Diseases were few, and Nature taught them the Use of Simples, to assist her when in Extremity: Temperance, Sobriety, and moderate Exercise, supplied the Place of Physicians to the Patriarchal Age'.[49] Times changed:[50]

> as Vice and Immorality gained Ground, as Luxury and Laziness prevailed, and Men became Slaves to their own Appetites, new Affections grew up in their depraved Natures, new Diseases, and till then unheard of Distempers, both chronick and acute, assaulted their vitiated Blood, and baffled the Force of their former natural Catholicons.

Health deteriorated, and so doctors arose:[51]

> Then Physicians became necessary; Nature grew weak, and sunk under the Load of various Evils, with which Vice, Lust, and Intemperance had loaded her; her Faculties became numbed, the Frame of the Human Constitution was shaken, and her Natural Powers debilitated.

Thanks to developments saluted by Enlightenment minds – e.g., the supersession of barbarism and boorishness by urbanity – heightened sensibilities and self-awareness were, many feared, actually rendering people hyper-conscious of sickness and less capable of bearing pain. 'Fashionable complaints' were proliferating, deplored A.F.M. Willich at the beginning of the nineteenth century:[52]

> The gout, formerly a regular but uncommon disease, which attacked only the external parts of persons advanced in years, has now become a constitutional indisposition, a juvenile complaint, torturing the patient in a thousand different forms.

This critique of the tendency of modernization – wealth accumulation, commercialization, urbanization, mechanization, industrialization, growing literacy, the accelerating pace of living, a communications revolution – to undermine health was extended, in Beddoes's day, by Thomas Trotter.

A baker's son from Melrose, Roxburghshire, Trotter was born in 1760, the same year as Beddoes.[53] At seventeen, he went to study medicine at Edinburgh University,[54] afterwards serving as a surgeon's mate in the Navy, before returning to Edinburgh and taking his M.D. in 1788 with a dissertation, *De Ebrietate* ('On Drunkenness').[55] Trotter then pursued a distinguished career in medicine, before finally settling as a medical practitioner in Newcastle, publishing his two most important works, the *Essay . . . on Drunkenness* (1804), and the *View of the Nervous Temperament* (1807), which advanced a social pathology in many ways parallel to Beddoes's.

Drunkenness, Trotter argued, was an appalling social evil,[56] but little understood, because it had been left to well-meaning but uncomprehending parsons and moralists. In truth, the *Essay . . . on Drunkenness* claimed, drink problems were properly the province of the 'discerning physician',[57] for inebriety was 'strictly speaking . . . a disease',[58] and not just a personal condition: the epidemiology of drunkenness would become clear, Trotter claimed, only within a wider socio-historical perspective. What a later generation would call 'alcoholism' was of a piece with worsening abuse of a range of other stimulants and intoxicants – opiates, tobacco, tea, coffee, cordials, and, most disturbingly, medicines – increasingly consumed in the emergent consumer society. The growing habit of consumption itself needed attention. The Ancients had been frugal and temperate; in his day, by contrast, Trotter noted, honour demanded that gentlemen drank each other under the table – even statesmen had to be three-bottle men.[59] Nor was the fair sex immune, being equally addicted, if usually furtively, to brandy-based cordials, laudanum and volatile spirits, to say nothing of their inordinate sipping of the slow poison of green tea.[60] The consequence? – a widening sickness horizon:[61]

> The last century has been remarkable for the increase of a class of diseases, but little known in former times, and what had slightly engaged the study of physicians prior to that period. They have been designated in common language, by the terms NERVOUS; SPASMODIC; BILIOUS; INDIGESTION; STOMACH COMPLAINTS; LOW SPIRITS; VAPOURS, &c.

To understand this novel socio-pathology, Trotter proposed, in his *View of the Nervous Temperament* (1807), a comprehensive historical sociology of health and sickness.

Against the backdrop of the enigmas of progress – debated by Montesquieu and Rousseau in France, and by the 'conjectural historians' with whose writings he must have become *au fait* while in Edinburgh[62] – Trotter pictured the epochal transformations from 'rudeness to refinement'. Man had developed the useful and the fine arts; through science and technology he had mastered Nature; wealth had multiplied leisure; social organization had grown more sophisticated, manners and morals brilliantly polished. Modern society boasted unrivalled opulence, refinements, and personal liberty, offering enticing opportunities and kindling boundless expectations.

But what consequences did these developments have in store for human nature and happiness, for man's permanent well-being, psychic and physical? Echoing Rousseau, Trotter looked back to the Old Testament Patriarchs, to the elemental civilizations of Antiquity, and even to Tacitus's gothic barbarians, and discovered peoples blessed with a noble 'simplicity'.[63] 'Our rude ancestors', he claimed, were sturdy, hardy, independent; they suffered few ills, because they had few needs: 'where the savage feels one want, the civilized being has a thousand'.[64] Above all, they 'had few bodily disorders', and none was 'brought to the grave by excess or debauch'.[65] It might be conceded of the 'primitive', that 'his enjoyments are limited'; nevertheless 'his cares, his pains, and his diseases are few'.[66]

On Trotter's balance-sheet, the march of civilization, with its vertiginous urbanization, its claustrophobic easy-chair existence, its 'refined life',[67] its sedentary occupations – or none at all![68] – signalled the spread of discontents and disorders, fuelled by spiralling opportunities, ambitions, and appetites. 'In a state of progressive improvement and civilization', mankind quits 'hunting and fishing for the town' and thereby crucially 'forsakes a mode of life that had been presented to him by nature, and in adopting a new situation he becomes the creature of art'.[69] And once a child of art, there was no curbing the spirit of inquietude, that restless, insatiable quest for intenser experiences, new gratifications, exquisite novelties, wilder excitements. Surplus wealth had brought idleness, indolence, and consequent 'low spirits';[70] moroseness in turn had spurred fresh cravings for 'excessive stimuli'.[71] Indulgence in luxuries begat 'debilitating pleasures';[72] and the cultivation by the 'voluptuary' of subtler tastes and exquisite sensitivities heightened pain susceptibility. In short, under the inevitable pressures of 'inordinate stimulation', stoicism yielded to sensibility.[73]

These morbid cravings in polite society for novel stimuli engendered a further search for sedatives, to deaden the pains of civilized restlessness – not least the 'hysteria' and 'hypochondriacism' resulting from the interplay of hothouse life styles with ultra-febrile imaginations.[74] Spurred by the allure of the new and the empire of fashion, the civilizing process thus created insatiable urges, first for 'inordinate stimulation',[75] and then for narcotics. More specifically – and here Trotter was absolutely of a mind with Beddoes – such artifices of modish living as over-sophisticated diet,[76] stifling rooms, and lack of exercise, necessarily bred ill-health and invalidism, and so automatically led (given new supersensitivities to pain) to the gulping of ever-greater quantities of analgesics, cordials and medicines. Since many of these were both harmful and habit-forming, they further destroyed the stomach and the nervous organization, debilitating the constitution, causing secondary biliousness, and requiring yet further spirals of medication to quell iatrogenic maladies.

All in all, judged Trotter, the much-trumpeted growth of freedom of choice was illusory. The pleasure of new pursuits rapidly evaporated, trapping the voluptuary on a treadmill, for 'the exhilarating powers . . . lose their fine zest and high relish, by being too frequently indulged'.[77] Thus modern man was trapped by his own great expectations, by self-induced physical and mental weaknesses. Britons who supposedly 'ruled the waves' had degenerated, bemoaned Trotter, into a 'nation of slaves',[78] civilization itself had become a mode of disease.

So, dizzy from that very 'nervous temperament' which the civilizing process had created, coveted even, modern man rode a morbid merry-go-round. To revive jaded appetites, the élite resorted to such stimuli as ardent spirits; to ease their pains and calm their jangled nerves, the highly-strung swallowed sedatives; but such desperate remedies merely gave new twists to the spiral of sickness. Medicines proper had the same deplorable side-effects, leading to further addiction. For, argued Trotter,[79]

> All nervous persons are uncommonly fond of drugs; and they are the chief consumers of advertised remedies, which they conceal from their medical friends. Among some well-meaning people, this inordinate desire for medicine has frequently become of itself a disease.

And all the while, Trotter emphasized, endorsing Lockean theories of habit- and character-formation through education and environment, these pathological facets of civilization were stamping themselves on human nature itself. Embossed as acquired characteristics upon the collective consciousness, such traits then descended down the generations. Far from being fixed, human nature was thus the product of self-development, or rather self-degeneration. And civilized man, that aetiolated, hothouse sapling, was above all, Trotter insisted, a '*creature of habit*',[80] victim of the 'nervous temperament' precisely because he was the '*creator* of his own *temperament*' – *homo faber*, self-made man with a vengeance![81] 'In the present stage of society', he underlined in his *Essay*, 'human kind are almost taken out of the hands of Nature; and a custom called *fashion* . . . now rules everything'.[82]

Within this process, the disposition to drunkenness, in individual, community and race, was both a symptom and a spur. Despite its apparent macho associations, the craving for strong liquor betokened a decadent, effeminate stage, for 'natural appetite requires no such stimulants'.[83] Trotter was not such a primitivist as to aim to repudiate stimulants entirely, but he deemed such substances as rum and hyson tea as, in their very essence, harmful; and he deplored the fact that stimulants like wine, safe and even beneficial if temperately deployed, had been reduced to necessities. Soda water likewise, which ought to be used strictly medicinally, had become a habitual beverage. They were sorry times when opium, God's greatest gift to the physician for pain relief, had become, in the shape of the laudanum phial, indispensable to every fashionable lady's reticule. People dosed themselves with potent medicines as though they were sweets.[84] In fact, Trotter concluded, Britain was being swamped with 'narcotics', including 'ardent spirits, opium, and all those articles commonly called anodynes, hypnotics, paregorics, &c.':[85]

> All the articles now enumerated, act very much alike on the human body. In small quantities, they induce vigor, activity and strength, and an increase of muscular power throughout the frame; at the same time are felt serenity, pleasure and courage of mind. In larger doses they bring on sleep, stupor and delirium; and when carried to the utmost quantity, insensibility, apoplexy and death. . . . When long continued, they are known to weaken the nervous system in a surprizing degree; disposing to amentia, epilepsy, palsy, tremors, convulsions, melancholy, madness, &c.

Thus, in both individual and society, there was a maelstrom of desire and dissatisfaction, sucking mankind down.

'Polished society' was so acting as to 'bring on its own dotage' and 'dig its own grave'.[86] Trotter was, of course, far from the first to point to the swings and roundabouts of the transition from 'rudeness to refinement'.[87] From both the authoritarian right and the populist left, critics offered comparable versions of pastoral, arcadian ages when life was simpler, happier, healthier. Trotter's own evocation of the maladies of rich and poor alike in Newcastle closely parallels Beddoes's contemporary bludgeoning of the Bristolians. But if his diagnosis of the diseases of civilization was hardly unique, there was something distinctive in Trotter's emphasis upon the symbiosis between physical and psychological dependency, both in the individual (increasingly hooked on his stimulants, whether alcoholic or medicinal, or both), and also in that 'creature of habit and imitation',[88] civilized man at large, in thrall to fashion and fantasy, 'wallowing in wealth and rioting in indulgence'.[89] Chemical stimuli such as alcohol excited the senses; this action in turn eroded the nervous system, producing the 'nervous temperament'; this disposition affected the psyche; and, finally, the imagination begat fresh desires, triggering chain-reactions of cravings. 'Are not habits of drunkenness', pondered Trotter, 'more often produced by mental affections than corporeal diseases? I apprehend few people will doubt the truth of this'.[90] Convinced thus of psychological enslavement, it was natural that Trotter explicitly cast habitual drunkenness as a mental illness, and diagnosed modernity itself as a kind of mental aberration.

Another great disorder that came to haunt the eighteenth-century imagination was tuberculosis. Traditional medicine had handled consumption, like other chronic, constitutional conditions, within an explanatory framework derived from Antiquity which saw the human body holistically, as a precarious equilibrium of vital fluids. Nutrition (inputs of food, etc.) had to be balanced against expenditures (activity) to preserve a golden mean. Waste matter had to be energetically expelled to avoid the build-up of poisons within the system. And, within a macrocosm/microcosm epistemology accustomed to juxtapose the body political against the body human, medical understanding of the springs of life, and its potential pathology, traded in idioms and images similar to those used in economic and political analysis of the principles of well-being in the state. In both, there was a dialectics of wealth, or well-being, and waste; in both, balance and moderation were valued. Yet the situation was complex.[91]

Traditional understanding of vitality likened it to a burning candle. In this decaying, sublunary sphere, the natural tendency of a flame to sink and die could be postponed – though not infinitely – by renewed external stimuli.[92] Eating and drinking fuelled the vital fires.[93] And in a milieu where hunger, dearth, and even famine[94] stalked the land, people needed little persuading that hearty eating and drinking provided fortification against disease, debility, and death. Traditional wisdom regarded 'living high' as a form of preventive medicine. The Englishman's cultic roast beef was not mere chauvinism, gluttony, or fantasy, but positively therapeutic, for it was believed that the stomach – Edward Jenner called it that 'grand Monarque of the Constitution'[95] – needed to be active and tonic, to digest the copious quantities of aliment required to concoct the blood, generating the spirits that enlivened the limbs.[96] Hence the most nourishing victuals were savoury and strong, and the red meat and wine diet of the rich evidently more invigorating than the insipid water-gruel of the poor.[97]

This model of the healthy body as a vital economy, thriving upon energetic stimulus, generous imput and unimpeded outflow, was widely accepted, not least by the medical profession itself. But this need for positive stimulus had to be squared with other age-old doctrines – both medical and moral – advocating temperance, moderation, and the golden mean. For the fear was that over-energizing the system might precipitate pathological excess. Gluttony was parlous, and toping constitutionally lethal. Drunkards 'died by their own hands', opined the *Tatler*. Intoxication, judged Samuel Richardson, was 'the most destructive of all vices: *asthma's, vertigoes, palsies, apoplexies, gouts, colics, fevers, dropsies, consumptions, stone,* and *hypochondriac diseases,* are naturally introduced'.[98]

And therein, with the listing of consumption, lies the point. Just as, in the body politic, wealth easily turned to waste, so in the individual, consumption, carried to excess, could, seem- ingly paradoxically, produce not strength but physical dissolu- tion. Late seventeenth-century medicine was alarmed by the apparently rapid spread of the various 'cachexies' or wasting diseases – scurvy, cancers, scrophula, *tabes dorsalis,* venereal infections, ascites, catarrhs, dropsy, asthmas and a galaxy of hysterick fevers and hypochondriack melancholias. Over a generation before Cheyne labelled nervous disorders as *The English Malady,* Gideon Harvey had designated scurvy the 'disease of London' and consumptions as the 'morbus anglicus',[99] and Benjamin Marten was shortly to pronounce that there was 'no Country in the World more Productive of Consumptions than this our Island'.[100]

Such scurvies were diseases of wasting, exhibiting symptoms including general malaise, weight loss, flaccid flesh, and a general 'rottenness' of health. Collectively known as 'the consumptions', and including, but far from exclusively confined to, tuberculosis, this congeries of chronic constitutional conditions[101] was largely blamed upon excess.[102] Feasting, toasting, and 'sporting in the Garden of Venus' were identified as prime causes of such 'wasting diseases', resulting in premature enfeeblement and what Thomas Willis called the 'withering away of the whole body'.[103]

Precisely how did 'consumption' create 'consumptions'? On this matter, such post-Restoration authorities as Christopher Bennet, Gideon Harvey, Thomas Willis, Richard Morton and Benjamin Marten were substantially agreed in laying blame at the door of appetite. In his monumental *Treatise of Consumptions*, Morton ascribed wasting distempers to 'too plentiful and unseasonable gorging of meat and drink and also an imprudent choice of such meats and liquors as abound with excrementatious parts and are not easy to be digested'. When wasting was accompanied by jaundice, Morton believed that 'frequent and long debauches', laced with liquor, were to blame.[104] Dissolution occurred through various physiological processes. Over-burdening the guts, Marten indicated, brought on violent purging, diarrhoeas, and defluxions.[105] According to Bennet, the liver and kidneys were likewise unable to cope, resulting in 'dropsies'.[106] And above all, gastric overload impeded digestive processes, creating 'acid spittle' and inducing what Bennet called 'erroneous fermentation', which filled 'the blood with Corruption', and rendered it 'sharp' and 'incorrigible',[107] bringing on a 'morbid disposition'.[108]

Such inflammatory fermentations, it was feared, would provoke ulcerations, tumours, tubercles in the lungs, schirrosities and cancers. These in turn would precipitate further 'Obstructions' to the vital processes, which, through metastasis, would eat up the vitals. Stoppages of all kinds – e.g., amenorrhoea – must thus be heeded, Morton advised, as harbingers of consumptions.

In short, medical opinion argued that wasting conditions – manifest sometimes in emaciation, sometimes in bloating – followed from self-indulgence and living high. 'Consumptions prevail more in England than in any other part of the world', William Buchan explained, 'owing perhaps to the great use of animal food and strong liquors, the general application to sedentary employments, and the great quantity of pit-coal which is there burnt'. Wealth, ease, and urbanism were above all hazardous to 'the rich, who are not under the necessity of labouring for their bread'.[109]

Hence to prevent consumptions, the medical men of the late seventeenth and early eighteenth centuries urged moderation. If Addison and Steele taught *politesse* to the *nouveaux riches*, physicians such as Cheyne instructed its Tunbelly Clumsies in the art of civilized eating.[110] With wasting disorders as with nervous diseases, Cheyne challenged the credit of the 'high diet', by mounting a critique of corporeality, and replacing the carnal with an accent on light diet.[111]

So how did understanding of consumption change in the Georgian age? Late eighteenth-century doctors were appalled by the advance of chronic diseases. Above all, pulmonary tuberculosis became a veritable 'white plague'. Around 1700, one in ten deaths registered by the London Bills of Mortality had been attributed to consumption.[112] By 1800, the figure was one in four. The single largest killer of adults, tuberculosis had become, in Erasmus Darwin's phrase, a 'giant-malady . . . which . . . destroys whole families, and, like war, cuts off the young in their prime, sparing old age and infirmity'.[113]

Why this catastrophic spread of consumption? For late-Georgian doctors, it was not – contrary to the views of Willis, Morton, Bennet and Marten popular a century earlier – because of crass personal over-indulgence. It was due, rather, to a subtler phenomenon, to what Thomas Beddoes called changes 'in almost every circumstance of the manner of living'. Indeed, the factors he isolated in the spread of the disease of consumption are ones central to what, in the sphere of economic history, has been called the 'consumer revolution' of the early industrial age.[114]

Two cohorts, Beddoes suggested, formed its chief victims. On the one hand, sections of the labouring population: those so poor as to suffer from absolute 'want of food', especially 'pot bellied' youngsters, were desperately susceptible.[115] Hardly less vulnerable, however, were operatives in sedentary trades, labouring in workshops whose atmospheres were polluted with irritant fibres, dust, and particles – 'carpet-manufacturers, taylors and lace-weavers', 'casters of fine brass-work', 'needle-grinders' and so forth,[116] who succumbed not through a constitutional diathesis, but because of the 'nature of the occupation', with its 'chemical and mechanical irritating substances'.[117] Such workers were thus 'forced into the disease', through their own 'self-neglect' and the 'unconcern' of their masters.[118]

Further changes in manufacturing imperilled the industrial work-force. Men who abandoned physical hard labour, allured by good money in 'the almost feminine occupations of the cloathing manufacture', became 'frequently consumptive'.[119] Worse still, innumerable operatives had been seduced into wearing the new fashionable textiles they themselves wove – 'light cotton dresses, instead of the warmer plaid which was formerly worn'.[120] To these new fabrics, that provided no protection against cold and damp, 'no small share of the equally common prevalence of colds, fevers, rheumatisms, asthmas, consumptions, is owing'.[121] Thus the producers of the 'consumer revolution' often paid the tribute of their health, and even their lives.

But the consuming classes fared no better. Here Beddoes, as we have seen, indicted the affluent for pursuing pernicious life styles that sacrificed health to the household deities of fashion. The fetishism of belongings and appearances threatened well-being. Mad for the mode, high society was decking itself out in the 'light dress' all the rage in the Revolutionary '90s.[122] To accommodate themselves to this 'injudicious conduct',[123] they resorted to intense domestic heating. But the fug of stuffy rooms merely exacerbated constitutional delicacy; while the inevitable dramatic temperature changes involved in moving from room to room, or from indoors to outside, lacerated the lungs. Why not wrap up in thick woollens, like the Dutch, or wear flannel?[124]

Frivolous sartorial fashions were but the tip of the iceberg. For, as noted in Chapter Five, the modish 'method of education' fostered in polite circles was almost custom-built to turn children into weaklings.[125] Seduced by the new sensibility, parents pressed their infants into study, music and fine accomplishments. After serving time as 'poor prisoners' in draughty boarding schools,[126] adolescents, 'weak, with excess of sensibility',[127] were then allowed to loaf around on sofas, reading improving literature and 'melting love stories, related in novels'.[128] Diversions designed to 'exercise the sensibility' proved 'highly enervating'.[129] Not surprisingly, thanks to this 'fatal indolence', 'the springs of their constitution have lost their force from disuse'.[130] All such Lydia Languishes lived under 'hazard of consumption', triggered by no more than a cold or chlorosis.[131]

Banish such genteel accomplishments born of snobbish aspirations to sensibility! (Beddoes begged parents) – abandon the itch to turn your children into pampered objects of consumption! The young needed robust physical exercise. They should pursue 'Botany and gardening abroad, and the use of a lathe, or the study of experimental chemistry at home'.[132]

And Beddoes spied a further insidious danger in sedentariness: the solitary vice. Masturbation became the target of many Georgian writers, who exposed it not just as a sin, vice, or character weakness, but as ruinous to health, because it supposedly induced wasting conditions. As reproductive biology increasingly conceptualized semen as a vital fluid, its onanistic waste was made to shoulder the blame for adolescent consumptions. A youth who 'was observ'd to Manstrupate very often', shortly 'died of a deep Consumption, having lived till he became like a Ghost, or living Skeleton', reported *Onania*, the most popular of these sensationalist warnings.[133] Beddoes endorsed such denunciations of masturbation, which he judged the predictable outcome of the irresponsible mix of mollycoddling and neglect that passed for a polite upbringing.

Worse still, by being associated with smart sensibility, tuberculosis was itself becoming positively fashionable. 'Writers of romance (whether from ignorance or because it suits the tone of their narrative) exhibit the slow decline of the consumptive, as a state on which the fancy may agreably repose, and in which not much more misery is felt, than is expressed by a blossom, nipped by untimely frosts.'[134] The preposterous idea had taken root that 'consumption must be a flattering complaint', because decline from the 'valetudinary state' was so gradual, initially painless, and non-disfiguring. Conferring an intriguing, enticing languor, consumption had become associated with superior imagination, talents, and discrimination.

Hence in the process whereby a girl was 'manufactured into a lady',[135] parents positively delighted in delicacy. Because thin was in, such darlings were allowed to get away with finicky eating. Hoodwinked by pseudo-medical faddery – perhaps even by reading Cheyne! – parents were now encouraging vegetarianism, convinced that macrobiotics purified the blood and toned up the nerves: 'There are . . . among the higher classes, some who keep their children to the fifth, or even the seventh year, upon a strict vegetable and milk diet', revealed the appalled Beddoes, 'believing that they thus render the constitution a signal service', seduced by the 'false hope of rendering the blood of their children pure, and their humours mild'.[136]

All such foibles had to be abandoned. The Medievals could serve as models. These sturdy swain – their heavy armour proved their 'Herculean form' – hunted, fought, hawked, and did without 'effeminate' carriages. 'It seems probable, that the general diet of former centuries was more invigorating', for the 'opulent of both sexes, appear to have participated rather more largely of animal food',[137] often breakfasting 'upon a fine beef steak broiled', perfect for 'resisting cold'.[138] 'It is not, as Addison supposed, among high dishes, that gout and palsy lurk', asserted the Brunonian Beddoes: far better, 'to *use animal food freely*'.[139]

Thus the preciosities of the fastidious left them pathetically vulnerable: 'it is upon the lilies of the land, that neither toil nor spin, that the blight of consumption principally falls'.[140] They were too weak, being fixed 'immoveably upon well-cushioned chairs and sofas, in hot, close apartments', to 'receive and digest a proper quantity of aliment'. Far healthier were labourers who pursued heavy physical exercise, drank with gusto (Beddoes denied that 'excess in respect to wine, directly of itself induces consumption, even in the predisposed'),[141] and above all, were lusty carnivores. 'The persons most free from consumption are precisely those that consume most animal food'.[142]

As is obvious, Beddoes's arguments spell a remarkable reversal of earlier medical discourse. Late-Stuart doctors blamed consumption upon excess; Beddoes indicted deficit. How far, one wonders, had Cheynian salvoes against 'high living' helped induce the transformation in dietary habits Beddoes supposedly saw and abhorred?

Above all, Beddoes denounced the tendency, particularly amongst parents, to be *blasé* about consumption through subscribing to that archetypal consumerist belief that money would put everything to rights.[143] The foolish idea had grown up – it will be examined in the next chapter – that one could buy back health, by a trip to a spa, the sea-side, or the South. Here mercenary doctors were culpable, for consumption was keeping many in clover.

What was to be done? In his early, optimistic days, Beddoes felt confident that pneumatic chemistry would provide sure cures for consumption. But, with his 'try anything' approach, he also experimented with foxglove or digitalis. One wonders whether he endorsed this old folk cure, recently touted by William Withering, because of its populist connotations.[144] Certainly his most touted tuberculosis treatment involved almost a blatant repudiation of the ways, a blunt assault upon the sensibilities, of fashionable urban society. This was the 'cow-house method'. Beddoes urged consumptives to live in barns, with cattle for companions, till cured. 'Stabling with cows' is 'not unpromising',[145] Beddoes insisted, while prophylactically adding, anticipating the chortles of latter-day Swiftians, 'I feel that I am preparing a feast for those who resort to ridicule'.[146]

The philosophy of the cow-house was two-fold. The beasts themselves would yield regular, steady warmth, twenty-four hours a day, the best mode of central heating alive. Moreover, the volatile alkaline fumes of their excreta would purify the patient's lungs. Beddoes devoted much of his *Observations on the Consumptive* to evaluating this treatment which he had 'long been in the habit of recommending',[147] even though (he confided) 'not unfrequently did I forfeit the good opinion of my patient'.[148] It had enjoyed signal success. He thus relayed the 'narrative of Madame —', who had, predictably, gadded around as a bright young thing, 'continuing to go out, to keep late hours, and in *every thing* to live in a manner too agitated for my state of health', until her consumption worsened, when she finally opted for the cow-house treatment. So strong was the vapour, 'that every thing white which was brought in, became reddish in a very short time', and, worse, she had to endure idling gawpers who 'came to see me as an object of curiosity'. Nevertheless, she improved,[149] as too did Mrs Finch, none other than Joseph Priestley's daughter, who, in a letter datelined 'Cow-House, *Oct* 8', explained that 'she has found a cow-house a much more comfortable abode than she had formed an idea of', though the stench was 'nauseous', and 'successive generations of flies were a considerable nuisance': 'I am', she concluded, 'more than ever a friend to the cows'.[150]

Consultations were not always so smooth, however, for certain patients 'spoke of the *disgrace* of being in such a situation', a 'fellow-lodger with the cows'.[151] A scaled-down alternative to being physically 'closeted in a cow-house' was fortunately, available.[152] For, Beddoes explained, 'Vessels containing the fermentable substances could easily be introduced into a warm apartment'.[153]

Beddoes anatomized the 'giant-malady' of tuberculosis as the product of an economy and a life style, a disease of civilization. 'Consumption may be regarded as a vast pit-fall, situated on the high road of life, which we have not sense enough of our common interest to agree to fill up, or fence round. Heedless fathers and mothers are for ever guiding their sons and daughters directly into it'.[154] Proceeding 'from domestic mismanagement, and not from the inalterable dispositions of nature', it was preventable.[155] The mentality of 'opulent families' must seem 'paradoxical' indeed, to those convinced that 'health is the first of blessings',[156] for they appeared indifferent to the fact that 'our chronic maladies are of our own creating'. Obsession with objects and neglect of health were together responsible for the 'tribute of lives we render to consumption'.[157]

Beddoes was, thus, not the only diagnostician of social ills; his analysis formed part of a growing concern in Enlightenment England with the maladies of modernity and the paradoxes of progress amongst doctors shifting their attention from individual ailments and habits to the deleterious tendencies of society itself, plotting the imprintation of society's tempo and temptations, its fashions and consumption patterns, upon the body, through the physiology of the nervous system.

Médecins-philosophes worried that 'the civilizing process' was actually exacerbating sickness. The prime proof of these fears were, it seemed, the epidemics of hypochondria and hysteria, maladies originally defined as regular somatic disorders, but apparently undergoing a mutation in nature and significance to become the marks of supersensitive souls who (it might punningly be said) thought and felt themselves sick – 'hippish' folks such as James Boswell, who signed his newspaper column, 'The Hypochondriack'. Such disorders became badges of identity and media of social intercourse, for, as Dr James Makittrick Adair remarked, *à propos* of such *malades imaginaires*, 'mutual communication of their ailments is often a topic of conversation [and] the imagination frequently suggests a similarity of disease, though none such really exists'.[158]

The hyper-sensitivity to health identified by Beddoes and others as signs of the times is not hard to explain. Polite society esteemed self-awareness and introspection. But where did responsible individualism stop and morbid brooding take over? In his *Treatise of the Hypochondriack and Hysterick Diseases* (1730), the leading Enlightenment physician, Bernard Mandeville, thus pondered the fictional case of a liberally educated man of letters, 'Misomedon', possessed of sufficient leisure to dwell upon his pains, and of book-learning to be adept at fantasizing the workings of disorders and drugs. Partly thanks to unscrupulous physicians, his life became a battle with 'diseases' which, though initially imaginary, in time materialized, as reckless physicking and self-medication took their toll.[159] Some might scoff, Mandeville conceded, but hypochondria could be the death of people and deserved both sympathy and – herein lay Mandeville's mandatory paradox! – expert doctoring.

Disillusioned doctors like Beddoes blamed the spread of hypochondria upon that democratization of information perpetrated by popularizers such as Buchan: too many self-dosing opportunities existed amongst those (mocked Dr Adair) 'who are sick by way of amusement and melancholy to keep up their spirits'.[160] Yet 'no disease is more troublesome', Adair added,[161]

> either to the Patient or Physician, than hypochondriac Disorders; and it often happens, that, thro' the Fault of both, the Cure is either unnecessarily protracted, or totally frustrated; for the Patients are so delighted, not only with a Variety of Medicines, but also of Physicians.

Catch 22! For hypochondria's revenge was that the doctor's intervention would, all too easily, merely reinforce the hypochondriac's dependence. Hence, as John Hill stressed,[162] 'Though the physician can do something toward the cure, much more depends upon the patient'.

An Enlightenment mutation, hypochondria is a mark of the enculturing of sickness into sickly sensibility. Hysteria evolved similarly – indeed, the two conditions were often represented as brother and sister.[163] Classically an organic malady of women, a disease of the womb, by the eighteenth century 'hysteria' was being deployed to label the volatile physical symptoms associated with hyper-sensitivity, a lability thought especially common in the sex, though – significantly, in a culture in which 'Enlightenment' was blamed for making men 'effeminate' – not exclusively so.[164] In hybrid coinages such as 'hysteric cholic', the epithet signalled a rather superior malady, while also marking the mysterious *je ne sais quoi* of ailments that were intermittent, unpredictable, and without palpable physical causes.

This 'coming-out' of the hypochondriac and hysteric marks an important cultural juncture, the pathologization of Enlightenment individualism. Polite society encouraged a certain narcissism. Within the permitted degrees of conventional polish, the literati were expected to dazzle, be different, even a touch prima donna-ish. Yet individual freedom took its toll. The tensions between distinction and polite conformity bred anxieties, in turn somatized into physical complaints, which, through the manipulation of the sick-role, could be simultaneously owned and disowned. Sickliness thus provided social alibis, while suffering purchased the right to be different. Such pres- sure complexes are, of course, superbly illustrated in the exem- plary 'nervous breakdown' of David Hume.[165]

But the new prominence of hypochondria also highlights a health culture increasingly engrossed in the dynamics of commercialization. Sick people, it seemed, were consulting more doctors more often, paying them fatter fees, while still patronizing quacks and irregulars; obtaining mountains of medication, stimulants and sedatives, from apothecaries, nostrum-mongering itinerants, and druggists;[166] devouring books offering *Physick for Families*; and, finally, investing in well-stocked proprietary medicine-chests.[167] The profession ritualistically wrung its hands as it pocketed its fees.[168] 'Fashionable physicians, from Asclepiades the Bithynian to Warren the Briton', cashed in, Beddoes claimed, as will be shown in the next chapter, on poorly ladies whose 'comfortless existence renders them in every sense the best friends of the medical fraternity. . . . To have half a dozen such patronesses has always been better than to discover a remedy for the most cruel of human diseases'. 'No single cause, perhaps', Beddoes clinched his tirade, 'has so effectually retarded the progress of medicine'.[169]

The commercialization of health-consciousness brought a further turn of the screw. People had always, doctors alleged, eaten and drunk themselves to destruction. Now, critics complained, sufferers were newly *medicating* themselves to death – or at least consuming a pandora's box of *soi-disant* stimulants and pain-killers to relieve their distempers, only to become dangerously habituated. Enlightenment culture is seminal for both the idea, and the actuality, of addiction.[170]

Beddoes was not the only physician to denounce doctor- and

drug-dependency as prime evils of the age. The irony is that, precisely because of their advanced involvement with chemistry, with experimentation, and, indeed, their ardent humanitarianism, such 'experimentalists' as Beddoes were themselves particularly responsible for drug-induced human tragedies. Beddoes's circle was prone to experiment with untried narcotics, from nitrous oxide (laughing-gas) to opiates. 'We will have a fair trial of Bang', Coleridge promised Tom Wedgwood on one occasion, 'Do bring down some of the Hyoscyamine pills, and I will give a fair trial of Opium, Henbane, and Nepenthe'.[171] Tom Wedgwood's addiction had itself been triggered by Erasmus Darwin's prescription of large doses of opium ('3/4 of a grain, or a grain, of opium, taken every night for many months')[172] for the relief of a tubercular cough. Wedgwood ended up hopelessly hooked:[173]

> I am very low at present having had constant fever & headache since I have been here & have lost 4lbs. of flesh. This is the third attempt I have lately made to reduce my opium. I cannot do it – my spirits become dreadful – the dullness of my life is absolutely unsupportable without it.

Under such circumstances – when, to recur to a statement of Trotter's, the 'inordinate desire for medicine has frequently become of itself a disease' – the putatively clear-cut distinction between disease and medicine melted like spring snow. Medicating habits caused pain, and the craving for artificial stimulants was viewed, by Trotter and others, as a species of 'disease of the mind'. If utilitarianism was the philosophical expression of desire for a consumer society, it is surely no accident that it was Coleridge who defined addiction as 'the desire of a desire'.[174]

This chapter has argued that alongside the medical optimism Gay found in the Enlightenment, *philosophes* and doctors alike were also profoundly troubled by what they saw as the counterproductive consequences for health of the spread of progressive ideas, refined culture, and commercial, urban values. An intellectual movement that had promised the healthy critique of *ancien régime* malaises and the emancipation of the self, readily turned into that narcissistic, morbid self-absorption medicalized under the disease labels of hypochondria and hysteria, nervous and wasting disorders. Enlightenment fascination with consciousness – with exposing traditional false-consciousness and creating new sciences of the mind for a new society – led to postulation of new categories of disorders rooted in the psyche: madness construed as a psychiatric disorder, masturbation, alcoholism, nymphomania, and addiction. The conscription of mind as the engine of liberation itself unveiled the self-imprisoning, morbific potential of the psyche. It is no accident that Beddoes was fond of the epigraph: 'Physician: heal thyself'.[175]

Notes

1. P. Gay, 'The Enlightenment as Medicine and as Cure'; *idem, The Enlightenment*; for discussion, see R. Porter, 'Was There a Medical Enlightenment in Eighteenth Century England?'.
2. Gay, *Enlightenment,* II, 19. I cite the book version, since its situation at the outset of the second volume (*The Science of Freedom*) signals its centrality to Gay's vision.
3. Gay, *Enlightenment,* II, 18.
4. Gay, *Enlightenment,* II, 19.
5. Gay, *Enlightenment,* II, 12.
6. Gay, *Enlightenment,* II, 22.
7. Gay, *Enlightenment,* II, 23.
8. Gay, *Enlightenment,* II, 12.
9. Gay, *Enlightenment,* II, 21.
10. Gay, *Enlightenment,* II, 16.
11. C. Rosenberg, 'The Therapeutic Revolution'; E. Shorter, *Bedside Manners*; W.F. Bynum, 'Health, Disease and Medical Care'.
12. E.A. Wrigley, 'No Death Without Birth'; *idem* and R.S. Schofield, *The Population History of England 1541–1971*; David Levine, *Family Formation in an Age of Nascent Capitalism*; *idem, Reproducing Families.*
13. For today's revisionism see G. Risse, *Hospital Life in Enlightenment Scotland.*
14. For childbirth and -rearing see especially A. Wilson, 'Participant or Patient?'; *idem,* 'William Hunter and the Varieties of Man-midwifery'; E. Shorter, *A History of Women's Bodies*; V. Fildes, *Breasts, Bottles and Babies*; *idem, Wetnursing.* See Edward Shorter, 'The Management of Normal Deliveries and the Generation of William Hunter'; Judith S. Lewis, *In the Family Way.*
15. J. McManners, *Death and the Enlightenment*; Ruth Richardson, *Death, Dissection and the Destitute*; C. Gittings, *Death, Burial and the Individual in Early Modern England*; Roy Porter and Dorothy Porter, *In Sickness and in Health,* ch.13; Dorothy Porter and Roy Porter, *Patient's Progress,* ch.9; P. Ariès, *The Hour of our Death.*
16. For such conjectural histories, see J.A. Passmore, *The Perfectibility of Man*; David Spadafora, *The Idea of Progress in Eighteeenth Century Britain.*

17. K.M. Baker, *Condorcet: From Natural Philosophy to Social Mathematics.*

18. T. Beddoes, *Letter to Erasmus Darwin, M.D., on a New Method of Treating Pulmonary Consumption and Some Other Diseases Hitherto Found Incurable* (1793), 59.

19. W. Buchan, *Observations Concerning the Prevention and Cure of the Venereal Disease,* xxvi. Buchan is quoting Benjamin Rush.

20. W. Buchan, *Observations Concerning the Prevention and Cure of the Venereal Disease,* xxvi. See C.J. Lawrence, 'William Buchan'; C. Rosenberg, 'Medical Text and Medical Context'. Buchan's views parallel the *Encyclopédie.* See W. Coleman, 'Health and Hygiene'.

21. Buchan, *Observations Concerning . . . Venereal Disease,* 9.

22. Cf. Henry Vyverberg, *Historical Pessimism in the French Enlightenment.*

23. G. Cheyne, *The English Malady.* For Cheyne's life see H.R. Viets, 'George Cheyne, 1673-1743'; extremely perceptive is G.S. Rousseau, 'Mysticism and Millennialism: "Immortal Dr Cheyne"'; and see also the 'Introduction' by Roy Porter to G. Cheyne, *The English Malady.* Cheyne's other works offer similar outlooks. See *An Essay on Regimen; idem, The Natural Method of Cureing; idem, The Method of Cureing Diseases of the Body and the Disorders of the Mind.*

24. Trotter, *View of the Nervous Temperament,* xvi.

25. Trotter, *View of the Nervous Temperament,* xvii.

26. Trotter, *View of the Nervous Temperament,* xvii.

27. Trotter, *View of the Nervous Temperament,* xvii.

28. For the most recent and best biographical study of Cheyne see G. S. Rousseau, 'Mysticism and Millennialism: "Immortal Dr Cheyne"'.

29. Roy Porter, 'The Rage of Party'; O. Doughty, 'The English Malady of the Eighteenth Century'; J.F. Sena, 'The English Malady: The Idea of Melancholy from 1700 to 1760.

30. Cheyne, *English Malady,* 16, 26, 56, 66.

31. Cheyne, *English Malady,* 66.

32. Cheyne, *English Malady,* 56.

33. Cheyne, *English Malady,* 174 and 49.

34. Cheyne, *English Malady,* Preface, i–ii.

35. Cheyne, *English Malady,* 174.

36. Cheyne, *English Malady,* 174.

37. Cheyne, *English Malady,* 52.

38. Cheyne, *English Malady,* 54.

39. Cheyne, *English Malady,* 54.

40. Cheyne, *English Malady,* 181, 52.

41. Cheyne, *English Malady,* 188.

42. G.S. Rousseau, 'Mysticism and Millennialism: "Immortal Dr Cheyne"'.

43. Cheyne, *English Malady,* 34.

44. Cheyne, *English Malady,* iii.

45. For nerves, see G.S. Rousseau, 'Nerves, Spirits and Fibres'; *idem,* 'Science and the Discovery of the Imagination in Enlightenment England'; *idem,* 'Psychology'; J. Spillane, *The Doctrine of the Nerves;* C.J. Lawrence, 'The Nervous System and Society in the Scottish

Enlightenment'; *idem*, 'Medicine as Culture: Edinburgh and the Scottish Enlightenment'; R. French, *Robert Whytt, the Soul and Medicine.*

46. Cheyne, *English Malady*, 14.

47. Cheyne, *English Malady*, 105.

48. Cheyne, *English Malady*, 60.

49. See R. Campbell, *The London Tradesman*, 37.

50. Campbell, *The London Tradesman*, 37.

51. Campbell, *The London Tradesman*, 37.

52. A.F.M. Willich, *Lectures on Diet and Regimen.*

53. For Trotter, see Roy Porter, 'Introduction', to *Thomas Trotter: An Essay, Medical, Philosophical and Chemical, on Drunkenness*; Roy Porter, 'Addicted to Modernity: Nervousness in the Early Consumer Society'.

54. The best accounts of Trotter's life are Ian Porter, 'Thomas Trotter, M.D., Naval Physician'; Sir Humphry Rolleston, 'Thomas Trotter, M.D.'. Hardly any manuscript material seems to have survived.

55. Thomas Trotter, *De Ebrietate, Eiusque Effectibus in Corpus Humanum.* There is a copy in Edinburgh University Library.

56. For the place of drinking within pre-industrial society see A.L. Simon, *Bottlescrew Days*; J.A. Spring and D.H. Buss, 'Three Centuries of Alcohol in the British Diet'; M.M. Glatt, 'The English Drink Problem: its Rise and Decline Through the Ages'; P. Clark, *The English Ale-House.* For the gin craze see J. Watney, *Mother's Ruin*; D.M. George, *London Life in the Eighteenth Century*; T.G. Coffey, 'Beer Street: Gin Lane'.

57. Thomas Trotter, *An Essay, Medical, Philosophical and Chemical, on Drunkenness and its Effects on the Human Body*, 6.

58. Trotter, *Essay . . . on Drunkenness*, 8, 179. For similar formulations, see *ibid.*, 128, 182 ('the habit of intoxication belongs to the mind'), 26 (drunkenness is 'a species of insanity'), and 186 ('are not habits of drunkenness more often produced by mental affections than corporeal diseases?'). For further discussion, see Roy Porter, 'The Drinking Man's Disease'. For histories of the idea of alcoholism, and Trotter's part therein, see W.F. Bynum, 'Chronic Alcoholism in the First Half of the 19th Century'; J. Hirsch, 'Enlightened Eighteenth Century Views of the Alcohol Problem'; H.G. Levine, 'The Discovery of Addiction'; John Romano, 'Early Contributions to the Study of *Delirium Tremens*'; J.-C. Sournia, *Histoire de l'Alcoolisme.* For Erasmus Darwin see *Zoonomia*: Darwin explicitly termed 'drunkenness' a disease (it was number I.1.2.2 in his classification, a disease of 'irritation').

59. Trotter, *Essay . . . on Drunkenness*, 165.

60. Trotter, *Essay . . . on Drunkenness*, 154, 174.

61. Trotter, *View of the Nervous Temperament*, xv.

62. See Gladys Bryson, *Man and Society*; David Spadafora, *The Idea of Progress in Eighteeenth Century Britain.*

63. Thomas Trotter, *View of the Nervous Temperament*, viii.

64. Trotter, *View of the Nervous Temperament*, 220.

65. Trotter, *View of the Nervous Temperament*, 20.

66. Trotter, *View of the Nervous Temperament*, 29.

67. Trotter, *View of the Nervous Temperament*, 35.

68. Trotter, *View of the Nervous Temperament*, 22.

69. Trotter, *View of the Nervous Temperament*, 70.
70. Trotter, *View of the Nervous Temperament*, 27.
71. Trotter, *View of the Nervous Temperament*, 142.
72. Trotter, *View of the Nervous Temperament*, 48.
73. Trotter, *View of the Nervous Temperament*, 27; see 69 for a discussion of the modern voluptuary.
74. Trotter, *View of the Nervous Temperament*, 39.
75. Trotter, *View of the Nervous Temperament*, 31.
76. Trotter, *View of the Nervous Temperament*, 24.
77. Trotter, *Essay . . . on Drunkenness*, 29.
78. Trotter, *View of the Nervous Temperament*, xi.
79. Trotter, *View of the Nervous Temperament*, 104.
80. Trotter, *View of the Nervous Temperament*, 31.
81. Trotter, *View of the Nervous Temperament*, 34.
82. Trotter, *Essay . . . on Drunkenness*, 153.
83. Trotter, *Essay . . . on Drunkenness*, 155.
84. Trotter, *Essay . . . on Drunkenness*, 38; *idem*, *View of the Nervous Temperament*, 312. See V. Berridge and G. Edwards, *Opium and the People*.
85. Trotter, *View of the Nervous Temperament*, 133.
86. Trotter, *View of the Nervous Temperament*, 106.
87. Trotter, *View of the Nervous Temperament*, 143.
88. Trotter, *View of the Nervous Temperament*, 233.
89. Trotter, *View of the Nervous Temperament*, 257.
90. Trotter, *Essay . . . on Drunkenness*, 186.
91. For the organic understanding of society, see W.J. Greenleaf, *Order, Empiricism and Politics*; L. Barkan, *Nature's Work of Art*; J.B. Bambrough, *The Little World of Man*; E.M.W. Tillyard, *The Elizabethan World Picture*; J. Broadbent, 'The Image of God or Two Yards of Skin'; F. Barker, *The Tremulous Private Body*; and, more conceptually, B. Barnes and S. Shapin (eds), *Natural Order*; A. Marcovich, 'Concerning the Continuity between the Image of Society and the Image of the Human Body'. On early modern economic theory, see Joyce Appleby, 'Ideology and Theory'; *idem*, *Economic Thought in Seventeenth-Century England*; Albert O. Hirschman, *The Passions and the Interests*. For background culture about the body see F. Bottomley, *Attitudes to the Body in Western Christendom*; J. O'Neill, *Five Bodies*; J.-P. Peter and J. Revel, 'Le Corps: L'Homme malade et son Histoire'; R. Cooter, 'The Power of the Body: the Early Nineteenth Century'; Roy Porter, 'Body Politics'.
92. For traditional medical concepts of the body system, decay, ageing and dying see L.M. Beier, *Sufferers and Healers*; O. Temkin, *Galenism*; *idem*, 'Health and Disease'. Important for the view of life as a flame are G. Rees, *Francis Bacon's Natural Philosophy*; and P. Niebyl, 'Old Age, Fever, and the Lamp Metaphor'.
93. The cultures of eating, drinking, and 'digestion' are admirably discussed in Francis McKee, 'The Earlier Works of Bernard Mandeville, 1685–1715'.
94. On dearth see A. Appleby, 'Nutrition and Disease'; *idem*, *Famine in Tudor and Stuart England*.
95. G. Miller (ed.), *Letters of Edward Jenner*, 7.

96. For spirits and blood see Valerie Grosvenor Myer, 'Tristram and the Animal Spirits'; M.M. Wintrobe, *Blood, Pure and Eloquent.*

97. S. Mennell, *Manners*, 182f.

98. R. Steele, *The Tatler*, 24 Oct., 1710; S. Richardson, *Familiar Letters*, 41.

99. Gideon Harvey, *Morbus Anglicus*, 4, 8, 22; *idem*, *The Disease of London.* On scurvy, see K. Carpenter, *The History of Scurvy and Vitamin C.* Quack doctors in particular made much of scurvy. See Roy Porter, *Health for Sale*, ch.5.

100. Benjamin Marten, *A New Theory of Consumptions*, 10; L. Stevenson, '"New Disease" in the Seventeenth Century'.

101. In our post-bacteriological age it is important not to assume that a single, fixed, specific 'ontological' disease was meant by the word 'consumption', its synonym, 'phthisis' – or, in fact, by most other diagnostic labels. Diseases were rather *sui generis*, marking states and symptoms, not things.

102. Harvey, *Disease of London*, 11. Harvey noted that smoke produced 'vitiated choler': 33. Thomas Sydenham attributed the high incidence of consumption in London to the fact that 'we live here in a perpetual mist': S.L. Cummins, *Tuberculosis in History*, 26; Richard Morton laid much blame on 'a foggy and thick air and that which is filled with the smoke of coals': see L.F. Flick, *Development of our Knowledge of Tuberculosis*, 100. On Morton, see R.Y. Keers, 'Richard Morton'; R.R. Trail, 'Richard Morton (1637–98)'.

103. For Willis, see Cummins, *Tuberculosis in History*, 16.

104. For Morton, see Flick, *Development of our Knowledge of Tuberculosis*, 99, 155.

105. Marten, *New Theory of Consumptions*, 22, 36.

106. Christopher Bennet, *Theatrum Tabidorum*, 19.

107. Bennet, *Theatrum Tabidorum*, 33–5.

108. See Flick, *Development of Our Knowledge of Tuberculosis*, 134.

109. Buchan, *Domestic Medicine*, 218. For the impact of the atmosphere see J. Arbuthnot, *An Essay Concerning the Effects of Air on Human Bodies.*

110. F. Childs, 'Prescriptions for Manners in Eighteenth Century Courtesy Literature'; Norbert Elias, *The Civilizing Process.*

111. Extremely perceptive is G.S. Rousseau, 'Mysticism and Millennialism: "Immortal Dr Cheyne"'.

112. For histories of tuberculosis, see René Dubos and Jean Dubos, *The White Plague*; L. Bryder, *Below the Magic Mountain*; F.B. Smith, *The Retreat of Tuberculosis 1850–1950*; L.S. King, *Medical Thinking. A Historical Preface*, 16–69; H.D. Chalke, 'Some Historical Aspects of Tuberculosis'; R.M. Burke, *A Historical Chronology of Tuberculosis*; G.N. Meachen, *A Short History of Tuberculosis*; W. Pagel, 'Humoral Pathology: A Lingering Anachronism in the History of Tuberculosis'; G.A.M. Milkomane, *The Conquest of Tuberculosis*; P.J. Bishop, 'Blackmore on Consumption'; *idem*, 'Thomas Young and his "Practical and Historical Treatise on Consumptive Disorders"'.

113. Darwin's phrase is to be found in T. Beddoes, *Letter to Erasmus Darwin*, 61.

114. Thomas Beddoes, *Essay on the Causes, Early Signs, and Prevention of Pulmonary Consumption for the Use of Parents and Preceptors* (1799), 11. For the idea of a consumer revolution, see N. McKendrick, John Brewer and J.H. Plumb, *The Birth of a Consumer Society: The Commercialization of Eighteenth-Century England* (London: Europa, 1982).

115. Beddoes, *Essay on . . . Consumption*, 178–9.

116. Beddoes, *Essay on . . . Consumption*, 62–4.

117. Thomas Beddoes, *Hygëia: or Essays Moral and Medical, on the Causes Affecting the Personal State of our Middling and Affluent Classes*, 3 vols (1802), vol.1 essay ii, pp. 24–25 [future references will be given in the form 1 ii 24–25].

118. Beddoes, *Hygeia*, 1 ii 24–5.

119. Beddoes, *Essay on . . . Consumption*, 85. Beddoes is quoting Sir John Sinclair.

120. Beddoes, *Essay on . . . Consumption*, 87–8.

121. Beddoes, *Essay on . . . Consumption*, 89.

122. Beddoes, *Essay on . . . Consumption*, 80. On flimsy fashions, see E. Ewing, *Dress and Undress*.

123. Beddoes, *Essay on . . . Consumption*, 80.

124. 'Flannel should be worn': Beddoes, *Essay on . . . Consumption*, 128–9. Beddoes also recommended 'a tin *foot-warmer*', 'manufactured of a convenient form, by Lloyd, near Norfolk Street, Strand, London': pp.132–3.

125. Beddoes, *Essay on . . . Consumption*, 90. For aspirant middle-class lifestyles, see L. Davidoff and C. Hall, *Family Fortunes*; L. Stone, *The Family, Sex and Marriage in England 1500–1800*; R. Trumbach, *The Rise of the Egalitarian Family;* Peter Earle, *The Making of the English Middle Class.*

126. Beddoes, *Essay on . . . Consumption*, 121.

127. Beddoes, *Essay on . . . Consumption*, 219.

128. Beddoes, *Essay on . . . Consumption*, 190.

129. Beddoes, *Essay on . . . Consumption*, 121.

130. Beddoes, *Essay on . . . Consumption*, 190.

131. Beddoes, *Essay on . . . Consumption*, 124.

132. T. Beddoes, *Observations on the Medical and Domestic Management of the Consumptive*, 185. *Cf.* K. Figlio, 'Chlorosis and Chronic Disease in Nineteenth-Century Britain'; I.S.L. Loudon, 'Chlorosis, Anaemia and Anorexia Nervosa'.

133. *Onania*, 22; E.H. Hare, 'Masturbatory Insanity: the History of an Idea'; J. Stengers and A. Van Neck, *Histoire d'une Grande Peur: La Masturbation*; L.J. Jordanova, 'The Popularisation of Medicine: Tissot on Onanism'. The linkage of onanism and consumption pervades Laurence Sterne's *Tristram Shandy.*

134. Beddoes, *Essay on . . . Consumption*, 6.

135. Beddoes, *Essay on . . . Consumption*, 119.

136. Beddoes, *Essay on . . . Consumption*, 114. For the wider sensibilities of 'anorexia', see R.M. Bell, *Holy Anorexia*; J.J. Brumberg, *Fasting Girls*; Hillel Schwartz, *Never Satisfied.* Shelley offers a good example of the pursuit of vegetarianism to prevent scurvy. See N. Crook and D. Guiton, *Shelley's Venomed Melody.*

137. Beddoes, *Essay on . . . Consumption*, 162, 167.
138. Beddoes, *Essay on . . . Consumption*, 156.
139. Beddoes, *Essay on . . . Consumption*, 116. On Beddoes's Brunonianism, see W.F. Bynum and Roy Porter (eds), *Brunonianism in Britain and Europe*; C.J. Lawrence, 'Cullen, Brown and the Poverty of Essentialism'.
140. Beddoes, *Hygëia*, 1 ii 43, 44, 68.
141. Beddoes, *Essay on . . . Consumption*, 125.
142. Beddoes, *Essay on . . . Consumption*, 112, 103. Beddoes reported hearing from Dr William Withering that butchers also kept themselves healthy by inhaling the steam of newly slaughtered carcasses.
143. Beddoes, *Hygëia*, 1 ii 89.
144. Beddoes, *Essay on . . . Consumption*, 55, 264. On foxglove see J.K. Aronson, *An Account of the Foxglove*.
145. Thomas Beddoes, *Observations on the Medical and Domestic Management of the Consumptive; on the Powers of Digitalis Purpurea; and on the Cure of Scrophula* (1801), 22. Beddoes's cow-cure raises issues regarding the juxtaposition of man and beast, and the transgression of their proper 'separate spheres', in a culture increasingly sensitive about man's unique status (highly relevant is the fate of Gulliver, once finally returned to England). At almost the same time, Jenner's cowpox 'vaccine' raised profound popular fears. For a broad background see K.V. Thomas, *Man and the Natural World*; and P. Stallybrass and A. White, *The Politics and Poetics of Transgression*, which contains a fascinating discussion of the pig as an intruder into human culture.
146. Beddoes, *Observations on the . . . . Consumptive*, 22.
147. Beddoes, *Observations on the . . . Consumptive*, 23.
148. Beddoes, *Observations on the . . . Consumptive*, 23.
149. Beddoes, *Observations on the . . . Consumptive*, 28–34.
150. Beddoes, *Observations on the . . . Consumptive*, 50.
151. Beddoes, *Observations on the . . . Consumptive*, 66.
152. Beddoes, *Observations on the . . . Consumptive*, 85.
153. Beddoes, *Observations on the . . . Consumptive*, 86.
154. Beddoes, *Hygëia*, 1 ii 100–1. For this idea, see B. Inglis, *The Diseases of Civilisation*.
155. Beddoes, *Essay on . . . Consumption*, 120.
156. Beddoes, *Essay on . . . Consumption*, 120.
157. Beddoes, *Hygëia*, 1 ii 98.
158. J. M. Adair, *Essays on Fashionable Diseases*, 73.
159. B. Mandeville, *A Treatise of the Hypochondriack and Hysterick Diseases*.
160. Adair, *Essays on Fashionable Diseases*, 95.
161. Adair, *Essays on Fashionable Diseases*, 73.
162. J. Hill, *Hypochondriasis*, 24.
163. E. Trillat, *Histoire de l'Hystérie*; I. Veith, *Hysteria*; E. Showalter, *The Female Malady*.
164. E.g., Joseph Farington reported how his friend Hone had 'been in a very nervous Hysterical state, the effect of anxiety of mind': K. Cave (ed.), *The Diary of Joseph Farington*, X, 3705.
165. See the discussion in Roy Porter and Dorothy Porter, *In Sick-*

ness and in Health, ch.12, 210–12.

166. See Dorothy Porter and Roy Porter, *Patient's Progress*, chs 7–9; Joan Lane, '"The Doctor Scolds Me"'; I.S.L. Loudon, 'The Nature of Provincial Medical Practice in Eighteenth-Century England'; *idem*, *Medical Care and the General Practitioner 1750–1850*; G. Holmes, *Augustan England: Profession, State and Society, 1680–1730*; Roy Porter, 'William Hunter: a Surgeon and a Gentleman'; C.H. Brock, 'The Happiness of Riches'; Roy Porter, 'Lay Medical Knowledge in the Eighteenth Century: the Evidence of the *Gentleman's Magazine*'.

167. See Roy Porter, 'The Patient in the Eighteenth Century'.

168. Beddoes, *Essay on . . . Consumption*, 260.

169. Beddoes, *Essay on . . . Consumption*, 127. Richard Warren was the darling of Whig salons, patronized by the Regent (and hated by George III, who called him 'Richard Rascal').

170. See Roy Porter (ed.), 'Introduction' to Thomas Trotter, *An Essay on Drunkenness*; Thomas Trotter, *A View of the Nervous Temperament*, 105.

171. B. Wedgwood and H. Wedgwood, *The Wedgwood Circle*, 127.

172. D. King-Hele, *Erasmus Darwin*, 248; Darwin was very free in his recommendation of opium.

173. Quoted in Wedgwood and Wedgwood, *Wedgwood Circle*, 129.

174. Discussed in M. Lefebure, *Samuel Taylor Coleridge*, 375.

175. These paradoxical developments of the mind/body problem and the emergence of ideology are further explored in Roy Porter, 'Barely Touching'; *idem*, 'Love, Sex and Madness in Eighteenth-Century England'; *idem*, 'Monsters and Madmen in Eighteenth-Century France'; *idem*, 'The Drinking Man's Disease'; *idem*, '"Under the Influence": Mesmerism in England'; *idem*, *Mind Forg'd Manacles*; *idem*, 'Body Politics: Approaches to the Cultural History of the Body.

7

Cashing in on vulgar errors

We see men in stays where they saw men in armour.
(Peacock, *Nightmare Abbey*)

I have been scrutinizing Thomas Beddoes's dread that modernity was creating a sickness culture in which illness became a modish language of self and of social exchange. This chapter will touch upon other commentaries on the new world of the 'valetudinarian', before examining in greater detail Beddoes's *exposés* of the institutions created by the collusion of the sick and the medical profession to articulate its sickness culture.

Self-dramatizing hypochondriacs and mercenary doctors long pre-date Beddoes, of course, in reality and in literature. In mid-Georgian England, the spa, Bath especially, became the venue for satire, whether gentle, as in Christopher Anstey's *The New Bath Guide* (1757), or, biting, as in Smollett's *Humphry Clinker* (1771).[1] By the close of the century, valetudinarian Mr Woodhouse figures were moving stage-centre, and the sea-side, as *Persuasion* (1818) indicates, had become a prime site for the *beau monde* to congregate for the convenience of physicians milking and bilking them. Vulgar preoccupations with gout and 'taking the waters' were becoming *passé*, being replaced by more refined anxieties about the nerves.[2] The supreme literary expression – indeed, debunking – of this culture is Jane Austen's *Sanditon*, left unfinished when the author died in 1817 of Addison's Disease.[3]

The fragility of health – at least that of the denizens of the new world of fashion – is accentuated from the novel's very first sentence. 'A gentleman and lady travelling from Tonbridge towards that part of the Sussex coast which lies between

Hastings and Eastbourne, being induced by business to quit the high road, and attempt a very rough lane, were overturned in toiling up its long ascent, half rock, half sand. The accident happened just beyond the only gentleman's house near the lane'. Mr Parker has suffered a 'sprained foot'; he begs the handy gentleman to summon the surgeon. 'The surgeon, sir!' – replied Mr Heywood – 'I am afraid you will find no surgeon at hand here, but I dare say we shall do very well without him'; for, he adds, 'we are always well stocked with all the common remedies for sprains and bruises'.[4]

Heywood serves in Austen's novel as a spokesman for the old order: rustic, rooted, hale and hearty. Parker heralds the new economy depicted by Beddoes – febrile, restless, energetic, on the make. He is travelling through the Weald in search of a surgeon, to grace and promote his new speculative development: Sanditon, a sea-side hamlet in the process of being commercialized into a modish health resort, adorned with promenades, circulating libraries, trinket shops and all the palaver of modernity. Parker is a booster for the sea. It is sure to heal his ankle. As soon as he gets home, he assures his wife, 'we will have our remedy at hand you know. – A little of our own bracing sea air will soon set me on my feet again. – Depend upon it, my dear, it is exactly a case for the sea. Saline air and immersion will be the very thing. – My sensations tell me so already'.[5] Indeed, he[6]

> held it as certain, that no person could be really well, no person (however upheld for the present by fortuitous aids of exercise and spirits in a semblance of health) could be really in a state of secure and permanent health without spending at least six weeks by the sea every year. – The sea air and sea bathing together were nearly infallible, one or the other of them being a match for every disorder, of the stomach, the lungs or the blood; they were anti-spasmodic, anti-pulmonary, anti-sceptic, anti-bilious and anti-rheumatic. Nobody could catch cold by the sea, nobody wanted appetite by the sea, nobody wanted spirits, nobody wanted strength. They were healing, softening, relaxing – fortifying and bracing – seemingly just as was wanted – sometimes one, sometimes the other. – If the sea breeze failed, the sea-bath was the certain corrective; – and where bathing disagreed, the sea breeze alone was evidently designed by nature for the cure.

Austen's fragment is set chiefly in Sanditon itself, where, alongside Lady Denham, the local landowner, who is angling for consumptive visitors so that she can put her two milch-asses to profit, we meet Parker's two utterly Beddoesian invalid sisters, Diana and Susan ('I do not believe', remarks their brother, 'they know what a day's health is').[7] Diana suffers from 'spasmodic bile' (by the late eighteenth century, it had become highly fashionable to be 'bilious').[8] Susan, who resembles her sister though 'more thin and worn by illness and medicine',[9] is a victim of nerves (by then *démodé*). Having run without benefit through 'the whole medical tribe', the sisters have taken to self-medication. 'Six leeches a day for ten days' have not, however, improved Susan's headaches, and so Diana has decided that her troubles lie in the gum, and has persuaded her to have three teeth extracted.[10]

There is additionally an invalid brother, Arthur, troubled by a 'cough', which inevitably suggests a consumption. But it is another sort of consumption by which he is chiefly characterized.[11] Assuredly, he endlessly complains of lethargy, feebleness and lack of stomach ('I am very nervous. – To say the truth, nerves are the worst part of my complaints in my opinion. My sisters think me bilious, but I doubt it').[12] But it is implied that his debility follows mainly from a Trotterian drinking habit – which he himself excuses as medicinal – 'the more wine I drink (in moderation) the better I am'.[13] Indeed, Austen caustically observes that 'Mr Arthur Parker's enjoyments in invalidism were very different from his sisters' – by no means so spiritualized',[14] noting how he hogs the fire and lards his toast with butter ('so far from dry toast being wholesome', he rationalizes his grossness, 'I think it a very bad thing for the stomach. Without a little butter to soften it, it hurts the coats of the stomach'),[15] while explaining earnestly how a couple of dishes of green tea would 'entirely take away the use of my right side, before I had swallowed it five minutes'.[16]

Austen plants the Parkers in a cultural landscape. The sisters were endowed with 'some natural delicacy of constitution'; this, combined with 'an unfortunate turn for medicine, especially quack medicine, had given them an early tendency at various times, to various disorders; – the rest of their sufferings was from fancy, the love of distinction and the love of the wonderful'.[17] In short, the cult of delicacy, as anatomized by Beddoes, was both the making and the ruin of such impressionable gentlefolk; and they in turn were the making of such places as Sanditon, that throve upon myths about the special virtues of location and habitat, and the sensitive individual's obligation to search out and sustain a healthsome environment.

Such views were ubiquitous, and not just in fiction. One of the most deeply entrenched dicta of traditional medicine, both learned and lay, was that health depended upon milieu. The notion, of course, had its philosophical roots in the Hippocratic teachings of 'Airs, Waters and Places', in the doctrine of the 'non-naturals', in astrology, and in the correspondences linking the macrocosm of Nature and the microcosm of man. The external elements governing climate – air, earth, fire, and water – were reflected and registered by the internal humours; the body, one might anachronistically say, acted as a kind of barometer. Given that a healthy constitution required maintenance of an optimal humoral balance – the right mix of the hot and the cold, the moist and the dry – was it not evident that such equilibriation depended upon adroit adjustment of the individual to the atmospheric environment?[18]

Such teachings applied, across the centuries, to the *minutiae* of day-to-day living, as 'Every Man His Own Physician' advice books and private letters made plain.[19] Readers of Pepys's *Diary* are continually brought face-to-face with his dread of damp – for cold would lead to colds, and colds, by clogging the pores, could precipitate internal poisoning by peccant humours.[20] Draughts, damp sheets, the hazards of sudden entrances from cold to warm rooms, or exits from clammy houses into night air, watermark the pages of all manner of writings about health, professional and lay, fact and fiction. Dean Clerke had just expired. Edmund Pyle, prebendary of Salisbury Cathedral, explained his friend's sad fate:[21]

> He died of an ague; caught by living in that vile damp close of Salisbury, which is a mere sink; and going to a church, daily, that is as wet as any vault; and which has destroyed more, perhaps, than it has saved.

And expertise in gauging the meteorological parameters of health was also meant to inform life's big decisions. Was North more salubrious than South, East than West? Where was it safe to set up home – town or country, hill or vale, coast or plain? Who could doubt the Tropics might prove deleterious to those of choleric temperament?[22] Or that, for sufferers from phlegmatic or melancholic distempers, the misty, murky British winter was a health hazard? By the eighteenth century, it was becoming the done thing for delicate gentlefolk – especially the 'phthisical' or consumptive – to fly south with the birds in winter, making pilgrimages to Montpellier, Nice, or Livorno in search of purer and milder air. Keats and Shelley followed suit.[23]

The quest for sanative climes also offered a further advantage: the medical benefits of travelling. No prescription, perhaps, was touted more enthusiastically, more insistently, and (one surmises) more desperately by pre-modern practitioners. Riding – colloquially, 'Dr Horse' – was best for recuperating a sound system, but even a smart bowl in a chaise would do. Rhythmic motion would aid digestion, change of scenery would raise the spirits of those disordered with the vapours or spleen. 'I must be on horseback for life, if I would be healthy', claimed John Wesley.[24] On one occasion, David Garrick attributed his own recovery to 'that excellent *physician*, a *horse*',[25] and Betsy Sheridan said of her sick father that 'Riding is to him of more service than all the Phisicians'.[26]

The desiderata of travel and salubrious air coincided at the health resort. Especially, perhaps, with the new Georgian affluence, the benefit of travelling for health was said to be clinched by making one's destination a spa or watering-place, although increased favour was being shown to sea-side stations, such as Margate, Brighton, Weymouth, or fictive Sanditon.

This was the recipe for health adopted by the propertied and the polite of Georgian Britain. Some may have tried spas as a last resort, when all else failed. Many, of course, inhaled the air and drank the waters incidentally to the social round, making health the pretext for holiday, and taking advantage of the ample facilities – for gambling, gossip and gawping – at Cheltenham, Scarborough or Bath Spa itself, albeit grumbling, like Smollett's Matt Bramble, at the expense and fatigue of it all (you had to be exceedingly fit, ran the old joke, before risking convalescence at Bath). But it is beyond dispute that Georgian polite society was genuinely anxious about damp, unwholesome winds, dewy mornings, nippy evenings, miasmata and other morbific affluvia, and possessed of an authentic – though not blind – faith in the tonic properties of favoured prospects, a good lie of the land, wholesome atmospheres, and balneological regimens. 'Wherever there is water, there is *malaria*', dogmatizes Mr

Firedamp in Peacock's *Crotchet Castle* – yet he has the answer: 'The great object of a wise man should be to live on a gravelly hill'.[27]

Collapsing in 1753 from all manner of constitutional maladies, above all, gout and dropsy, Henry Fielding quit his London house and decamped to Ealing. Why? Because, he wrote, it had 'the best air, I believe, in the whole kingdom, and far superior to that of Kensington Gravel Pits [for] the place [is] higher and more open towards the south, whilst it is guarded from the north wind by a ridge of hills, and from the smells and smoke of London by its distance'.[28] He didn't improve, however, and soon his physician was urging him to winter in Aix-en-Provence; eventually he set sail, as is recorded in his posthumous *Voyage to Lisbon*, on a last, lonely trip to much-favoured Portugal. Tobias Smollett, practitioner as well as novelist, and racked by asthma and probably consumption,[29] spent much of the 1760s scurrying round the South of France and the Ligurian Riviera trying to recruit his lungs. At the same time, his arch-rival, Laurence Sterne, was also travelling in France in hopes that the mild air would arrest encroaching tuberculosis. Volume Seven of *Tristram Shandy* opens with Death rapping on the door, and the panting hero giving him the slip through flight.[30] Good iatro-mechanists, Smollett and Sterne both set great store by keeping matter in motion.[31]

The correspondence of the Georgians abounds with neighbourly advice for negotiating the pains and pitfalls of the environment, or where to go to convalesce. When Samuel Johnson heard his acquaintance, John Perkins, was taking a break from his brewing business, he despatched him a tabulation of health advice.[32] 'I am much pleased that You are going on a very long Journey', he announced, a trifle ambiguously, 'which may by proper conduct restore your health and prolong your life':[33]

Observe these rules

1. Turn all care out of your head as soon as you mount the chaise.
2. Do not think about frugality, your health is worth more than it can cost.
3. Do not continue any day's journey to fatigue.
4. Take now and then a day's rest.

5. Get a smart seasickness if you can.
6. Cast away all anxiety, and keep your mind easy.

The advocacy of sea-sickness, which might appear a peculiarly Johnsonian asperity, was in fact traditional; back in 1538 Edward Corbett noted that Thomas Cromwell was about to embark on a return trip to Calais, 'because he would purge and scour his stomach'.[34]

Satirists rallied the foibles of those who ruined their constitutions and purses in pursuit of hot air. Nevertheless, the literature on environment and weather continued to multiply, evidently in response to demand from valetudinarians. Big-city atmosphere (it advised) was sure to be vitiated; ponds, marshes and estuaries exuded exhalations. Summers bred gastric infections and such low fevers as typhus; the ague came with the autumn. Exposure to biting east winds was fatal to the aged. Everyone touted his own pet theory about the rival virtues of mountain or dale, cliff or strand, North or South, sun or cloud, and belvederes balmy, breezy or bracing. In short, it was not the twentieth century that invented that great British institution: talking about the weather.[35]

Few were so sceptical as to puncture this hot-air balloon of theory and practice concerning climate and travel. One such was Beddoes, ironically – or, perhaps, *significantly* – so, in view of his own early enthusiasm for applying pneumatic chemistry to such lethal diseases as consumption through the inhalation of laboratory-produced gases. Beddoes left it to others to accumulate thermometric and barometric readings and correlate them against the rise and fall of epidemics.[36] Deafened by the medical claptrap about airs, Beddoes, however, took a rather different turn, confronting the corpus of traditional meteorological health lore, and treating it as a kind of mental monster: whence had this excrescence arisen? Did it possess any particle of validity, or was it wholly spurious, as vapid as gossip, and as devoid of meaning as the asininities of exploded scholasticism?

Addressing popular doctrines of airs, waters, and places, Beddoes set out to show they were so much piss and wind, blindly built upon the *ipse dixits* of ignoramuses and lacking solid factual grounding. Worse still, they provided legitimacy for corrupt medical practice and shameless profiteering. Truth was, medical meteorology was barely out of the cradle. Ideally, the discipline should aim to elucidate the laws of health; at present, however, one might be forgiven for thinking that its practice was 'merely to furnish indefatigable dulness with the creation of cyphering throughout all generations'.[37]

Despite the reams written on the subject of healthy and unhealthy seasons, the impact of seasonal variability upon health had been grotesquely exaggerated. Beddoes favoured dividing up the English year into five: starting at the new year, the frosty, the early mild, the cold dry, the hot, and finally the raw wet season.[38] Common experience taught that some of these weather patterns were more hazardous than others. But only a fool would so neglect his constitution as to leave himself prey to the, in truth, not very daunting effects of English draughts and chills. Susceptibility to the vagaries of climate could be dramatically curtailed by cultivating a sturdy constitution, and by building reserves of stamina. Above all, regular habits were essential. Proper nutrition would provide doughty protection against cold. 'Our shivering race' insisted Beddoes, harping on an old theme, must abandon tea and toast, and return to the 'meat breakfast of our ancestors'.[39] Sensible clothing was needed too, to replace the 'too thin a dress', lamentably *à la mode*, flimsy muslins in particular.[40] Attention should rather be paid to designing 'dress and habitations that afford sufficient shelter against the intensity of the cold'. The stalwart health of the Dutch, swathed in layers of winter woollies, proved that the well-insulated body generated ample heat to combat colds, chills and catarrhs.[41]

Finally, inner warmth should be developed by hardening, accustoming the constitution to cold, and sustaining it by exertion. For this, Beddoes deemed the 'task exercises' of gym training – for instance, dumbbells – a mistake, because, being mindlessly boring, they would soon be abandoned. Better to develop such activities as engaged mind and body simultaneously: such as botanizing, carpentry, or, best of all, predictably, chemistry.

Popular talk of health lying at the mercy of the weather was just displacement activity, all words not deeds. 'As we end our letters with your *most obedient humble servant*', he griped, 'so there is a set of opinions, rehearsed by people *pro forma* on particular occasions, but not acted upon, though universally accepted and relating to points of practice. Such is that which respects the danger of neglecting colds'.[42]

People delighted in showering others with admonitions about the healthy life. They didn't like following it themselves. 'This is the best piece of advice in the whole book', Beddoes confided at one point in his *Manual of Health*, 'and therefore it will be the least followed. . . . It is simply sitting a good deal during winter in a room without a fire'[43] – for in this way 'the mucous membrane of the chest grows less susceptible to cold, [and] the skin will increase in vital power'.[44] In nippy weather, there was no substitute for self-generated inner warmth, though palliatives, like mustard baths, might be helpful till one could 'make the constitution supply heat enough for itself'.[45] And if the mystique of the weather gripped the British imagination, there was also a magic in the air about atmosphere itself. Confessing he might one day write 'a little dictionary of medical nonsense', to be offered, naturally, to the faculty on April Fools' Day, Beddoes bragged of the tome's superior utility, offering, as it would, 'a plentiful supply of words, relative to the art of physic. Amongst these words, I know none that promises to figure to more advantage than the simple monosyllable air, with its adjuncts – *a charming air – a fine air – a pure air – a soft air*'.[46]

Utterly disarming! 'How can a poor devil of an invalid, by long suffering rendered credulous to other advisers, in proportion as the regulars have disappointed his hopes, resist such magic terms, uttered in a certain tone, in recommendation of any spot?' Unscrupulous practitioners cared little that it was all *vox praeterea nihil*. A few generalities about the environment Beddoes admitted, were, indeed, copper-bottomed. 'It is allowed that our fens and swamps produce agues. The atmosphere of a city probably contains exhalations unfavourable to all, and particularly, as we have seen, pernicious to the young. Hospitals perhaps from this, certainly from some cause, favour gangrene and foulness in sores; they injure hectic [that is, consumptive] patients'.[47] But beyond that, ignorance reigned. 'It makes one's head turn to behold upon what a narrow base of fact they have reared all this doctrine concerning the wholesomeness of this and that air. I know not how many Scotch Montpelliers are talked of by the clergy-men who corresponded with Sir John Sinclair!'[48]

All such claims smacked of empty chauvinism.[49] Till evidence proved otherwise, 'the summer of one hill and one valley is as good as that of another'.[50] 'People will, I know, strenuously contend for the superior salubrity of this and that place', the sceptic admitted, but they did so on the 'the faith of facts', not their demonstration.[51]

Beddoes was here writing, perhaps, from painful experience: once bitten, twice shy. Reflecting on his own unguarded youthful enthusiasm for the virtues of artificial airs in curing diseases, he noted that 'in the early days of chemical discovery respecting gases, when it was imagined that an apparatus for breathing oxygen was every thing necessary towards attaining the age of Methusalem, some agreeable dreams were related of the superior purity of the sea breezes'[52] – but all these visions had been dispelled in the cold light of the lab. The same must apply to suppositions about the salubrity of the environment. A good finding was hard to find: 'how far do our *facts* really carry us? They warn us of the neighbourhood of swamps. They are far from recommending great towns: though nothing has been demonstrated in the atmosphere of the one or the other, different from that of the driest and clearest country. Farther than this our facts hardly go'.[53]

Why, then, such inflated pretence to assurance? Know-alls amongst the laity advanced claims for the superior virtues of this air or that resort, largely to gratify their intellectual vanity as 'private practitioners'. Their doctrines also served as a body of serviceable obfuscating fictions, excuses to *avoid* constructive but troublesome action to protect one's health in the first place. Beddoes thus mocked Edward Gibbon's rationalization of his migration from London to Lausanne, as being necessary on health grounds (truth was, the historian could no longer afford Mayfair). Swiss mountain air would be better for his gout, Gibbon tried to convince himself (and others), adding that the great Dr Tissot 'assures me that in his opinion the moisture of England and Scotland is most pernicious, the dry pure air of Switzerland most favourable to a gouty constitution'.[54] Once in Lausanne, Gibbon, of course, was soon back in bandages and on crutches – and complaining about the weather, and the folly of Tissot. What this episode proved, Beddoes concluded, was that the question of climate was just a smokescreen, clouding the issue, because the real source of Gibbon's gout, as Gibbon well knew, lay not in the clouds but in the claret. 'I still suspect', judged Beddoes, 'that but for the Madeira "improved by age" for the safe arrival of which he repeatedly expresses so much anxiety, he might never have had such a cluster of unfortunate reasons for renouncing his faith in dry air and Dr Tissot'.[55]

Gibbon was just one of millions. Today the panacea, bemoaned Beddoes, prefiguring *Sanditon*, was sea air. 'A large part of the public has learned to look towards the sea as a resource, to which they may fly in case of need without further enquiry'.[56] By consequence, he continued, 'the effects of sea-water and of the sea-air seem to be confounded in many minds. And it is for the benefit of the latter that, in the maturity and towards the decline of the summer, the metropolis pours out part of its crowds to the Kentish coast'.[57] Beddoes was left sceptical: 'That the moral and physical effects of a journey and of fresh scenery will do much towards the restoration of certain invalids is a fact daily experienced in the practice of physic. But in scrophulous debility, or under any serious scrophulous ailment, no expectation of this kind ought for a moment to be entertained from mere removal either to the sea coast or into the interior of the country'. True, the coast may be pleasant, 'but what, in the name of common sense, is to be put to the score of air?'[58] Overall, the waste was appalling:[59]

> It is to be lamented that the rich should adopt such false measures, and waste a portion of time that perhaps cannot be retrieved. It is more to be lamented that those, who are not rich, should throw away, after the same hopeless chance, that money which they can ill spare, and of which a portion, expended upon proper means, would certainly accomplish the object they have at heart.

Because, at bottom, no particular climate was significantly healthier than another, and airs were never *specifics* for individual diseases, Beddoes suspected that the whole palaver was counter-productive.[60] People descanted about the value of the South in winter. Not a bit of it! 'The West of England, taking its milder and moister climate together, has no advantage worth a journey even of 50 miles'.[61] It was time for plain-speaking.[62] 'For my part, I have no hesitation in saying that to the question, *where shall I spend the winter?* the general answer as before ought to be – *at home*; and this both in respect to health, oeconomy and comfort'. Above all, Beddoes judged that in obviously terminal cases of consumption, the torture of the turnpikes was the last thing the sick needed. 'Persons in confirmed consumption ought not to be sent from home for the sake of any air or water we have'.[63]

Perhaps all this climatological mummery amounted to a sort of collective delirium. 'I never in my life knew an old woman prone to talk about medicine, that had not a whole rosary of cases ready to count over in behalf of her favourite bathing place'. A few interferers, charity compelled him to admit, were merely credulous – nor did he deny that *some* sufferers did, indeed, recover in Bath, Devon or wherever – they would, however, equally have got better in 'the fens of Lincolnshire, or . . . the city sewers'.[64] What truly riled Beddoes was the sight of 'polite practitioners' perpetuating, and, worse still, cashing in upon, such false ideas and forlorn hopes. Nor were these sordid practices confined to quacks – in the promotion of watering-places and resorts, regulars and irregulars were like as two peas in a pod.[65] Reading 'the fine things which medical men put into their pamphlets about the air and water of the places where they constantly reside', Beddoes wondered whether these were 'to be received with grains, scruples, drams, ounces, pounds, hundreds or tons of allowance?'[66] For their statements read just like so many quack bills – in the entire *scala naturae* you could not find 'two links in the chain more closely connected than various specimens of watering-place literature and the productions of quacks'.[67]

Tireless crusader against the seduction of medicine by the sirens of commercialization, Beddoes denounced health resorts as corrupters of medical morals. Of course, the weary should travel. 'In no country is there so large a proportion of individuals who can so well afford, or have so much desire, and', he added, 'in truth such pressing occasion to exchange the sear realities of business, and the scenes where art exhibits her bold creations, for the romance of feeling, so well known to those who travel in a fine season through a picturesque country'.[68] Holidays were healthy days: 'The medical philosopher must see them with satisfaction undertaking these pilgrimages of pleasure, leaving the load of their affairs behind, breaking loose from the restraints of etiquette, and renovating their existence in some degree by recalling the associations of their youth'.[69] But at the end of the road, the health resort often undid all that benefit. For, argued Beddoes, 'the design is often frustrated by injudicious arrangements at our places of resort for invalids'. For one thing, they had – their commercial viability depended on having – too much high life: 'I would therefore advise those who are in earnest to get rid of indisposition, to shun places of glitter, parade and jostling. If there could be a paradise for loungers, BEAU NASH might perhaps have laid it out. But neither he nor his imitators could be expected to have talents to plan for the sick'.[70]

Worse, such resorts were a medical racket. Was it any accident that 'retreats for the consumptive' were always 'remote places, where desperate cases can be sent away from notice': might they not, therefore, be better described as 'receptacles for the dying, corresponding to charnel houses'? Such institutions were 'undoubtedly very convenient for the baffled practitioner', forming part of an elaborate rigmarole, enacted by the profession, essential for fulfilling one of the great ends of the art of medicine itself.[71]

For, Beddoes paused and quizzed his readers, 'what, I ask, is this art?' Of course, all the latest luminaries such as Hoffman and Cullen had advanced their own high-flown definitions of the *ars medendi*, couched in terms of diagnostics and therapeutics.[72] They were wrong. For medicine, Beddoes archly revealed, was truly 'the art of amusing those patients, whose diseases it can neither remove nor palliate. . . . Those who can amuse the patient succeed much better in the world than those who have a greater talent for curing the disorder; and deservedly'. In short,[73]

> the medical attendants upon the sick frequently aim more at amusing than curing; and, in many cases, never dream of the latter purpose at all, the object of visits being to divert the mind of the patient from the effect of the treatment altogether. Accordingly how often do we see that the presence of the doctor has quite a magical operation, when his prescriptions have none at all. Hence it is that such numbers of invalids, though they do not find themselves in the least better, are ever exclaiming what a fine man their physician is!

Everybody, concluded Beddoes, had heard of 'a *placebo* prescription'. The point was, 'among prescriptions, how many are there penned wholly, or in part, without the *placebo* intention!'[74]

Now all this had a deep bearing upon the fashionable treatment of the consumptive – whom the physician assuredly knew to be incurable. First, the practitioner ran through his repertoire of 'amusing prescriptions . . . stories, compliments, the small talk . . . the whole magazine of expedients by which the patient is diverted from the contemplation of his declining state'.[75]

This game could be spun out only so long. When the pantomime was exhausted, and the patient ominously began to sink, it was time to suggest the magic word of travel. For 'it would be cruel to leave a dying person without resource' – how could a tender family doctor in London 'bear to think, that the son or daughter of a dear friend of his should die at home, just under his nose'?[76] And so the patient was sent west – 'recommended to go to Dawlish, Exmouth, the Land's End, or God knows how much further off still. At all these places new scenes of amusement begin, and continue as long as they can.'[77] Not least, they flocked to Bristol, as 'Hotwells cases', a genteelism for a corpse – so much so, that one might fix up a sign 'upon Temple gate Bristol, reading "*Lasciate ogni speranza, voi ch'entrate*"'.[78]

This black comedy of transportation for the terminally sick was managed by the crew of practitioners thriving at such watering-places, whose job it was to keep up the amusements. These 'physicians and apothecaries . . . do not fall short in the great talent of simpering and bowing. Our medical brethren from the other side of the Tweed are reputed to be the greatest proficients here.'[79] Moreover, such sycophants were gratuitously given helping hands by lay decoy ducks, who, as it were, pimped for them. Never a watering-place without its 'dowager of quality encamped. Here they officiate as mistresses of the ceremonies of medicine, in virtue of their own appointment.'[80] Such Quality ladies gaily instructed new pilgrims in the medical pecking-order – saying '*Surely, my dear, you won't think of consulting any body but Dr. Such-an-one*' – by consequence of which 'you may always discover that their interference has in view the benefit of the doctor and not that of the patient'.[81] Without such *aides-de camp*, it might have been necessary to publish 'a *watering-place nursing and doctoring book*', to give instructions in the right sort of 'amusing medication'.[82]

So it was all a decorous *danse macabre.* 'Medical practitioners . . . squeeze as long and as hard as they can, and then toss the patient, all skin and bone, to a watering place correspondent, to be wrung to the very dregs'.[83] Your Baths and Scarboroughs and Margates were best viewed as 'institutions of convenience for one part of the faculty and of charity for another', it being handy for the family physician to have a sort of charnel-house ready provided into which he may toss a half-animated carcase'.[84] The scandal would have been mitigated, if the air, or waters, in these places, had any authentic healing properties.[85] But what proof was there? Of the Hotwells on his very doorstep, much-puffed as curative for tuberculosis, Beddoes complained that no one even seemed sure 'whether it be the water, the air of the valley, or that of the hill, which performs the miracle of healing ulcers of the lungs'.[86] The Hotwells were but a hotbed of quackery, exploited by regulars and irregulars alike. Beddoes always professed to be mystified at the outrage provoked by his suggestion that quack doctors be outlawed.[87]

> For what, I pray you, could invalids lose by the suppression of all quack medicines for consumption, while the regular faculty is in snug possession of the Hotwell here by the side of the Avon? What is there in Godbold's balsam that this water cannot replace? and (faith in the gift of St Vincent failing) have we not the air of Clifton close at hand, offering itself to us as presumptive heir to the reputation of the water?

Spa medicine had a vaudeville all its own. 'The Hotwell art of physic may be acquired in three days by a person of the most moderate capacity, what the worse is it when practised by a doctor in form, rather than by an old nurse, or unlicensed practitioner?'[88]

In his own treatment of consumptives, Beddoes was as good as his word: he urged them – prefiguring Jane Austen's Mr Heywood – to stay at home. Committed, unlike most nineteenth-century tuberculosis doctors, to the virtues of warmth, Beddoes, as we have seen, recommended the 'cowhouse method'.[89] At least it avoided the trauma of travelling: 'I had been endeavouring to persuade a gentleman who had resided two or three winters at Lisbon without the smallest advantage to try the cowhouse, rather than return to Portugal'.[90] Staying home was easier, and 'the article of oeconomy speaks for itself'.[91]

Not everybody, however, took kindly to being deprived by this Beddoesian ban of the traditional medical justifications for getting away and going abroad. The doctor's friend and patient, the genius, hypochondriac and opium addict, Samuel Taylor Coleridge, found his negatives about the value of travel hard to stomach.[92]

By the late 1790s, Coleridge was regularly sick with bilous disorders, gout, chronic neuralgia, insomnia, and who knows what else. '*Sinking, sinking, sinking*! I feel, that I am *sinking*', he wailed to Humphry Davy in May 1801.[93] 'My medical attendant says that it is irregular Gout with nephritic Symptoms – Gout in a young man of 29!! Swoln knees, and knotty Fingers, a loathy stomach, & a dizzying head – trust me, Friend! I am at times an object of moral Disgust to my own Mind.' Coleridge, a man with some of the traits of Austen's Arthur Parker, went on to propose to his friend that the real answer to his appalling health problems lay – not, of course, in actually reforming his own lifestyle – but in cruising off to the Canaries. 'But that this long long Illness has impoverished me', he explained, 'I should immediately go to St Miguel's, one of the Azores – the Baths & and the delicious climate might restore me – and if it were possible, I would afterwards send over for my Wife and children, & settle there for a few years'.[94]

Generous as always with advice, Coleridge proffered the same recommendations to his sick brother, James, telling him 'I have not the least doubt, that you would be completely renovated by a year passed in a warm & even climate, without those *Drafts* of air, & those irritating particles of sea coal, which make an English Fire-side . . . a very stepmother to pulmonary patients'.[95] Obviously he still had his own case on his mind. 'As to myself', he confided, 'I am determined to pass the next year or two of my Life either at Madeira, or Teneriffe, or Lisbon – with my Family'. In any case, he advised James to 'write a detailed account of your Health to Dr Beddoes. You and I, I dare say, think much alike of Beddoes's general mind. He is a very ingenious man, of great Learning & a very extensive Practice – but precipitant & bold, even to daring – a passionate Innovator'.[96]

Yet this mention of Beddoes brought the soaring idealist down to earth with a bump, reminding him of the doctor's dampener on this subject, for shortly afterwards Coleridge had to relay to Southey Beddoes's opinion that 'climate is no remedy'.[97] How exasperating! What dreadful dogmatism from the doctor! – 'this is in the teeth of every medical writer of Note on the gout, who have all prescribed hot climates for gouty people – & what weighs more with me, in the teeth of particular facts in my own knowledge'. Anyway, expostulated Coleridge, he'd already tried everything without a glimmer of success:[98]

> What gouty Medicines are there that I have not used? What gouty regimen? . . . What can I want more decisive than my own experience – in hot rooms I am well – in hot weather I am well – Cold, wet & change of weather uniformly disease me. It is astonishing how well I was three hot weeks last summer – a cold rain came on, & I was ill as instantly as if it had poisoned me . . . Heat in a hot climate is the only regular & universal Stimulus of the external world; to which if I can add Tranquillity, the equivalent, & Italian climate, of the world within, I do not despair to be a healthy man.

It was a bone Coleridge could not drop. 'I am sure', he was soon telling Southey:[99]

> if Dr Beddoes lived near me, or in the same house with me, he would soften down his opinions respecting the inefficiency of Climate in gout cases. The effects of weather are to the full as palpable upon me, as upon the little Old Lady and Gentleman in the weather box – or on the sea weed in the Barber's shop . . . my dear Southey, do call on Dr Beddoes – & read such parts of this Letter to him, as you think fit.

He would make one last try with medicines, he promised – Welles's gout medicine as recommended by Beddoes[100] – but if that didn't work, 'I then, by God, go off to Malta or Madeira. Madeira is the better place.' Malta, however, it was to be. Coleridge landed a post as secretary to the Governor; just to twit his doctor – another case of the patient proved right! – he proceeded to mend.[101]

Beddoes's attitudes are worth pondering. His indignation on behalf of assaulted humanity, common sense, and, of course, health and life were wholehearted. He was outraged at the squandering of the health and lives of those who had more money than sense, furious that physicians were colluding in the farce of spas and seaside. All reason and science were against it.

One is, of course, tempted to probe further. Why such inordinate anger? How do we interpret it? Was it essentially the frustrated rage of the friend of humanity, unable to save those beyond hope? Or was there more to Beddoes's habitual denigration of and resentment towards his own profession? These are issues the next chapter addresses.

Notes

1. C. Anstey, *The New Bath Guide*; Tobias Smollett, *The Expedition of Humphry Clinker*; G.S. Rousseau, *Tobias Smollett*; A. Barbeau, *Life and Letters at Bath in the Eighteenth Century*; Roy Porter (ed.), *The Medical History of Waters and Spas*; Phyllis Hembry, *The English Spa, 1560–1815. A Social History*.

2. For this aetherialization, see Roy Porter, 'Barely Touching'; see also Janet Todd, *Sensibility*.

3. There is suberb discussion of Jane Austen's handling of all these issues in John Wiltshire, *Jane Austen and the Body*.

4. Jane Austen, *Sanditon*, 157.

5. Jane Austen, *Sanditon*, 158. For Austen's interest in the new world of consumerism see Edward Copeland, 'Jane Austen and the Consumer Revolution'; *idem*, 'Fictions of Employment: Jane Austen and the Woman's Novel'; *idem*, 'Money Talks: Jane Austen and the *Lady's Magazine*'. See further N. McKendrick, John Brewer and J.H. Plumb, *The Birth of a Consumer Society*; and John Brewer and Roy Porter (eds), *Consumption and the World of Goods*. For the sea and holidays, see J.A.R. Pimlott, *The Englishman's Holiday*.

6. Jane Austen, *Sanditon*, 163.

7. Jane Austen, *Sanditon*, 174.

8. Jane Austen, *Sanditon*, 175. On the fashion for biliousness, see Roy Porter, '"Expressing Yourself Ill"'.

9. Jane Austen, *Sanditon*, 199.

10. Jane Austen, *Sanditon*, 175. For the resort to self-medication see Roy Porter, 'The Patient in the Eighteenth Century'; *idem*, 'Health and Wealth'; Dorothy Porter and Roy Porter, *Patient's Progress*, chs 1–4.

11. Jane Austen, *Sanditon*, 176. For the pun on consumption, see Roy Porter, 'Consumption: Disease of the Consumer Society?'.

12. Jane Austen, *Sanditon*, 201.

13. Jane Austen, *Sanditon*, 201.

14. Jane Austen, *Sanditon*, 203.

15. Jane Austen, *Sanditon*, 203.

16. Jane Austen, *Sanditon*, 203.

17. Jane Austen, *Sanditon*, 198.

18. G. Miller, 'Airs, Waters and Places in History'; P. Niebyl, 'The Non-Naturals'; O. Temkin, *Galenism*. For planetary influences, see Patrick Curry, *Prophecy and Power. Astrology in Early Modern England*.

19. For the history of advice literature see Ginnie Smith, 'Prescribing the Rules of Health'; *idem*, 'Cleanliness'; C.J. Lawrence,

'William Buchan: Medicine Laid Open'; C. Rosenberg, 'Medical Text and Medical Context'.

20. For Pepys see Roy Porter, 'The Patient's View'; L.M. Beier, *Sufferers and Healers.*

21. Quoted in Roy Porter and Dorothy Porter, *In Sickness and in Health,* 21.

22. W. Ernst, *Mad Tales from the Raj.*

23. N. Crook and D. Guiton, *Shelley's Venomed Melody*; D.C. Goellnicht, *The Poet-Physician.*

24. R.A. Knox, *Enthusiasm,* 425.

25. D. Little and G. Kahrl (eds), *The Letters of David Garrick,* i, 236.

26. W. LeFanu (ed.), *Betsy Sheridan's Journal,* 95.

27. D. Garnett (ed.), *The Novels of Thomas Love Peacock,* 661.

28. H. Fielding, *A Voyage to Lisbon,* 197.

29. G.S. Rousseau, *Tobias Smollett.*

30. Laurence Sterne, *The Life and Opinions of Tristram Shandy,* 459f.; W. Cross, *The Life and Times of Laurence Sterne*; D. Furst, 'Sterne and Physick: Images of Health and Disease in *Tristram Shandy*'; Roy Porter, 'Against the Spleen'; *idem,* '"The Whole Secret of Health"'.

31. Carol Houlihan Flynn, 'Running out of Matter'.

32. R.W. Chapman (ed.), *The Letters of Samuel Johnson,* iii, 498–9.

33. Chapman (ed.), *Letters of Samuel Johnson,* iii, 498–9.

34. Muriel St Clare Byrne (ed.), *The Lisle Letters,* v, 186.

35. For the importance of atmosphere in Georgian thinking about health see Roy Porter and Dorothy Porter, *In Sickness and in Health,* esp. chs. 9 and 15.

36. For the popularity of medical meteorology, see U. Tröhler, 'Quantification in British Medicine and Surgery 1750–1830'; and Simon Schaffer, 'Measuring Virtue: Eudiometry, Enlightenment and Pneumatic Medicine'.

37. T. Beddoes, *Manual of Health: or, the Invalid Conducted Safely through the Seasons* (1806), 262.

38. Beddoes, *Manual of Health,* 164.

39. Beddoes, *Manual of Health,* 238.

40. Beddoes, *Manual of Health,* 239.

41. Beddoes, *Manual of Health,* 166.

42. Beddoes, *Manual of Health,* 180–1.

43. Beddoes, *Manual of Health,* 228.

44. Beddoes, *Manual of Health,* 229.

45. Beddoes, *Manual of Health,* 230.

46. Beddoes, *Manual of Health,* 318.

47. Beddoes, *Manual of Health,* 319.

48. Beddoes, *Manual of Health,* 319. Sir John Sinclair's *Statistical Survey of Scotland,* which was interested in questions of health, was built upon replies by Scottish ministers to a questionnaire.

49. Beddoes, *Manual of Health,* 321.

50. Beddoes, *Manual of Health,* 323.

51. Beddoes, *Manual of Health,* 323.

52. Beddoes, *Manual of Health,* 323. For Beddoes's early faith in the healing powers of airs, in particular in connection with his Pneumatic

Institution, see L.S. Gottlieb, 'Thomas Beddoes M.D. and the Pneumatic Institution at Clifton 1798–1801'; T.H. Levere, 'Dr Thomas Beddoes and the Establishment of his Pneumatic Institution'; *idem*, 'Thomas Beddoes, The Interaction of Pneumatic and Preventative Medicine with Chemistry'; A.H. Miller, 'The Pneumatic Institution of Thomas Beddoes at Clifton'.

53. Beddoes, *Manual of Health*, 321.

54. T. Beddoes, *Hygëia: or Essays Moral and Medical, on the Causes Affecting the Personal State of our Middling and Affluent Classes*, 3 vols (1802–03), vol. 1, Essay ii, p.61. Hereafter references to this work will be in the form *Hygëia*, 1 ii 61. For Gibbon see P. Craddock, *Young Edward Gibbon*.

55. Beddoes, *Hygëia*, 1 ii 62.

56. Beddoes, *Hygëia*, 2 vi 80.

57. Beddoes, *Hygëia*, 2 vi 80.

58. Beddoes, *Manual of Health*, 324.

59. Beddoes, *Hygëia*, 2 vi 81.

60. Beddoes, *Manual of Health*, 345.

61. Beddoes, *Manual of Health*, 385.

62. Beddoes, *Manual of Health*, 385.

63. Beddoes, *Manual of Health*, 348.

64. Beddoes, *Manual of Health*, 325.

65. For Beddoes's hatred of quacks see Roy Porter, *Health for Sale*, 200f. For his belief that all medicine was pervaded by quackery see Roy Porter, 'Reforming the Patient'. For the 'polite practitioner' see Beddoes, *Manual of Health*, 389.

66. Beddoes, *Manual of Health*, 337.

67. T. Beddoes, *A Letter to the Right Honourable Sir Joseph Banks . . . on the Causes and Removal of the Prevailing Discontents, Imperfections, and Abuses, in Medicine* (1808), 105.

68. Beddoes, *Manual of Health*, 316–17.

69. Beddoes, *Manual of Health*, 316–17.

70. Beddoes, *Hygëia*, 3 ix 112.

71. Beddoes, *Manual of Health*, 328.

72. Beddoes, *Manual of Health*, 328.

73. Beddoes, *Manual of Health*, 329.

74. Beddoes, *Manual of Health*, 330.

75. Beddoes, *Manual of Health*, 330.

76. Beddoes, *A Letter to the Right Honourable Sir Joseph Banks*, 102.

77. Beddoes, *Manual of Health*, 331.

78. Beddoes, *A Letter to the Right Honourable Sir Joseph Banks*, 104. For the Bristol medical milieu, see M.E. Fissell, *The Physic of Charity*; M.R. Neve, 'Natural Philosophy, Medicine and the Culture of Science in Provincial England'.

79. Beddoes, *Manual of Health*, 331.

80. Beddoes, *Manual of Health*, 332.

81. Beddoes, *Manual of Health*, 333.

82. Beddoes, *Manual of Health*, 332–3.

83. Beddoes, *Manual of Health*, 335.

84. Beddoes, *Manual of Health*, 337.

85. Beddoes, *Manual of Health*, 337.
86. Beddoes, *Manual of Health*, 337.
87. Beddoes, *Manual of Health*, 330.
88. Beddoes, *A Letter to the Right Honourable Sir Joseph Banks*, 103.
89. See above, ch.6.
90. Thomas Beddoes, *Observations on the Medical and Domestic Management of the Consumptive; on the Powers of Digitalis Purpurea; and on the Cure of Scrophula* (1801), 48.
91. Beddoes, *Observations on the . . . Consumptive*, 85.
92. J. Cottle, *Reminiscences of Samuel Taylor Coleridge and Robert Southey*; N. Fruman, *Coleridge, the Damaged Archangel*; M. Lefebure, *Samuel Taylor Coleridge: A Bondage of Opium*; Richard Holmes, *Coleridge: Early Visions.*
93. E.L. Griggs (ed.), *Collected Letters of Samuel Taylor Coleridge*, no. 397, p.726, Monday 4 May 1801.
94. Griggs (ed.), *Collected Letters of Samuel Taylor Coleridge*, no. 397, p.726, Monday 4 May 1801.
95. Griggs (ed.), *Collected Letters of Samuel Taylor Coleridge*, no. 475, p.896, letter to James Coleridge.
96. Griggs (ed.), *Collected Letters of Samuel Taylor Coleridge*, no. 475, p.896, letter to James Coleridge.
97. Griggs (ed.), *Collected Letters of Samuel Taylor Coleridge*, no. 491, p.930.
98. Griggs (ed.), *Collected Letters of Samuel Taylor Coleridge*, no. 491, p.930.
99. Griggs (ed.), *Collected Letters of Samuel Taylor Coleridge*, no. 513, p.976.
100. See A. Welles, *An Account of the Discovery and Operation of a New Medicine for Gout*, which contains a recommendation by Beddoes.
101. D. Sultana, *Samuel Taylor Coleridge in Malta and Italy.*

8

Reforming the profession

> He now became troubled with the *passion for reforming the world.*
>
> (Peacock, *Nightmare Abbey*)

Beddoes urged radical reform of the medical profession.

He was not, of course, the only one: reform was on the agenda for many British medical men around the turn of the nineteenth century, and a rousing rhetoric of moral outrage was widespread. The body medical had grown corrupt. There was a surplus, or, maybe, a shortage, of practitioners; too many doctors were too old, or, perhaps, too young, or under-trained, or over-qualified; some were too opulent, others too poor; and anyway practice was infested with a 'vile race of quacks', impostors, mountebanks and itinerants. Much of the blame for this was to be laid squarely upon the shoulders of the sick – for playing fast and loose with poor, honest, long-suffering practitioners – but the responsibility for remedying this parlous situation had to rest with the profession itself, which needed to put its own house into order, probably with the aid of Parliament.[1]

This reformist rhetoric was a call to arms that flowed like quicksilver from Beddoes's pen. Beddoes, however, couched his protests not in the language of careers open to talent, fair-trading, professional closure, of the fine-print of parliamentary statutes and legal powers, but in the idiom of public virtue. Indeed, Beddoes wrote in a moral language far more hard-hitting than the 'dearly beloved' pieties that fill the pages of the formal works of medical ethics penned at this time.[2] If John Gregory and Thomas Percival saw the ills of medicine as superficial, Beddoes thought them systemic, constitutional, terminal even. Many reformers around 1800 looked to change through tinkering; Beddoes espoused the radical philosophy of moral renewal.

For the malaise, in Beddoes' view, was not just a question of collegiate corruption, oligarchic blight, or charlatan voracity; rather, it was structural and endemic. The root of the evil was quackery. Like his regular colleagues, Beddoes detested quackery with all his heart, deploring the despoliations of ignorant hucksters who were cashing in hand-over-fist from the ever-gullible public, and wrecking the nation's health into the bargain.[3] Time and again he warned readers against such saturation-advertised nostrums as mercurial vermifuges for infants, which he regarded as little short of criminal poisons. 'In consequence of money expended on their purchase', he fumed, 'families above the poorest class are frequently deprived of the necessaries of life; . . . there are instances where people have sold the bed from under them (the rage for quack medicines, in some familiar instances, being just the habit of dram-drinking)'.[4]

More incensed, and maybe more *dirigiste* than many of his peers, Beddoes was for public action against such quacks. Bodies should be established – presumably like the Parisian Société Royale de Médecine – to assay proprietary preparations; not least, bare-faced and impenitent quacks should be punished by Parliament:[5] 'a scheme for the reform of medicine without the abolition of quack medicines, is about as hopeful as one for making the rattle-snake harmless'.[6] No compromise was possible. 'The advertising and sale of secret medicines ought to be entirely suppressed.'[7]

Fulminations against quack doctors, ten-a-penny in the medical press of the day, need no elaboration here.[8] The true radicalism of Beddoes's attack lies in the fact that he indicted the profession itself of practising not healing but quackery – a palpable hit scored already, of course, by Grub Street satirists galore,[9] but rare enough as a *je m'accuse* from the pen of an august Oxford M.D. Time and again in his syllabus of medical errors, Beddoes pinpointed the parallels between quacks and regulars – or 'medical Jesuits' and 'medical Jansenists', as this ferocious foe of priestcraft was pleased to dub his fellows.[10]

Regulars vilified empirics – yet was this not a brazen case of the pot calling the kettle black? Quack was as quack did. Quacks were lambasted for self-publicizing; but, begged Beddoes, did not they, in so doing, merely 'manifest the spirit of the trade'[11] – for surely regulars were no laggards in touting for clients, albeit behind a genteel veneer: 'Indeed to coquet for custom in an equipage beyond his circumstances is considered as altogether essential to his success'.[12] In the same way, the novice practitioner was always 'advised to give so many *dinners of business* per annum', a tactic whereby he arranged for his wife – his 'serjeant Kite in petticoats' – to 'recruit for patients'. 'The good lady crams them with her dainties, in sure and certain hopes, that the turn of her doctor will come to cram them equally with his drugs'. So wherein lay the essential difference between regulars and their 'bastard brethren'?[13] In treatments and remedies, they were like as two peas in a pod. 'Of quack compositions we regulars cannot in honesty but confess that they are excellent, being, in fact, the very same which we use ourselves'.[14]

This device of superimposing regulars and quacks as doubles was Beddoes's graphic demonstration that practitioners had turned from healing to dealing, rather than practising their art as an exalted calling. Disregarding lofty ideals, modern physicians had become market-place higglers, their sights trained not upon health but wealth.[15]

Modern medical mercenariness hardly bothered to wear a fig-leaf. 'Physicians are often as needlessly prodigal of their visits', Beddoes huffed, 'as apothecaries of their potions' – a damning comparison indeed![16] A *bon mot* going round the salon: 'there is no getting doctors and workmen out of a house, once they get in'.[17] Time was when physicians had cultivated the arduous art of regimen. Gone were those days, now they treated only by doling out drugs, reducing healing to commodity-exchange. 'The public has learned to expect scarce any thing beyond particular prescriptions; and to minds little inured to reasoning, scarce any thing else is acceptable'.[18] And was not this lucrative vulgarization of the *ars medendi* the product of an unholy alliance 'between doctor and apothecary', or rather 'drench dealers' and vendors of 'medicated wash'?[19] 'The desire of the apothecary to swell his bill, and the complaisance of the physician towards the apothecary', Beddoes regretted, 'are justly believed to create infinite abuse in our profession'.[20]

Survey the topography of medical practice. Did one find that orderly tripartite, incorporated hierarchy, College of Physicians at the apex, which royal charters seemed to have mapped out? Not a bit of it. Instead of an established church-medical, there was a seething stew of activity,[21] in which it was quite impossible to draw dividing lines separating the sheep from the goats, men of principle from men on the make. Popularity and reputation would certainly never serve as litmus tests:[22]

> Without going a hundred miles from Clifton, Bristol and Bath, you may meet with practitioners, whose genius has transported them at a single bound from the side of the mortar to the bedside; and who go about distributing their *poudres de succession* through town and country, with as much professional gravity, as if they had gone through the longest course of study, and stood the severest trials of skill. As to consumption-doctresses, cancer-curers, mechanics professing to treat divers disorders, and particularly those of the female sex, there have arisen within my short memory, several, in whose behalf to speak with the cricket players, one might safely challenge all England; nay, in this favoured district, do we not behold the splendid seats of solemn, regular, respected quackery, methodized, as you shall hear, if you do not know it, according to the most approved forms of a foreign merchant's counting house.

Even esteemed physicians owed their clientele and credit to the world's applause, and the public recognized fortune as the sole yardstick of worth. 'Our dignity', Beddoes wailed, 'is unfortunately placed in the quantity of our gains, not of the good we do'.[23]

Gold had become the *primum mobile*, the very *archaeus* of medicine. 'Money, I perceive, can put all the members of the faculty and all its appendages into busy motion.'[24] Hence medics tailored their performances to public demand. 'But to what purpose? Very frequently, not to the purpose of deferring, one hour, the fatal crisis. If indeed, all this bustle console the sick, or the survivors, then must it be considered as well purchased, at whatever price'. But in truth, 'the doctor's pomp and apothecary's mysterious hurry' actually achieved nothing of therapeutic value, 'so impracticable has it been found to reduce health to the state of a mere article of commerce, and so entirely does HYGEIA disdain to become the slave of PLUTUS'.[25]

Beddoes was not above hurling an occasional bolt at individual practitioners whose love of lucre was grotesque. 'I understand that a fashionable physician in town is not to bestow above ten minutes under the peril of being deemed not sufficiently hurried'; and 'I have been assured, by a curious observer', he informed Sir Joseph Banks, 'that the late Dr Warren often bestowed but three minutes on a case' – the courtly Warren was so obsessed with lucre, rumour had it, that as he inspected his own tongue in the mirror in the morning, he automatically transferred a guinea from one pocket to another.[26] But Beddoes's prime aim was not personal vilification, but to lay bare the structural features promoting and perpetuating the perversion of medicine into 'the sick trade'.[27]

Beddoes, as we have seen, was a trenchant critic of the ascendancy of commercial capitalism wherein 'WEALTH, the most general object of power, becomes the most general object of desire',[28] and a 'chain of destructive vanity'[29] linked class and class in a cash nexus, presided over by that 'fawning, treacherous divinity', fashion[30] – which in turn, of course, made work for the medics, for 'does not gold bring with it its plagues'?[31] Disposable income had mushroomed, and goods and services were undergoing industrial commodification, becoming standardized products, each with its price-tag.[32] This was the new manufacturing system, and Beddoes viewed medical practitioners as cogs in its wheels – indeed, they had eagerly accommodated themselves to the enterprise ethos driving the *laissez-faire* economy. Since doctors traded like shopkeepers, might it be no bad idea, pondered Beddoes, with *caveat emptor* in mind, if 'medical certificates should . . . have written on them CAVEANT AEGROTI'?[33]

The seduction of doctors by market-place *mores* was bad enough. But there was a further facet to the problem, reflecting another evil of manufacturing society. Supply and demand had become the sovereign law. Doctors had set themselves up as medical traffickers in diagnostics and drugging. Today's economic historians make much of the demand factor in industrial expansion, and certainly Beddoes believed that medicine had become demand-driven (if supply-induced), stimulated by the whims of the sick – or, too frequently, the pseudo-sick.[34] Beddoes routinely portrayed doctors as suppliers subservient to customers and all their footling fads and foibles.

Beddoes protested against the reduction of medicos to mongers in a system in which the sick person always knew best, and as the paying piper called the tune.[35] Grandees and gentlefolks demanded deference from their physicians, as from butchers, bakers and candlestickmakers. At bottom, therefore, doctors were conditioned to operate as high-grade flunkeys in a service economy – one in which the Quality paymasters had not the slightest reason for treating regulars preferentially to quacks (where, to repeat, lay the difference?). The names of peers and parsons, Beddoes observed, were always to be found in newspaper quack bills, 'dangling by dozens, to the tail of frauds at half a guinea the bottle'.[36]

Practitioners were obviously impotent to challenge the patronage system pervading unreformed society. They had, however, Beddoes regretted, needlessly made a bad situation worse. For one thing, the profession must shoulder the blame for positively encouraging their paymasters to entertain exaggerated – and utterly destructive – conceptions of lay medical capabilities. Above all, they had been prominent in writing medical handbooks for popular consumption. Such prostitution of medicine by 'the projector of a new domestic medicine' was 'a scheme perfectly in the spirit of our literary traffick', Beddoes observed tartly, for 'to him, who has only in view the making of money, a grammar, a gazetteer, a medical compendium will appear identical, provided they prove equally saleable articles'.[37] On the whole, Beddoes concluded, do-it-yourself medical texts were more fatal than highwaymen: gentlemen of the road at least left victims a choice between 'your money or your life'. With books of auto-medication, by contrast, the rule was your money *and* your life. 'Quacking books are unquestionably the same evil wholesale which quack medicines are by retail'.[38] Of course, in defence of such practices, there was endless canting about the sovereign voice of public opinion, but what had that to do with healing? 'It is sometimes not impertinent to ask', Beddoes insisted, 'if there be any sense in the *vox populi*?'[39]

Apologists for market forces might insinuate that free choice would result in the cream of the profession rising to the top by spontaneous acclaim. But this was all baloney: informed choice was a myth – for who could deny that 'a great part of this very public is incapable of distinguishing square from round, black from white, in the forms and colours of medical character'?[40] Apply this criterion – 'the usual signs of public confidence in medicine' – and the most illustrious physician in Britain would manifestly be none other than the egregious Liverpool quack,

Samuel Solomon, vendor of the 'Balm of Gilead', 'a fellow who orders British gin from Bristol to Liverpool, colours and christens it balm . . . and who enjoys as much of this confidence as almost all the fellows of the three royal colleges put together'.[41] In sum, demand from below, articulated by a mis-educated and misinformed public seeking diversions in the medical bargain basement, could do nothing but reduce the art to travesty and whoredom.

Moreover, practitioners were further digging their own graves – or at least betraying their cloth – by their shameless acquiescence in an abject bedside farce, bowing and scraping to the jingle of guineas. Doctors' orders had given way to patients' orders. Serving patients whose 'minds are usually made quite up', the courtly doctor will often[42]

> listen with a face of sanctified wonder, protest that he was just thinking of the same thing, put his goose-quill under the guidance of their inspirations, and content himself with translating them into certain magical abbreviations, as *pilul.–pulv.–haust.*, which are the main support of his professional dignity and that grand mystery of the art, into which these his female prompters have not yet penetrated.

Beddoes was disgusted by the obsequious tuft-hunting of such courtier physicians as Thomas Gisborne, that notorious 'member of the *haute noblesse* of medicine'. 'One of the princesses being taken ill, and Dr. Gisborne in attendance', Beddoes maliciously related:[43]

> her royal highness enquired of the doctor if she might not indulge in the use of a little ice cream, as she thought it would greatly refresh her. Dr. G. who never contradicted his royal patients, answered that he '*entirely agreed with her royal highness*;' and the ice was accordingly provided. His Majesty, visiting the chamber and observing the glass, with some of the ice still remaining in it, seemed alarmed, on the supposition that it might be improper; but her royal highness assured him that she had the doctor's permission for what she had done. His Majesty ordered the doctor into his presence, and observing to him that he had never heard of ice being recommended in such cases before, expressed his apprehension that it was on some new

> system. The doctor seemed at first a little confounded, but quickly recovering himself, replied, '*Oh no, please your Majesty, it may well be allowed provided it be taken warm*' – '*Oh well, well, doctor, very well, very warm ice, warm ice.*'

– 'thus', concluded Beddoes, at his treasonable best, 'are the pretensions of the vulgar and the stupid fostered by flattery'.[44] Yet such complicity and rapacity amongst the '*petits maîtres* of physic that figure as favourites of the great'[45] must spell bad medicine, even if, Beddoes disarmingly avowed, 'I would not be so rash as absolutely to affirm that complaisance destroys more lives than contagion'.[46] The pantomime of deference was a perversion, patient-led medical demand had got out of hand, and the modern practitioner of physic was 'forced to prescribe for the alarms of patients, when there is no call upon him from their danger', in the knowledge that to 'treat their false fears lightly would be attended with the certain effect of forfeiting their confidence'.[47]

In short, patient patronage and purse power cast long, dark shadows over medicine. Practitioners performed as tradesmen. Such, of course, presumably came naturally for hundreds, perhaps thousands, of journeyman surgeon-apothecaries out in the sticks, whose training through apprenticeship had never inclined them to think that they were following a calling nobler far than that of butcher or sow-gelder.[48] But it also applied higher up the tree, where bewigged, cane-carrying, chariot-riding physicians gleefully acquiesced in Aesculapian prostitution because they were doing very nicely out of it. Who could be surprised at the 'lukewarmness towards improvement', Beddoes hectored, 'which so commonly arises when the physician has got upon the full scent of profit, and still less of the apathy which overtakes him as soon as he "has feathered his nest"'?[49]

Yet if Beddoes despised his mercenary brethren, he was not entirely without qualms about the motives of some of the more vociferous critics and reformers. Their blitz on quackery and insistence upon paper qualifications as the *sine qua non* of practice, seemed themselves to smack of an ominous monopolistic spirit. New reformer might be old oligopolist writ large, purifying zeal a new rationalization of a time-honoured 'jealousy of intruders'[50] on the part of those 'galled by their competition' and seeking to hog the 'privilege of lucrative homicide'?[51] So, if the text of the times must be 'Take physic, physic', how was that to be achieved?[52]

Medicine, Beddoes believed, would regain its honour as a liberal, ethical profession only if it escaped the seductions of trade. He entertained severe doubts as to whether some of the most touted reform proposals would actually accomplish this – suspecting, by contrast, they would merely perpetuate the commercial spirit perverting the profession. Take medical education. One influential reform voice contended that all practitioners within a purified profession should have graduated from a three-year medical training on the model afforded by Edinburgh University.[53]

Beddoes granted many virtues to the Edinburgh school.[54] For long, 'our [i.e., the English] supine and almost criminal neglect of our own advantages suffered Edinburgh to continue almost the only place in the three kingdoms, where at once degrees were conferred and lectures systematically read'.[55] Yet such were the 'extravagant assumptions of Edinburgh',[56] broadcast by the university's own self-service propaganda lobby, that it was easy to forget its crying evils, not least its nepotism in high places, or what Beddoes called its 'system of hereditary professorships'[57] – a system with 'every reputed disadvantage of hereditary monarchy, and not one of its advantages'.[58]

Edinburgh, judged Beddoes, offered a poor model for medical education. For one thing, its three-year course was far too brief. It was (and here Beddoes spoke from personal experience, having studied there, as well as Oxford and London), all rush and cram, with hordes of students hurtling from lecture to lecture, and many of these superficial – 'May Esculapius protect his votaries from ever again depending on *demonstrations* in the style of the elder Dr *****' [i.e., Monro].[59] Students had no time to read, but what matter? – for they could easily scrape through the farcically stereotyped finals thanks to the ministrations of external coaches aptly nicknamed 'grinders'. All was thus mechanical; as a consequence, 'do not blockheads enough pass through the Edinburgh sieve?'[60] In short, in an industrial age, Edinburgh was the new model medical degree-factory *par excellence*, grinding the maximum number of students off the production line at minimal cost, mirroring the Bell and Lancaster system in elementary schools.

Because students went up to Edinburgh as little more than schoolboys, and graduated while still striplings, the nation, Beddoes feared, was being filled with 'half-drilled medical recruits' – tyros still in their salad days, too raw to be fit to practise, though so what? – since it was easy enough for such a lackbeard 'to persuade some credulous knot of old ladies, that he come from Scotland full charged with healing virtue'.[61] 'I suspect', guessed Beddoes, 'that a good judge of medical stock would find many physicians educated during the greatest splendour of the Edinburgh school . . . among the sorriest sheep in the whole flock of Esculapius'.[62] He was bound to incur accusations of illiberality, Beddoes confessed, yet in conscience he had to state that it was no bad thing that the Royal College of Physicians of London had continually cold-shouldered these medics on-the-make.[63]

Medical education should not be organized on the factory system. More time was needed.[64] Rather than the Caledonian 'triennial manufactory', a full six years should be allotted for study.[65] Seventy-two months would allow the student an even chance of digesting 'from 500 to 800' volumes of medicine – such Beddoes, ever the voracious reader, judged the minimum fit to acquaint him with the art and science – to cultivate a well-stocked mind, and to permit the maturation of a tempered clinical judgement. Medical erudition was not to be despised. Who, after all, had been the acutest clinician of the older generation? William Heberden, a soul 'singularly learned'.[66] Heberden was, of course, a product of the Cambridge system. There was, assuredly, little enough to praise about contemporary Oxbridge tuition – did it even exist? – but Beddoes was an ardent enthusiast for the philosophy enshrined in the ancient universities, designed as it was to foster independence of judgement and a liberal spirit, and ensuring that the student ripened in years and character before embarking upon practice.

Not least – and one may be excused for thinking these remarks ring somewhat strangely, coming as they do from such a sworn foe of place, privilege and snobbery – the promotion of a liberal, Oxbridge-style medical education would decisively attract into the profession men of rank, family and breeding, who would thereby endow it with *éclat*. 'Medicine', Beddoes deplored, 'is the most servile of the professions, and still bears so strongly the marks of the ancient condition of its members. One has heard of fawning divines, fawning courtiers, and the like. But these spaniels in the human form have only to caper at the whistle of a single master; whereas the supple carcase of the physician must perform its cringes to a whole circle every day'.[67] Why was this? It had not a little to do with the fact that medicine was entirely composed of 'us plebeians'.[68] If only more of the Quality, generally perched upon the higher boughs of the Bar and the Church,[69] were to enter the healing art, and if only the Crown would further help by knighting or ennobling the top notch, the profession's prestige would inevitably soar, and with that, its independence.

Thus Beddoes's alternative to Edinburgh's 'too rapid manufacture of physicians'[70] was a revitalization of the Oxbridge educational philosophy, designed to confer upon medical graduates the intellectual eminence accorded by a liberal education. Herein, he was confident, lay the antidote to vulgar commercialism: being an Oxford B.A. and M.D., he knew it from his own experience. 'Having in early life been altogether a stranger to medicine as a trade', he confided, 'I naturally acquired the habit of regarding it purely as a body of doctrine, productive of certain advantages to society, and as respectable or the contrary, in proportion to the amount of those advantages'.[71]

Once medicine was peopled – or at least led and leavened – by practitioners of high intellectual calibre, displaying the accompanying ethos of medico-scientific authority, independent clinical judgement and honest practice could reassert themselves. The cash nexus, which – polite pretences to the contrary – dominated medical practice, would wither away, to be replaced by medically appropriate and truly respectful doctor–patient relations. The grateful sick would defer to the physician's superior wisdom, the physician would address himself to ailments, not advancement. The danger, Beddoes feared (O! His prophetic soul!), was that medical reform would get sidetracked by endless memoranda about certificates, courses, examinations, degrees, portals of entry, and professional associations. All such matters were peripheral, in contrast to the crying need for medicine – were it to fulfil its ends – to stand outside and rise above the imperatives of the commercial rat-race. The market-place was the place for quacks. Beddoes wanted to set the profession upon a new footing beyond the fringe.

Notes

1. And this, despite the fact that it seemed to many doctors to be a world of 'legislators equally unacquainted with the subject of national health': T. Beddoes, *Hygëia: or Essays Moral and Medical, on the Causes Affecting the Personal State of our Middling and Affluent Classes*, 3 vols (1802–03), vol. 1, Essay ii, p.81 [henceforth references will appear thus: 1 ii 81]. For the quoted phrase see Irvine Loudon, '"The Vile Race of Quacks With Which This Country is Infested"'. For the state of the medical profession, see *idem*, 'The Origins of the General Practitioner'; *idem*, 'The Nature of Provincial Medical Practice in Eighteenth-Century England'; *idem*, *Medical Care and the General Practitioner 1750–1850*; J. Lane, 'The Medical Practitioners of Provincial England in 1783'; I. Waddington, 'General Practitioners and Consultants in Early Nineteenth Century England'; *idem*, *The Medical Profession in the Industrial Revolution*; N. Parry and J. Parry, *The Rise of the Medical Profession*; M.J. Peterson, *The Medical Profession in Mid-Victorian London*. For the theory of the perverting effects of commerce, and the language of civic humanism, see J.G.A. Pocock, *Virtue, Commerce and History*; and John Sekora, *Luxury*.

2. We lack a good history of medical ethics in the Enlightenment. For a spirited interpretation see I. Waddington, 'The Development of Medical Ethics'. See also J. Gregory, *Observations on the Duties of a Physician*; T. Percival, *Medical Ethics*. For revaluations of seminal figures see Robert Baker, Dorothy Porter and Roy Porter (eds), *The Codification of Medical Morality in the Eighteenth and Nineteenth Centuries*, vol. i.

3. For contemporary attacks upon quackery see Irvine Loudon, '"The Vile Race of Quacks With Which This Country is Infested"'; Roy Porter, *Health for Sale*; R. Cooter (ed.), *Studies in the History of Alternative Medicine*.

4. T. Beddoes, *A Letter to the Right Honourable Sir Joseph Banks . . . on the Causes and Removal of the Prevailing Discontents, Imperfections, and Abuses, in Medicine* (1808), 98.

5. For the French situation see M. Ramsey, 'The Repression of Unauthorized Medical Practice'; *idem*, *Professional and Popular Medicine in France, 1770–1830*; *idem*, 'Property Rights and the Right to Health'.

6. Beddoes, *A Letter to . . . Banks*, 98.

7. Beddoes, *A Letter to . . . Banks*, 99.

8. Roy Porter, *Health for Sale*.

9. See for instance Gregory Glyster [pseud.], *A Dose for the Doctors*.

10. Beddoes, *A Letter to . . . Banks*, 105.

11. Beddoes, *A Letter to . . . Banks*, 108.

12. Beddoes, *A Letter to . . . Banks*, 106.

13. Beddoes, *A Letter to . . . Banks*, 107. The reference is, of course, to Farquhar's *The Recruiting Officer*.

14. Beddoes, *A Letter to . . . Banks*, 130. For this market-minded commercialism of the regulars see Dorothy Porter and Roy Porter, *Patient's Progress*, esp. chs 1 and 2.

15. See Andrew Wear, 'Medical Practice in Late Seventeenth Century and Early Eighteenth Century England'.

16. Beddoes, *A Letter to . . . Banks*, 110.
17. Beddoes, *A Letter to . . . Banks*, 110.
18. Beddoes, *Hygëia*, 1 ii 48.
19. Beddoes, *A Letter to . . . Banks*, 108, 110.
20. Beddoes, *Hygëia*, 2 viii 75.
21. Beddoes deplored the prevalence of sharp practice and competition between regulars themselves. *Cf. A Letter to . . . Banks*, 96.
22. Beddoes, *A Letter to . . . Banks*, 9.
23. Beddoes, *A Letter to . . . Banks*, 111. For Bristol see M. Neve, 'Natural Philosophy, Medicine and the Culture of Science in Provincial England'; J. Barry, 'The Cultural Life of Bristol, 1640–1775'; M.E. Fissell, *The Physic of Charity*.
24. Beddoes, *Hygëia*, 1 i 72.
25. Beddoes, *Hygëia*, 1 i 73. More stringent were the ethical prescriptions of the Revd Thomas Gisborne. See Roy Porter, 'Thomas Gisborne: Physicians, Christians, and Gentlemen'.
26. Beddoes, *A Letter to . . . Banks*, 128.
27. Beddoes, *A Letter to . . . Banks*, 100.
28. Beddoes, *Hygëia*, 1 ii 52, 54.
29. Beddoes, *Hygëia*, 1 ii 62.
30. Beddoes, *Hygëia*, 1 ii 62.
31. Beddoes, *Hygëia*, 1 ii 57.
32. For background on the development of consumer society see N. McKendrick, John Brewer and J.H. Plumb, *The Birth of a Consumer Society*; John Brewer and Roy Porter (eds), *Consumption and the World of Goods*.
33. Beddoes, *A Letter to . . . Banks*, 71. See Introduction to John Brewer and Roy Porter (eds), *Consumption and the World of Goods*.
34. David Cannadine, 'The Present and the Past in the English Industrial Revolution, 1880–1980'; Maxine Berg, *The Age of Manufactures*; N. McKendrick, 'Home Demand and Economic Growth'; Eric Robinson, 'Eighteenth Century Commerce and Fashion'; D.E.C. Eversley, 'The Home Market and Economic Growth in England 1750–1800'; E.L. Jones, 'The Fashion Manipulators'. There are interesting insights in Alan Macfarlane, *The Culture of Capitalism*.
35. N. Jewson, 'Medical Knowledge and the Patronage System in Eighteenth Century England'; *idem*, 'The Disappearance of the Sick Man from Medical Cosmology, 1770–1870'.
36. Beddoes, *Hygëia*, 1 ii 8, 16.
37. Beddoes, *Hygëia*, 1 ii 35.
38. T. Beddoes, *Manual of Health: or, the Invalid Conducted Safely Through the Seasons* (1806), 24.
39. Beddoes, *Manual of Health*, 26.
40. Beddoes, *A Letter to . . . Banks*, 26.
41. Beddoes, *A Letter to . . . Banks*, 26. On Solomon see Roy Porter, *Health for Sale*, 177–8.
42. Beddoes, *A Letter to . . . Banks*, 114.
43. Beddoes, *A Letter to . . . Banks*, 115. For courtier doctors see Vivian Nutton (ed.), *Medicine at the Courts of Europe*.
44. Beddoes, *A Letter to . . . Banks*, 116.

45. Beddoes, *Hygëia*, 2 v 66.
46. Beddoes, *Hygëia*, 1 i 71.
47. Beddoes, *Hygëia*, 1 i 60.
48. J. Lane, 'The Role of Apprenticeship in Eighteenth-Century Medical Education in England'; J.G.L. Burnby, *A Study of the English Apothecary from 1660 to 1760.*
49. Beddoes, *Hygëia*, 1 i 60.
50. Beddoes, *A Letter to . . . Banks*, 9.
51. Beddoes, *A Letter to . . . Banks*, 97.
52. Beddoes, *A Letter to . . . Banks*, 11.
53. Beddoes, *A Letter to . . . Banks*; *cf.* E. Harrison, *Remarks on the Ineffective State of the Practice of Physic in Great Britain.*
54. On medicine in Edinburgh see C.J. Lawrence, 'Medicine as Culture'; and more broadly on medical education, see S.W.F. Holloway, 'Medical Education in England, 1830-1858'; Roy Porter, 'Medical Education in England Before the Teaching Hospital'.
55. Beddoes, *A Letter to . . . Banks*, 55.
56. Beddoes, *A Letter to . . . Banks*, 56.
57. Beddoes, *A Letter to . . . Banks*, 79.
58. Beddoes, *A Letter to . . . Banks*, 78. G. Risse, *Hospital Life in Enlightenment Scotland*; *idem*, 'Hospital History'.
59. On Monro see Lawrence, 'Medicine as Culture'.
60. Beddoes, *A Letter to . . . Banks*, 38.
61. Beddoes, *A Letter to . . . Banks*, 41.
62. Beddoes, *A Letter to . . . Banks*, 36.
63. Beddoes, *A Letter to . . . Banks*, 39.
64. Beddoes, *A Letter to . . . Banks*, 59.
65. Beddoes, *A Letter to . . . Banks*, 72.
66. Beddoes, *A Letter to . . . Banks*, 74. Ernest Heberden, *The Life of William Heberden.*
67. Beddoes, *A Letter to . . . Banks*, 114. On Oxbridge see John Gascoigne, *Cambridge in the Age of the Enlightenment*; C. Webster, 'The Medical Faculty and the Physic Garden'.
68. Beddoes, *A Letter to . . . Banks*, 50.
69. Beddoes, *A Letter to . . . Banks*, 49.
70. Beddoes, *A Letter to . . . Banks*, 52.
71. Beddoes, *Hygëia*, 1 i 55.

9

Instructing the people

Build lecture rooms and schools for all.

(Peacock, *Crochet Castle*)

I have earlier discussed, especially in Chapter Five, Beddoes's salvoes against the pernicious folklore of health circulating amongst the 'gentlefolk', and their over-confident self-diagnosing and -dosing practices. There was also, it goes without saying, a parallel folklore amongst the 'commonfolk'. Indeed the two were largely coterminous. Historians have claimed that 'high' culture was seceding from 'low' culture during the age of the Enlightenment, and increasingly seeking to reform and police it. Patrick Curry, for instance, has convincingly demonstrated that, whereas 'everybody' believed in astrology in 1650, a century later, such beliefs had been relegated to the 'vulgar'.[1] This cultural bifurcation model, however, applies only very partially to medicine, as any manuscript remedy book compiled by a gentry family will show.[2] The hotchpotch of cures found in such collections – some deriving from family secrets, some from eminent physicians, some from lords and ladies, some from kitchen maids and stable lads, some from learned texts, newspapers, or such time-tried works as Culpeper's *Herbal*, and many from who knows where – bespeaks the enduring eclecticism of medical care in the pre-modern world.[3]

This routine openness to all manner of medical knowledges – what else made sense in an age before medicine could be relied on to work? – was reflected in, and reinforced by, medical practice itself. Candid practitioners admitted that key breakthroughs owed much to folk beliefs and practices. In developing vaccination, Edward Jenner drew upon village awareness that milkmaids who suffered cowpox escaped smallpox.[4] The Midlands practitioner, William Withering, picked up the properties of digitalis from countryfolk. 'In the year 1775', he wrote:[5]

> my opinion was asked concerning a family receipt for the cure of dropsy. I was told that it had been kept a secret by an old woman from Shropshire who had sometimes made cures after the more regular practitioners had failed. I was informed also that the effects produced were violent vomiting and purging, for the diuretic effects seem to have been overlooked. This medicine was composed of 20 or more different herbs; but it was not very difficult for one conversant in these matters to perceive that the active herb could be no other than foxglove.

And if the Quality and regular doctors still drew upon popular medical beliefs, the poor, for their part, were being increasingly exposed to the ministrations of regular, even graduate, practitioners, thanks to the opening of scores of charitable hospitals and dispensaries, the philanthropic activities of well-to-do physicians, and the growth of medical aid under the old Poor Law.[6]

Did these developments consitute a 'medicalization' movement, or in other words, the hegemonic imposition of élite medicine as one prong of a wider programme of the neutralization or suppression of village culture?[7] Certainly, magic was being pooh-poohed,[8] and the élite undeniably felt uneasy at certain elements of 'folk medicine'. Village midwives were often suspected of involvement with contraception, abortion, and infanticide;[9] propaganda campaigns encouraged genteel mothers to suckle their own babies, lest ignorance and superstition be caught from wet-nurses; and the polite often lost patience with the medical follies of their inferiors. When smallpox broke out in Eliza Pierce's household, one of the maids had to be confined to bed. The other, fortunately, had been inoculated, and so Mistress felt confident the outbreak would spread no further. Not so the stupid Abigail! – for 'she has taken it into her Head that she should have the disorder, tho' she was inoculated about three years ago, and had them very thick'. Mistress was mad: 'this has provoked me & done me more harm then any thing else, as she wou'd sit like a dead thing, and no reasons had any effect on her. [I] am convinced that had she had the least real complaint, or any feverish disorder that the College of

Physicians could not have saved her Life, so strongly was she prepossessed she would have the small Pox'.[10]

Relations between learned and vulgar medical beliefs were not, in other words, tension-free. Yet it would be anachronistic and simplistic to imply that there was a concerted alliance of élite opinion and the medical profession to suppress all healing activity amongst the poor. After all, economic and social trends were conspiring in the opposite direction. Education, literacy, and surplus wealth, for one thing, were offering greater opportunities for common people to pick up knowledge of regular medicine from books. Joseph Gutteridge, for instance, an artisan born near the close of the Georgian era, began by studying herbals and ended up a lay healer. 'My father gave me an old edition of Culpeper, with coloured plates', he explained: 'By the aid of this book I soon found out not only the common names of plants but their uses and medical properties'.[11] He started making drawings of medicinal leaves, and 'I experienced great delight in delineating the forms and colours of plants and flowers. The ability to do this proved to me in after times a ready means of fixing in my mind the peculiar characteristics of plants that otherwise might slip my memory'.[12] Gutteridge's first step towards abandoning doctors altogether was taken when his eldest son fell sick, and he could not afford a practitioner,[13]

> We were obliged to fall back upon our own resources. To succeed in this I procured by loan or purchase all the medical and physiological works I possibly could, especially books treating on the eyes, including Fyfe's 'Anatomy', Grainger's 'Elements of Anatomy', Southwood Smith's 'Philosophy of Health', and two or three Dictionaries of Medicine, but the work most suited to my wants was Gray's 'Supplement to the Pharmacopoea'.

Gutteridge was a happy medical autodidact: 'It is said that "A little knowledge is a dangerous thing"', he noted, but 'The sentiment would perhaps be more accurate if it read "*Too* little knowledge, or knowledge mis-applied, is a dangerous thing"'.[14]

Given men like Gutteridge – working people sufficiently literate, intelligent, and motivated to want to cull regular medicine from books – the appeal of works of popular physic is not surprising. The best-seller was John Wesley's endlessly-reprinted

Primitive Physick (1747), which listed disorders and offered brief and easy remedies. Drawing upon traditional lore, and mindful of poor folks' pockets, Wesley limited his *materia medica* to a basket of everday items – honey, onions, garlic, cold water, herbs and other hedgerow ingredients. The Methodist leader trusted to Providence and Nature's healing powers, deprecating complex drug cocktails, quack potions, and the professional ramp.[15]

The 'Family Physic' texts produced at this time commonly embraced a progressive, populist ideology. The empire of disease and death, readers were told, had been prolonged by vulgar ignorance and professional mumbo-jumbo. Now, thanks to printing and the liberty of the press, a new age of practical help for sufferers was dawning; medical enlightenment would consolidate improvements in the arts and sciences. Yet, such works presented a doctor's dilemma: how far was it desirable that common people be encouraged to be their own physicians? I shall examine Thomas Beddoes's opinions on this question; but to contextualize his outlooks, I shall first discuss two of his contemporaries eminent for their contributions to this diffusionist genre: William Buchan and James Parkinson, both, like Beddoes, belligerent socio-political radicals no less than medical enlighteners. So what were the ties, and what the tensions, between political and medical radicalism?[16]

William Buchan, a Scots-born Edinburgh graduate who settled as a practitioner, first in Sheffield, then in London, was the author of the evergreen *Domestic Medicine*, first published in 1769, and reprinted well into the nineteenth century, and also of *Observations Concerning the Prevention and Cure of the Venereal Disease* (1796). Sympathetic to the American and the French Revolutions, Buchan became a ferocious critic of the medical establishment.[17]

James Parkinson, a talented scientific polymath, general practitioner and parish doctor in London's East End, was a political activist of real stature. In the 1790s he was to the fore of the pro-Jacobin London Corresponding Society – the Privy Council quizzed him on his alleged involvement in the so-called 'pop-gun plot' – making a name as a fiery political pamphleteer. He also wrote numerous health advice books, including *The Budget of the People* (1793), *Medical Admonitions to Families, Respecting the Preservation of Health, and the Treatment of the Sick* (1801), *The Town and Country Friend and Physician . . . with Cursory*

Observations on the Treatment of Children (1803), and *The Villager's Friend and Physician* (1802) – this last also being condensed into a handbill, entitled *The Way to Health, Extracted from the Villager's Friend and Physician* (1802), designed to be pasted up in workshops, taverns, etc.[18]

Like Beddoes, Buchan and Parkinson railed against Old Corruption, denouncing despotism, oligarchy and aristocracy, and parading their contempt, medical and moral alike, for High Society corruption. Drawing especially upon the idiom of liberal individualism and natural rights, they embraced the cause of the people, propounding an Enlightenment faith in human betterment, to be achieved by the progress of science, the diffusion of useful knowledge, and the defeat of sinister interests. Each diagnosed ill-health as symptomatic of the rottenness of the *ancien régime* body politic,[19] and exacerbated by the nepotism, toadyism, and incompetence of medical corporations animated by love, not of health but wealth. All believed the rights of man included the right to health, indeed, the right to its self-management. Beyond such consensus, however, their views sharply diverged, in ways indicative of the wider ideological polarities of medical politics. I shall examine them in turn.

Buchan's *Domestic Medicine* (1769) was the age's best-selling text written by a medical regular; it reputedly partnered the Bible on the shelf of every Scottish crofter. Unlike Wesley's *Primitive Physick*, *Domestic Medicine* went beyond do's-and-don'ts and bare recipes, expounding a comprehensive philosophy of health to be achieved through temperance, hygiene, and intelligent abiding by Nature's dictates.

Most explicitly in his *Observations . . . on Venereal Disease* (1797), Buchan embraced a late-Enlightenment populism, aimed at 'rendering medicine more extensively beneficial to mankind'.[20] Medically speaking, the people were as yet but children: 'the credulity of mankind in regard to medicine is truly astonishing'. Hence sickness crises left them 'the easy dupes of every pretender to a secret medicine'.[21] Sufferers thus needed to be safeguarded against quackery, and those 'not able to employ' regular doctors, for reasons of cost or inaccessibility, required instruction in self-help.

Buchan had no Rousseau-tinted faith in folksy ways or wisdom. Often dirty and slovenly, the people also spouted bizarre medical prejudices, some of which – e.g., sex with a virgin as a cure for syphilis – boggled the understanding (was it more 'wicked or absurd'?).[22] Not least, they were feckless, and failed to comply with physicians' orders. 'He will seldom tell the truth, and perhaps never the whole truth' – thus began Buchan's character assassination of the venereal patient:[23]

> but what is still worse, he seldom implicitly follows the doctor's directions, with regard, either to regimen or medicines. . . . Some patients think it is the business of the doctor to find out their disorders, without being told any thing about them. They treat physicians as conjurors, and think they need no information.

Yet their ignorance was understandable, for the real cause of such benightedness was that 'Physic is still engrossed by the faculty'.[24] Physicians had long and cynically monopolized medicine as a mystery, a closed shop whose shop-talk was a dead tongue, simply to gratify the sordid greed of those who would 'make a trade of it'.[24] Popery had reduced religion to mumbo-jumbo and priestcraft; physicians had similarly sought to 'disguise and conceal the art', and had set up doctorcraft.[25]

'While men are kept in the dark, and told that they are not to use their own understanding, in matters that concern their health', Buchan explained, *à propos* of venereal disorders:[26]

> they will be the dupes of designing knaves; and a disease the most tractable in its nature, and almost the only one for which we possess a specific remedy [i.e., mercury], will be suffered to commit its ravages on the human race, and to embitter the most delicious draught that Heaven has bestowed for the solace of human life.

Monopoly had a vested interest in ignorance. Quoting the American physician, Benjamin Rush[27] – a man, Buchan stated, holding 'the same liberal sentiments concerning medicine as I entertain' – he vented his rage that[28]

> for a long while, air, water, and even the light of the sun, were dealt out by physicians to their patients with a sparing hand. They possessed for several centuries the same monopoly over many artificial remedies. But a new order of things is rising in medicine, as well as in government.

> Air, water, and light are taken without the advice of a physician, and Bark and Laudanum are now prescribed every where by nurses and mistresses of families, with safety and advantage.

So there were, at least, grounds for optimism in a groundswell of change: 'Human reason cannot be stationary on these subjects. The time must, and will come, when, in addition to the above remedies, the general use of Calomel, Jalap, and the lancet, shall be considered among the most essential articles of the knowledge and rights of men'.[29] Improvement was in the air. 'Many peasants at present know better how to use some of the most important articles in the *materia medica*, than physicians did a century ago'.[30]

The cause of popular politics thus entailed the democratization of medicine, and that meant openness and education.[31] 'It is no more necessary', Buchan wrote, again approvingly quoting Rush, 'that a patient should be ignorant of the medicine he takes to be cured by it, than that the business of government should be conducted with secrecy in order to insure obedience to just laws. Much less is it necessary that the means of life should be prescribed in a dead language, or dictated with the solemn pomp of a Necromancer'.[32] The goal? 'To bring medicine out of the schools, to lay open its hidden treasures.' The means? 'A code of laws for the preservation of health.' 'Properly digested, and duly executed', this would 'be of more use to mankind than all the efforts of the faculty'.[33] Above all, medical terms must be tailored to the popular idiom. The incomparable Thomas Sydenham had made notable medical breakthroughs, but, because he had written in Latin, it had proved easy for the faculty to impede the diffusion of his works. Buchan, by contrast, prided himself upon having 'addressed my publications to the people'.[34] Empowering the laity was his crusade. 'I shall never cease to give them all the information in my power, both with regard to the prevention and cure of diseases.'[35]

Because of oligarchic vested interests, however, progressives would necessarily meet fierce resistance. He had himself, he claimed, suffered persecution by the medical establishment for his popularizing pains. Publication of his *Observations* would, he predicted, inevitably draw 'fresh torrents of abuse from the faculty'[36] – especially from that 'sordid part', who 'think their trade in danger' if medical mysteries are exposed.[37] For medical monopolists abhorred open minds and free thought: 'whoever has dared to think for himself, in matters relating to health, and was not of the faculty, has been looked upon as an intruder, and held up to ridicule'.[38] Such a vile 'spirit of persecution' was sure to persist, till medicine's 'doctrines are laid open, and candidly submitted to the examination of all men' – until that day, 'medicine will be little better than a piece of mummery'.[39] Of course, such plain-speaking was 'not likely to lessen their malice', and persecution would continue, but 'I am prepared for the worst they can do', Buchan assured his readers, for, 'While the rest of mankind are on my side, I can laugh at the malice, and despise the resentment of the faculty'[40] – their 'censure will always constitute my highest praise'.[41]

So what future did Buchan foresee? He urged not the abolition of professional medicine but its reform. He had no desire to 'supersede the physician',[42] he insisted, for 'to talk of making all men physicians, is the extreme of folly'. But he did want the public to be well-informed, capable judges of medicine – the sure way to spike corporate mystification and knavish quackery. And he was confident that most disorders could actually be self-treated. Readers of *Domestic Medicine* could rest assured that few clinical problems, from diarrhoea to a dislocated neck, lay beyond the capacities of a sensible common man or woman. Nature would cure many disorders; nothing would cure some; and most of the rest could at least be relieved by following a simple regimen – above all, the use of fresh air, cleanliness, plain diet and plenty of rest – and by deploying a handful of drugs. Even with venereal disease, 'if men were taught to do what is in their own power, and had resolution to put it in practice, there would seldom be occasion for the physician, and little reason to dread the consequences of the venereal infection'. Indeed, in most sexual disorders, 'the patient may be his own physician'. In Buchan, the Enlightenment ideal of 'committing the care of . . . diseases to the people' – medicine for the people, by the people – receives its most triumphant flourish.[43]

Buchan's somewhat sentimental vignette of a (potentially) noble commons and a (potential) vanguard of doctors who were the people's friends also figures in the tracts of James Parkinson, who had extensive practical experience of treating the poor of London's East End.[44] Was lay medical activity desirable? On this, Parkinson was a pragmatist, less doctrinaire than Buchan. Like a ship without a pilot, self-medication was hazardous. Expert help was best. Hence *The Villager's Friend and Physician* instructed readers, when sick, to 'apply directly to the man of judgment and experience'.[45] If a regular could not be afforded, try a hospital, Parkinson advised, but never a quack or the neighbourly amateur who 'possesses a medicine chest and the small share of skill which is derived from the perusal of some treatise on domestic medicine'.[46]

Yet Parkinson was a realist, who knew people would willy-nilly undertake self-medication. So if the ship inevitably lacked a pilot, it should at least carry good charts. And it was in this light that Parkinson regarded such popularizing publications of his own as *Medical Admonitions to Families Respecting the Preservation of Health and the Treatment of the Sick*, which, 'convinced that many lives are lost by neglecting to apply sufficiently soon for medical aid, and by improper treatment of disease by domestic practitioners', was designed to enable readers to judge, from self-scanning of symptoms, which disorders required professional attention, and which could safely be handled by domestic first-aid.

Parkinson's most popular work was *The Way to Health*,[47] a body-maintenance guide for manual labourers that also appeared as a handbill. It painted an idyllic vision of manual labour: thanks to their routines of honest toil, labourers were potentially blessed with sound constitutional health, and, whereas the doctor's work involved endless responsibility and anxiety, their labour, by contrast, should be a joy. 'The All wise Disposer of all things has decreed the due exercise of our powers to be an inexhaustible source of pleasure; so that man returns to his daily toil with cheerful alacrity.'[48] Labourers must, however, avoid dissipating their God-given strength through the temptation to overwork, for, he warned 'all violent and long continued exertions, even in your wonted labours, may not only prove a serious injury to your health, but will also lessen, rather than increase, the weekly provision for your family'. Not least, overwork would encourage drinking, and by that fatal path, 'industry may become the mother of drunkenness',[49] and the alehouse 'the house of misery and disease'. 'He who being engaged in works of labour, flies to liquor for a spur, whenever nature droops from too great exertion, makes terrible havoc with himself', bringing on 'tremblings, sinking of the spirits', and finally some 'deadly malady'.[50]

No less pernicious to labouring men than drink, Parkinson continued, were the temptations of the table. Avoid fancy, spicy fare – it caused indigestion and ruined the stomach;[51] eat plain food instead: 'he that breakfasts on milk, dines one day on animal food, and the other on pudding etc., and sups lightly on milk, pottage, &c. may with reason hope for health'.[52] Furthermore, labourers should cultivate the mind not the palate – though, even here, 'moderation in the enjoyment of pleasure' was needed.[53] Workmen should pass their evenings instructing their youngsters in the 'advantages of industry, civility and sobriety; let them see the necessity and advantage of rendering themselves useful to those around them. Place before them particularly the policy of such conduct towards their employers.'

Medicine thus afforded Parkinson a means for imparting to the poor a homespun moralism that taught respectability, regularity and responsibility. The reward of steady toil was health. Idleness, or the frantic overwork induced by greed, would dissipate God's gifts by leading to alcoholism and debility. Writing about hygiene in the guise of a doctor enabled Parkinson to ignore any consideration of the actual conditions of life and labour unavoidably endured by the masses in the early nineteenth-century city. The laws of health, and the sanctions of disease, were invoked to promote self-control and moral reformation in his readers. If the unlettered poor were presently the authors of their own misfortunes, with instruction they could become guardians of their own health. In Parkinson's account, responsibility for health disorders rested ultimately in the individual's own hands, with due guidance from enlightened members of the medical profession.

This survey of radical physicians has revealed certain ambiguities, paradoxes even. Buchan, Beddoes and Parkinson criticized the powers-that-be in society and medicine alike. Like Beddoes, Parkinson damned the rich for callously standing by while the poor starved.[54] Buchan and Beddoes saw medicine as seduced by commerce and fashion. All three were convinced that because the public was ill- or mis-informed, quackery was rampant. Such indictments came easily to men steeped in Enlightenment radicalism.

Yet Parkinson was convinced that the masses would cease to be sick only when they ceased to medicate themselves and put their trust in the enlightened, expert practitioner. For, while tempted to paint a pastoral idyll of a sturdy peasantry, he also felt obliged to protect the people from their own vices, in the name of preventive medicine and doctors' orders. Ordinary people did not, and could not, know their own best medical interests. Only with guidance would they reach the promised land of Health. The altruistic physician would thus be the natural tutor of the new common man, who, seeking health, would also (it followed) adopt habits of sobriety, regularity, steadiness, and cleanliness.[55] Herein lay the radical doctor's classic dilemma: might not the people, to echo Rousseau, also need to be forced to be healthy?

Here we encounter a deep difference of opinion as to the capacity of the masses to treat their own disorders. Buchan was confident that medical enlightenment would lead to competent self-help and a whittling away of the medical profession. Parkinson, by contrast, had a bone to pick with Buchan.

Discussing 'vulgar errors', Parkinson noted that, in common households, Buchan's *Domestic Medicine* was a 'favourite book'.[56] Alas! For it was often 'more likely to be productive of harm than good'.[57] How so? Because Buchan's text encouraged excessive independence. In cases of ague, for instance, Buchan advised, the sick need not attend a doctor unless the fits were 'dangerous' – a course, Parkinson riposted, prejudicial to both patient and doctor. Buchan had suggested smallpox inoculation could be performed by a nurse or a family member: Parkinson demurred, counter-citing the eminent inoculator, Daniel Sutton.[58] With pleurisy and inflammation of the lungs, Buchan recommended home nursing. How irresponsible, fumed Parkinson: 'in a disease so dangerous in its nature, the vague and desultory practice of domestic medicine must be very hazardous'.[59] And so forth. Where, then, did Beddoes stand?

Beddoes believed health reform must go hand-in-hand with political change, and, like Buchan, he was adamant that people ought to be caretakers of their own health.[60] Yet there was no pure and pristine foundation of popular wisdom upon which to build. People had to 'unlearn' their mistakes. And the knowledge they ought then to acquire was emphatically *not* the principles and practice of medicine. In lay hands, Beddoes never tired of stating, medicine was a menace, lay physic was bad physic. For clinical treatment was so intricate an art, so dependent upon vast experience and tempered judgement, that only the trained physician should perform it.

Here Beddoes, of course, departed root-and-branch from Buchan's Jacobin dictum that medicine was properly a simple skill accessible to anyone, complexity a professional smoke-screen, and from his pledge to impart 'all the information in my power, both with regard to the prevention and cure of diseases'.[61] Indeed, Beddoes probably believed Buchan himself had done the people's health grave disservice. Unlike Parkinson and Adair, Beddoes never indicted Buchan by name.[62] But was not Buchan understood to be numbered among the 'adventurers', Beddoes believed were advancing themselves through 'attempts to popularize the practice of medicine'?[63]

A staunch radical, Beddoes naturally did not seek the perpetuation of popular ignorance. But the desideratum must be to teach plebeians, no less than patricians, skills in cultivating health. Passionately committed to sense-oriented pedagogics, Beddoes thought it best to start with 'teaching children accurately to distinguish the parts of the body. Such information will lead them to observe many important changes, which as they take place slowly, are apt to proceed unobserved'.[64] And not only youngsters: 'The ignorant of all denominations, and the poor and the young among the rest, we perpetually find unable to fix, with any tolerable accuracy, the seat of their maladies. Hence arises one great difficulty in their treatment'.[65]

Crucial to Beddoes's grand strategy was public health education by pamphlets and open lectures: courses in anatomy and physiology, and in general self-care. 'It must be', he insisted,[66]

> their aim to make fully sensible the mischiefs arising from systematic irregularity; from injudicious management after exposure to the inclemencies of the weather, and from the other innumerable ordinary errors of individual conduct. They must explain the origin and conduct, much more minutely than the treatment of diseases. They may be conveniently undertaken wherever there exists an infirmary.

Together with phrenology, elementary physiological education became, as Roger Cooter has shown, pivotal to the self-improvement campaigns of nineteenth-century artisan and petty bourgeois radicals.[67]

Betraying a sentimentalism akin to Parkinson's, Beddoes believed that the health prospects of common people were in some respects more promising than those of the polite. For their life style was perforce more robust, more manly, less vitiated. Through idleness and fashion, anxiety and luxury, the rich had wasted their natural constitutional vivacity. Genteel vices – sickly sensibility, faddish diet, sedentary occupations, morbid introspection – induced such class-specific diseases as gout. What could be more unhealthy than upper-class effeteness? 'No mortal would ever have thought of making apathy the mode, but a worn out beau'.[68] Worse still, nobs had money to squander on the dire health hazards of fashionable physicians, spa treatments, and the like! By contrast, necessity, labour, exposure to the elements, and basic rations – all these hardened the labouring poor, reinforcing resistance. 'If you would do well', Beddoes taunted the *ton*, 'you must eat and digest like a ploughman'.[69] Beddoes valued – romanticized even – a certain spartan health he identified with rustic habits. What then, precisely, were Beddoes's attitudes towards the popular politics and the people's health?

Beddoes was an unswerving, pugnacious, late-Enlightenment radical.[70] Everywhere, history showed, regimes had been conspiracies of princes, popes and prelates to rob the people of their birthright through military might and enforced tributes. Such views were broadcast with all the exuberance of a young man on the crest of the French Revolutionary wave in his early epic poem, *Alexander's Expedition down the Hydaspes and the Indus to the Indian Ocean*, privately printed in 1792.[71] In this work, versified in the manner of Erasmus Darwin, Beddoes partly endorsed the standard Augustan view of Alexander the Great as a power-crazed tyrant, and author of 'mad misrule'; but primarily used the Macedonian's conquests as a pretext for impassioned anti-imperialist tirades. Thanks to monarchical militarism, he suggested with an echo of Volney, 'plague and rapine' were everywhere rampant:[72]

But earth's fond hopes, how blasted in their bloom!
How feels a world convulsed by early doom!
What mingling sounds of woe and outrage rise!
How wide the eddying dust of ruin flies!

The conquered Indians – Beddoes's metonym for downtrodden peoples, past and present, the world over – deserve our 'pity', being 'degraded by oppression'.[73] Their plight would remain beyond relief, 'Till the last hour of their merciless tyrants from Europe shall arrive'; evils would multiply till we 'banish slavery and despotism of every species from the face of the earth'.[74] From Alexander to Warren Hastings, Indian history had been nothing but a chronicle of 'crime', 'carnage', greed ('the rage accursed of Gain'), and 'firebrand warfare'.[75] 'European soldiers' were even then giving 'loose to their rapacity, cruelty and caprice'.[76]

The human race had a boundless potential for progress, argued the poem's prose commentary, but its prospects had been blighted by tyrants. Beddoes ventured a characteristic conjectural anthropology. Civilization had been cradled in such favourable ecological niches as the Levant. 'Here the species would go on increasing, till it matched the natural and spontaneous resources of the soil. Very simple arts would afford new supplies in great abundance. By degrees, societies would be formed and' – here was the rub! – 'great empires established'.

This 'order of things' Beddoes suggested, had the potential for securing 'all the happiness of which man seems capable, a perpetual and unlimited extension of desires and gratifications, a boundless activity of mind and body'. It was not to be, for 'in this promising progress', he continued, man[77]

> was arrested by the rise of monarchies and hierarchies. The energy of human nature being repressed on all sides by the tyranny of priests and despots, the primitive nations sunk into languor.

Hence, judged Beddoes, refuting Malthus before he even wrote, and anticipating Shelley, it was not Nature, but potentates, that held peoples in thrall: *pace* Montesquieu, 'the comprehensive cause of Asiatic indolence' was not climate, but 'temporal and ecclesiastical despotism'.[78] Overall, Beddoes lamented the doom of India, subject first to Alexandrine and subsequent conquests, and then to capitalism[79]

> Mourn, India, mourn – the womb of future Time
> Teems with the fruit of each portentous crime.
> The Crescent onward leads consuming hosts,

And carnage dogs the Cross along thy coasts;
From Christian strands, the Rage accursed of gain
Wafts all the Furies in her baleful train:

Readers were invited to 'join in execrating despotism in all its forms and degrees whether mercantile or monarchical'.[80]

The French Revolution evidently concentrated Beddoes's political mind. He was from the first, as is shown by his extensive and expansive correspondence with his junior, Davies Giddy, an enthusiast for the rights of man, though, like so many 'friends of liberty', from late 1792 he began to deplore the slide from democracy into despotism.[81] Above all, after initial optimism about a new dawn, Beddoes bewailed the counter-revolutionary backlash in England. For, in his view, the wily William Pitt seized the chance afforded first by fear, and then by the outbreak of Anglo-French hostilities, to wage diabolical war on English liberties, through suspending Habeas Corpus, arresting Painite leaders, and introducing gagging bills. Pitt's opportunist war-mongering, despicably manipulating patriotism to consolidate personal and party power, disrupted trade, and proved ruinously expensive, leading to spiralling taxes and inflation, and hence mass distress and starvation. In a flurry of pamphlets – *Where would be the Harm of a Speedy Peace?* (1795), *An Essay on the Public Merits of Mr Pitt* (1796), *Alternatives Compared: or, What Shall the Rich do to be Safe?* (1797), and, most trenchantly, *A Word in Defence of the Bill of Rights against Gagging Bills* (1795) – Beddoes countered that Britain's greatness derived not from pestilential potentate-politicians like Pitt, but from having long secured to 'a superior degree the use of REASON and FREE SPEECH, the two great faculties by which the Almighty had distinguished MAN from the brute creation'.[82] By contrast, Pittite 'tyranny and oppression' were the harbingers of 'servitude'.[83] If the 'alternative is to speak or be enslaved', Beddoes roused his readers, recapturing patriotism for the people, 'our popular national song, Rule Britannia, rule the waves For Britons never will be slaves' should not be forgotten; the future must spell not 'servitude' but 'peace and plenty'.[84] While insisting, 'I deprecate all violence. I have no talents for pillage', vigilance alone (he reminded readers) would defeat the 'ferocious spirit of bigotry'.[85]

Beddoes pursued Pitt – almost his exact contemporary – with implacable venom, partly as a political pamphleteer, but largely in the guise of a doctor and sanitarian, appalled that Pittite adventurism was reducing the people to penury, dearth, and ill-health. His savagely ironical *Essay on the Public Merits of Mr Pitt* (1796) denounced the wicked window tax for forcing people to brick up their windows, diminishing light and ventilation and encouraging epidemics. For their part, 'tillers of the ground . . . [had been] doomed to the greatest hardship and the most scanty allowance [so that] they practise methods of preventing the increase of offspring'.[86] The Prime Minister had thus declared war on the living.

Beddoes's detestation of Pitt peaked in the savage *A Letter to the Right Hon. William Pitt, on the Means of Relieving the Present Scarcity, and Preventing the Diseases that Arise from Meagre Food* (1796), a work drawing on the sardonic spirit of Swift's *Modest Proposal*. Tongue in cheek, Beddoes assured readers that it was Pitt to whom he was addressing his thoughts, since he represented 'power in conjunction with genius'.[87] Callous indifference to 'plenty' had led to 'distress' and 'scarcity', ran Beddoes's *j'accuse*;[88] cold and starvation in turn had spawned 'disease'. 'Charity' was dead in a decadent aristocratic régime abandoned to conspicuous waste; hence resource-use must be rationalized, maximizing marginal utility. The answer? Food science. More potatoes should be grown (elsewhere, dropping the mask of irony, Beddoes argued that potatoes had ruined the nation's stomach),[89] and prudence dictated sowing varieties of fodder crops for swine that might, in time of emergency, be eaten by the swinish multitude. Above all, in a chillingly Gillrayan vision, Beddoes commended the installation of vast vats for boiling up bones, to provide soup for the poor at practically no cost to the rich, to be supplemented by opium handouts – if, that is, that powder were 'capable of supplying the place of food'.[90]

Thus Beddoes raged against Pitt's proto-Thatcherite policies of grinding the face of the poor. But what was positively to be done to improve their health? This was Beddoes's alternative. In a society riddled with medical errors and idiocies, only the upright doctor, his scientific expertise matched by his social conscience, could prescribe for the people's health.[91] The physician's duty, Beddoes contended, was to protect and sustain; the people should, reciprocally, defer to the benevolent physician. The ideal type of this paternal, even pastoral, contract between doctor and people was most guilelessly drawn in Beddoes's moral fable, *The History of Isaac Jenkins, and of the Sickness of Sarah his Wife, and Their Three Children* (1792), an improving fiction related as an entertaining, sentimental yarn, calculated to appeal to the labouring poor.[92]

It is the bleak mid-winter of 1783. Isaac Jenkins, a labourer, Sarah, his wife, and their three children, live in Titterstone, a Shropshire village known to Beddoes since childhood. Illness overtakes the family. Unable to afford the doctor, they buy some white powder off the local quack. When they can't pay him any more, the huckster naturally stops calling ('your quack doctors', asides Beddoes, in the persona of the narrator, 'care not a farthing whether they cure or kill, all they want is to fleece those that know no better').[93]

Luckily, one day Surgeon Langford rides past, *en route* to attend the parson, who had (typical Beddoesian touch!) been injured while out shooting. Langford gets talking to Sarah, hears the children are sick, treats them free, and listens to her tale of woe. Isaac has taken to drink. This lapse stems, interpolates the preachy Beddoes, not from any inherent depravity, but from a terrible accident which had befallen the family. Some louts had caused a horse to bolt; it had trampled the Jenkins's eldest son to death. Grief-stricken, Isaac is now drowning his sorrows. The family suffers. While condemning the 'heinous practice of drunkenness', the narrator judges Isaac is to be 'pitied' more than 'blamed': 'I believe for my part that the poor are well disposed, and do wrong oftener for want of knowing better than from wickedness'.[94]

Langford has a heart-to-heart with Isaac, prescribes medicines, and shames him into resuming his long-neglected family duties. A loan from Langford enables the family to pay off the publican. Abiding by doctor's orders, Isaac recovers – unlike his nasty master, Simcox, who (another Beddoesian class barb) comes to a disgustingly wretched end, his over-indulgence leading to death from dropsy. All ends happily, with Isaac learning the difference between 'plenty with sobriety and a light and cheerful heart, and beggary with drunkenness and discontent'.[95] An 'epilogue' for the 'refined reader' urges that, in the light of Lockian psychological theories, the poor should not be stigmatized as born reprobates, but viewed as victims of circumstances, capable of coming good, given proper education and instruction.[96]

The parable of Isaac Jenkins and Surgeon Langford pointed the way to the rescue of the labouring poor through enlightened medical succour. How did Beddoes himself practise what he preached? For one thing, he energetically published works of practical advice, in fulfilment of his heartfelt commitment to popular education. In his *Extract of a Letter on Early Instruction, Particularly that of the Poor* (1792), he insisted that universal education was desirable, feasible, and essential. Accepting Thomas Day's view that 'the soul of a child . . . essentially resides in his senses',[97] he contended that all knowledge must come from experience, hence notions not derived from the senses (instance: hellfire) were meaningless, and 'parrot' learning was brainwashing, a tool of despotism and obscurantism. Mass education was necessary for 'humanizing the minds of the people. Upon this the welfare of civil society immediately depends, for a savage spirit in the people and tyranny in the possessors of power are to one another cause and effect'.[98]

Idealistic about educability (to doubt the possibility of personal improvement is a 'calumny of the human race'), Beddoes also appealed, in the manner of Mrs Barbauld and Sarah Trimmer, to enlightened self-interest. 'A well digested system of public instruction will secure the peace of society more efficiently than the gallows and the bayonet'.[99] Not surprisingly, therefore, Beddoes himself penned cheap 'take care of yourself' booklets. Thus *Good Advice for the Husbandman in Harvest* (1808) was a pamphlet, based upon pieces first published in the *Bristol Gazette*, to be bought by employers for distribution to workmen (it included the disclaimer: 'how hard it is to persuade people to try to swim against the stream of custom!'). Steer clear of hard liquor, it told harvesters, drink milk and barley water instead; in any case, warned the friendly doctor, the idea that strong ale makes harvesters hale and hearty is a hoary myth, based on semantic sleight-of-hand.[100] Beddoes anticipated brickbats from suspicious readers, who might 'feel as if there were a design to deprive them of their dearest and most valuable perquisites'. Far from being a killjoy, he countered, his advice suited the interests of the pockets and stomachs of the farm-hands themselves.[101]

Diatribes against drink were, of course, ten-a-penny. More ambitiously, Beddoes also offered a broader vista of health in works such as *A Guide for Self Preservation, and Parental Affection; or Plain Directions for Enabling People to Keep Themselves and their Children Free from Several Common Disorders* (1793), a threepenny tract of two-dozen pages, containing 'directions for people respecting their health', designed 'to give the poor in particular, some instruction in the art of rearing their children, and to teach those who are grown up, how they may escape several serious disorders, as well as some of those lighter ailments which, in this fickle climate, often render the half of life uncomfortable'.[102] The *Instructions* comprised a commonplace advocacy of moderation, good temper, sensible diet, and so forth.

Beddoes thus aimed to enlighten the laity, both through print and from the podium. But his faith in literature and lectures was limited, as were his expectations of dispensaries and other mushrooming medical philanthropies for the ambulant poor which merely doled out bottles of jalap. 'The experience of former medical charities shows that the sick are constantly flying off before they have a chance of due benefit'.[103] If lessons were to sink in, it was crucial to indoctrinate the poor at really close quarters. For this Beddoes devised a new medical site, designed to unite clinical treatment with comprehensive instruction and screening of the sick: this was the Preventive Institution, or the 'Medical Institution for the Sick and Drooping Poor'.[104]

The Preventive Institution opened in 1802 in Dowry Square, Clifton. The poor could obtain advice, and usually medicines, gratis. In return, they were expected to leave a surety of 2s. 6d. (no small sum!), refundable upon discharge, a measure meant to ensure 'punctual attendance till regular dismissal'. 'In case of sickness', patients were to attend for one hour per week (absence to be excused by prior notes). Improper behaviour would be followed by dismissal and loss of deposit.[105]

The goal, explained Beddoes's *Rules of the Medical Institution, for the Benefit of the Sick and Drooping Poor* (1804), was prevention, or at least early treatment, especially in tubercular and scrophular cases. 'Early caught, early cured', he quipped, using proverbial lore to tune into his readers' wavelength ('I flatter myself', he boasted, that his text would be 'intelligible to the humblest reader').[106] Saying nothing about 'treatment', Beddoes aimed in the booklet, and doubtless also in face-to-face interviews, to alert readers to 'the dangers by which you are most likely to be surrounded . . . and where you may find safety', in particular by drilling them to recognize the symptoms of consumption.[107] Because it was mainly the young who were stricken, the early signs of lethal conditions like tuberculosis were shrugged off all too casually in the family circle. Beddoes wanted to raise the alarm, even suggesting commissioning artists to paint shockingly grisly portraits of consumptives.[108]

Reminding readers that 'a stitch in time saves nine', Beddoes argued for the Institution's preventive function.[109] Hence, when a consumptive child attended for treatment, the whole family was to be brought in for surveillance; proper questioning would disclose whether siblings had such telltale symptoms as weight loss.[110]

Securing disciplined compliance posed problems. The poor were inured to bearing maladies 'with stupid patience', but such fatalism too often proved fatal.[111] Parents failed to present consumptive children, excusing themselves because, they said, 'a child does not complain'.[112] Many lower-class patients were, in any case, delinquent; scared of 'being obliged to take physic', they played 'dumb' about their disorders.[113] To avoid taking Beddoes's medicine, they preferred to patronize quacks, and swallowed home brews, 'which good old ladies hawk about as sovereign remedies for consumption'. 'Refuse them', Beddoes commanded: they are 'offered free', but 'we should have to pay for them with our lives'.[114] Not least, such 'wise women' were radically unwise about diagnoses. They commonly diagnosed worms in children, and so 'the poor ailing creatures are jalapped, or dosed with some popular quack medicine, in the most unmerciful manner'. Actually, the infants were in the grip of incipient scrophula.[115] In short, everything conspired against nipping sickness in the bud: 'such calamities may in general be prevented, but they will certainly occur unless pains be taken for the purpose of prevention'.[116]

Folly fuelled fecklessness. However 'forewarned', patients rarely completed courses of physic.[117] Beddoes could take a charitable view of this delinquency, laying blame at the door of defective doctoring – 'All has hitherto been conducted in a style of authority. It has been too much mere dumb shew between doctor and patient'.[118] Too often, physicians lacked communication skills. 'Confidence is placed in ignorant neighbours', Beddoes opined, 'because they speak to the sick in their own language, and pretend to give some sort of reason for what they recommend'. Distant doctors left the patient with 'no conception of the turns his disorder must take before it can go off':[119]

> he is cast down without cause. He goes to another doctor, and from him to a quack. Nay, in some parts, poor sick people cannot be persuaded to go to any body but to the most silly old women. Here, in Bristol, I often find sad mischief done by some improper medicine, and it turns out nine times out of ten that the medicine has been advised by some ignorant neighbour.

Regulars must thus shoulder responsibility for medical mischief, and mend their ways ('Let them explain to the poor as much as the case will admit').[120] Yet not all Beddoes's bile fell the doctors' way: non-compliant patients got their share. All too often, patients defaulted (partly, he judged, because 'many among the poor are miserable cowards'). It was to reduce the ranks of such deserters that he introduced the deposit system; he also went to the extraordinary length of publishing a list of those patients who jumped ship![121]

In other words, Beddoes was, to say the least, ambivalent towards poor patients. Some of their shortcomings could be excused, but he also felt betrayed. Parents sometimes made a great to-do about their children's illnesses, but would rarely enforce a course of physick, because they thought they knew best.[122] They rejected medicines because they were too harsh, bizarrely preferring the pains of sickness to the pills of health.[123] Money better spent on meat and milk they squandered on tea ('just so much poison').[124]

In Beddoes's view, people and profession were equally indifferent to prevention.[125] Having looked to 'the discoveries in science of some of the ablest men of the last century', and thinking they 'offered a chance for accomplishing a part of that which everyone must acknowledge to be so wanting', it was to this end that he had established his Preventive Institution in the first place. His reward? – 'obloquy'.[126] Why? In part because his clinical practice had became the object of whispering campaigns.[127] For 'whenever attempts have been made to deliver mankind from the plague of sickness, it has almost always been noised abroad that improper trials or EXPERIMENTS were on foot'. The result? The sick kept away, especially after the introduction of the deposit system.[128]

Life and death were, however too important to be left to popular *mentalités*. A section entitled 'How to Act in Some Situations Where Health is at Stake' advised that, in case of sickness, so-called commonsensical remedies should be shunned and people should summon the doctor.[129] Calling the doctor – to save the individual, the community, indeed, society at large – seemed to Beddoes, trapped between corrupt patricians and stupid plebeians, the only way forward. The author of *Rules* would become the new ruler of the people's health.

Beddoes was a complex man, in some ways critically self-aware about the nature of knowledge as a double agent. He characteristically concluded his *Rules* by musing whether, like other projectors, he might have fallen a 'dupe to self deception'.[130] Yet he also conceived his mission as the replacement of self-deception by enlightenment. The sick, rich and poor, were often desperately mistaken about their health, fancying 'themselves but a trifle out of sorts, though really pining under some deadly disorder': 'we propose to undeceive and rescue them'.[131]

The sick had certainly deceived themselves; they had been further deceived by quacks, and unscrupulous regulars; above all, though clouds of misinformation had circulated, they remained in the dark. That model Enlightenment optimist, William Buchan, aimed to lay medicine open to the people; in large measure, the sick could become their own doctors.[132] Though championing the people against their political oppressors, Beddoes had no confidence in democratizing medicine. Proper healing hinged on technical expertise and professional judgement. Doctors' orders required authority relationships. The old sickness regime had to be reformed, and replaced by a new professionalism. Beddoes was a champion of the people, a political radical, a democrat even, but he staunchly insisted that medicine was one domain for an élite of guardians. Medicine should be *for* the people, but it should never be *by* the people.

Some of these complexities will be raised, if not resolved, in the final chapter.

Notes

1. Patrick Curry, *Prophecy and Power*. For the general relations of the cultures, see J.M. Golby and A.W. Purdue, *The Civilization of the Crowd*; Peter Burke, *Popular Culture in Early Modern Europe*; *idem*,

'Popular Culture between History and Ethnology'; *idem*, 'Revolution in Popular Culture'.

2. L. Guthrie, 'The Lady Sedley's Receipt Book, 1686'; M. Chamberlain, *Old Wives' Tales*, discusses remedy books, of which there is a fine collection in the library of the Wellcome Institute for the History of Medicine, London.

3. The case for such pluralism is made in Dorothy Porter and Roy Porter, *Patient's Progress*, esp. chs 1 and 2. For the interchange of different sources of knowledge, see Roy Porter, 'Lay Medical Knowledge in the Eighteenth Century'; *idem*, 'The Patient's View'; *idem*, 'Laymen, Doctors and Medical Knowledge in the Eighteenth Century'; *idem*, 'The Patient in Eighteenth-Century England'. A superb regional study is Mary E. Fissell, *The Physic of Charity*.

4. J.R. Smith, *The Speckled Monster*, P. Razzell, *The Conquest of Smallpox*; J.K. Aronson, *An Account of the Foxglove*.

5. Quoted from William Withering's *Account of the Foxglove* in Chamberlain, *Old Wives' Tales*, 175. *Cf.* Aronson, *Account of the Foxglove*. On women healers, lay and professional, see Roy Porter, *Health for Sale*, ch.4; *idem*, 'Female Quacks in the Consumer Society'; A.L. Wyman, 'The Surgeoness. The Female Practitioner of Surgery, 1400–1800'; P. Crawford, 'Printed Advertisements for Women Medical Practitioners in London, 1670–1710'.

6. E.G. Thomas, 'The Old Poor Law and Medicine'; J. Lane, 'The Provincial Practitioner and his Services to the Poor 1750–1800'; *idem*, 'A Provincial Surgeon and his Obstetric Practice'; A. Wear, 'Caring for the Sick Poor in St Bartholomew's Exchange: 1580–1676'; Roy Porter, 'The Gift Relation'.

7. For medicalization, see J.-P. Goubert, *La Médicalisation de la Société Française 1770–1830*; *idem*, 'Twenty Years On'; R. Muchembled, *Popular Culture and Elite Culture in France, 1400–1750*; M. Foucault, *The Birth of the Clinic*; I. Illich, *Limits to Medicine*; for a sensitive attempt to evaluate the applicability of the idea of 'medicalization' in a local context see Fissell, *The Physic of Charity*.

8. See, e.g., R. Malcolmson, *Popular Recreations in English Society 1700–1850*; Patrick Curry, *Prophecy and Power*.

9. A. MacLaren, *Reproductive Rituals*.

10. V.M. Macdonald (ed.), *The Letters of Eliza Pierce*, 89.

11. V. Chancellor (ed.), *Master and Artisan in Victorian England*, 95. Gutteridge is more fully discussed in Dorothy Porter and Roy Porter, *Patient's Progress*, ch.11. See more generally, David Vincent, *Literacy and Popular Culture*.

12. Chancellor (ed.), *Master and Artisan*, 95.

13. Chancellor (ed.), *Master and Artisan*, 131.

14. Chancellor (ed.), *Master and Artisan*, 131.

15. J. Wesley, *Primitive Physick*; G.S. Rousseau, 'John Wesley's *Primitive Physick* (1747)'.

16. Themes such as these have been examined for the nineteenth century by R. Cooter, 'The Power of the Body'; *idem*, 'Interpreting the Fringe'; *idem* (ed.), *Studies in the History of Alternative Medicine*.

A. Marcovich, 'Concerning the Continuity between the Image of Society and the Image of the Human Body'.

17. For the career of Buchan, see C.J. Lawrence, 'William Buchan'; C. Rosenberg, 'Medical Text and Medical Context'.

18. For Parkinson see A.D. Morris, *James Parkinson*; and for the background of his radicalism, see E.P. Thompson, *The Making of the English Working Class*; S. Deane, *The French Revolution and Enlightenment in England 1789–1832*; Albert Goodwin, *The Friends of Liberty*.

19. We do not yet have a definitive study of the interplay of medical and political metaphors in this period. For some suggestive writings see S. Sontag, *Illness as Metaphor*, *idem*, *AIDS as Metaphor*, C.J. Lawrence, 'The Nervous System and Society in the Scottish Enlightenment'; R. Cooter, 'The Power of the Body: the Early Nineteenth Century'.

20. Buchan, *Observations Concerning . . . Venereal Disease*, iv.

21. Buchan, *Observations Concerning . . . Venereal Disease*, xvii.

22. Buchan, *Observations Concerning . . . Venereal Disease*, iv, xv.

23. Buchan, *Observations Concerning . . . Venereal Disease*, xxii.

24. Buchan, *Domestic Medicine*, xx.

25. Buchan, *Domestic Medicine*, xvii.

26. Buchan, *Observations Concerning . . . Venereal Disease*, 3. As will be evident, Buchan's characterization of the *status quo* – e.g., his conspiratorial vision of the medical establishment, the 'Faculty' – should not be taken at face value as historically accurate. The radical rant is rather a self-serving exercise.

27. The best source for Rush's radicalism is his letters. See L.H. Butterfield (ed.), *The Letters of Benjamin Rush*.

28. Buchan, *Observations Concerning . . . Venereal Disease*, xxiii, xxvi.

29. Buchan, *Observations Concerning . . . Venereal Disease*, xxvi.

30. Buchan, *Domestic Medicine*, xii. See generally David Spadafora, *The Idea of Progress in Eighteeenth Century Britain*.

31. Buchan, *Observations Concerning . . . Venereal Disease*, xxvii. For political context see John Brewer, 'Commercialization and Politics'.

32. Buchan, *Observations Concerning . . . Venereal Disease*, xxvii.

33. Buchan, *Observations Concerning . . . Venereal Disease*, xxiii.

34. Buchan, *Observations Concerning . . . Venereal Disease*, xxviii. For this theme, see Roy Porter, '"Expressing Yourself Ill"'.

35. Buchan, *Observations Concerning . . . Venereal Disease*, xxviii.

36. Buchan, *Observations Concerning . . . Venereal Disease*, xxiii. To reiterate, it hardly needs to be said that Buchan's portrait of persecution at the hands of a united, vindictive Faculty was essentially a self-serving fantasy on his part.

37. Buchan, *Domestic Medicine*, xx, xxi.

38. Buchan, *Domestic Medicine*, xxi.

39. Buchan, *Domestic Medicine*, xxix.

40. Buchan, *Domestic Medicine*, xxix.

41. Buchan, *Domestic Medicine*, xxxii.

42. Buchan, *Observations Concerning . . . Venereal Disease*, 2.

43. Buchan, *Observations Concerning . . . Venereal Disease*, 9.

44. A.D. Morris, *James Parkinson*. James Parkinson, *The Villager's Friend and Physician*, 2nd edn., 5.

45. James Parkinson, *The Villager's Friend and Physician*, 66.

46. James Parkinson, *The Villager's Friend and Physician*, 44. Parkinson insists, 'admit no tamperings, lest you have to accuse yourself of having thereby sacrificed the child of your heart'. He was deeply hostile to quacks. 'It would undoubtedly be rendering a great benefit to society, if some medical man were to convince the ignorant, of the pernicious consequences of their reliance on advertised nostrums: but unfortunately, the situation in which medical men stand is such, that their best intentioned, and most disinterested exertions for this purpose, would not only be but little regarded, but frequently would be even imputed to base and invidious motives': Parkinson, *Medical Admonitions*, 327.

47. James Parkinson, *Medical Admonitions*, 4th ed., 5. Parkinson then emphasizes the duty of obedience to the doctor: without 'strict compliance with orders', calamities would follow. James Parkinson, *The Way to Health*.

48. Parkinson, *The Villager's Friend and Physician*, 9.

49. Parkinson, *The Villager's Friend and Physician*, 10.

50. Parkinson, *The Villager's Friend and Physician*, 11.

51. Parkinson, *The Villager's Friend and Physician*, 15.

52. Parkinson, *The Villager's Friend and Physician*, 16.

53. Parkinson, *The Villager's Friend and Physician*, 16.

54. [James Parkinson], *A Sketch by Old Hubert*. This one-penny, four-page pamphlet goes on in a jeering way about how well the government and the rich are all eating, 'whilst the honest poor are wanting bread' – a phrase reiterated some half a dozen times.

55. Thus Beddoes discovered, on setting up his Preventive Institution, designed to relieve cases of tuberculosis amongst the poor, that his clients rarely came regularly for treatment. This cast him down. In order to overcome this fecklessness, he instituted systems of caution money and fines. Attendance dropped off. Thomas Beddoes, *Rules of the Medical Institution, for the Benefit of the Sick and Drooping Poor; with an Explanation of its Peculiar Design and Various Necessary Instructions* (1804). Note the foregrounding of the 'necessary instructions' in the very title.

56. Parkinson, *Medical Admonitions*, 20. Parkinson notes in *Introduction to the Table of Symptoms* that all too commonly 'the treatment of some dangerous disease is confided to anyone who possesses a medicine chest and the small share of skill which is derived from the perusal of some treatise on domestic medicine'. For discussion of medicine chests, see Roy Porter, 'The Patient in the Eighteenth Century'.

57. Parkinson, *Medical Admonitions*, 20.

58. Parkinson, *Medical Admonitions*, 286.

59. Parkinson, *Medical Admonitions*, 158.

60. T. Beddoes, *Hygëia: or Essays Moral and Medical, on the Causes Affecting the Personal State of our Middling and Affluent Classes*, 3 vols (1802–3), vol. 2, Essay vi, p.64 [henceforth references to *Hygëia* will appear thus: 2 vi 64.]

61. Buchan, *Observations Concerning . . . Venereal Disease*, 28.

62. J.M. Adair, *Essays on Fashionable Diseases*, accuses Buchan of causing untold evil by his attempts to popularize medicine: e.g., p.97.

Adair offers what he sees as a typical case of hypochondria. He visits a man's house, and 'I was shewn into the library, and found on his table *Tissot's Avis au Peuple* and *Buchan's Domestic Medicine*'; Adair insists that though he respects Buchan's own probity, 'I will venture to pronounce such publications to be very injurious, because they have a manifest tendency to encourage a dangerous species' (p.105).

63. Beddoes, *Hygëia*, 1 ii 33; 1 ii 30.

64. Beddoes, *Hygëia*, 2 vi 46; D.A. Stansfield, 'Thomas Beddoes and Education'; D. Clarke, *The Ingenious Mr Edgeworth*; W.A. Campbell Stewart and W.A. McCann, *The Educational Innovators, 1750–1880.*

65. Beddoes, *Hygëia*, 2 vi 47.

66. Beddoes, *Hygëia*, 2 vi 92.

67. R. Cooter, 'The Power of the Body'.

68. Beddoes, *Hygëia*, 2 viii 49.

69. Beddoes, *Hygëia*, 2 viii 6.

70. For Beddoes's type of political radicalism, see Albert Goodwin, *The Friends of Liberty*. The steadfast consistency of Beddoes's radicalism is worth emphasis, since many of his early radical associates, notably Coleridge, later turned conservative or reactionary. Beddoes became a target of the *Anti-Jacobin Review*, see e.g., vi (1800), 109–18, 'The Pneumatic Revellers', which alleged that Beddoes had finally demonstrated how far natural philosophy may be carried 'by the force of a flaming imagination' (p.109).

71. Thomas Beddoes, *Alexander's Expedition down the Hydaspes and the Indus to the Indian Ocean* (1792).

72. Beddoes, *Alexander's Expedition*, vi. For ambiguities towards 'greatness', see Isobel Grundy, *Samuel Johnson and the Scale of Greatness*; Leo Braudy, *The Frenzy of Renown*. While partly thinking of Alexander as a megalomaniac, Beddoes also partly self-identified with him as a fellow young man of genius: 'His character may be delineated in a very narrow compass; and of him as of other great men, he should think it sufficient to say, that his mind was discriminated by exquisite sensibility. By whatever object they were touched, the springs of his nature bent deeply inwards; but they immediately rebounded with equal energy into action'.

73. Beddoes, *Alexander's Expedition*, 13.

74. Beddoes, *Alexander's Expedition*, 13.

75. Beddoes, *Alexander's Expedition*, 32.

76. Beddoes, *Alexander's Expedition*, 34.

77. Beddoes, *Alexander's Expedition*, 57.

78. Beddoes, *Alexander's Expedition*, 57. Compare N. Crook and D. Guiton, *Shelley's Venomed Melody*.

79. Beddoes, *Alexander's Expedition*, lines 275–284.

80. Beddoes, *Alexander's Expedition*, 9.

81. See the Beddoes/Giddy correspondence in the Cornwall Record Office.

82. Thomas Beddoes, *Where Would be the Harm of a Speedy Peace?* (1795); *idem*, *A Word in Defence of the Bill of Rights against Gagging Bills* (1795), the text quotation coming from this broadsheet; *idem*, *An Essay on the Public Merits of Mr Pitt* (1796); *idem*, *Alternatives Compared: or, What*

Shall the Rich do to be Safe? (1797). On Beddoes as political radical, see T.H. Levere, 'Dr Thomas Beddoes at Oxford, Radical Politics in 1788–93'; *idem,* 'Dr Thomas Beddoes (1760–1808): Science and Medicine in Politics and Society'.

83. Thomas Beddoes, *A Word in Defence of the Bill of Rights,* 6.

84. Thomas Beddoes, *A Word in Defence of the Bill of Rights,* 8.

85. Thomas Beddoes, *A Word in Defence of the Bill of Rights,* 8: 'To abolish the Bill of Rights under the pretext of altering it, is to cut by one cruel stroke the nerve of affection by which each Englishman feels for the welfare or adversity of all. An unskilful minister engaged in a pernicious war, and trying, like a desperate gamester, to retrieve his original rashness, may go on staking our property, our lives, till the last guinea and the last man capable of bearing arms, be sacrificed. The more pernicious the measures, the more strenuous will the junto in power be, in maintaining throughout the kingdom the mournful silence of despair'.

86. Thomas Beddoes, *An Essay on the Public Merits of Mr Pitt* (1796).

87. T. Beddoes, *A Letter to the Right Hon William Pitt, on the Means of Relieving the Present Scarcity, and Preventing the Diseases that Arise from Meagre Food* (1796), 17. I am not claiming that this tract is wholly ironical. Beddoes may well be seriously recommending more efficient use of land and resources, and a rationalization of diet. But he is indignant that such measures may be forced upon the people by naked class legislation.

88. Beddoes, *A Letter to the Right Hon William Pitt,* 8.

89. See Roy Porter, 'Consumption: Disease of the Consumer Society?'.

90. Elsewhere, Beddoes writes of the deleterious effects of opium on the poor. 'Whether opium was first taken to recruit the labourer after excesive toil; or occasionally to cheer the gloom of despondence; or to make up the deficiences of that abominable water gruel and potatoe diet, by which the joyless being of so many pale, meagre, shivering women and children is prolonged, I am not informed. I lately received the following account from a medical observer. "The use of opium as a cordial, is very general among the poor of Sunderland, and I believe of the other sea-ports on this coast; and they all agree that it enables them to support a longer abstinence from food than they otherwise could. Its use seems, unfortunately as bewitching as that of spiritous liquors, and a gradual increase of the dose, as certainly induces a state of debility of the whole frame, as the other baneful habit. Nothing can be more wretched than the appearance of some whom I have seen; their skin of almost a leaden hue, the abdomen tumid, the limbs shrunk, and a countenance expressive of infinite anxiety and wretchedness"'. See J.E. Stock, *Memoirs of the Life of Thomas Beddoes MD,* 123.

91. The importance of science to Beddoes as the basis of medical authority is argued above in ch.4.

92. Thomas Beddoes, *The History of Isaac Jenkins, and of the Sickness of Sarah his Wife, and Their Three Children* (1792; the following

quotations are from the 1796 edition). This work, sold cheaply or given away, went through numerous editions. Already in 1793, a fifth edition had appeared. In 1796 Beddoes claimed that 40,000 copies of this tract had been sold or distributed. As late as 1830, freebie versions of it were still being produced.

93. Beddoes, *The History of Isaac Jenkins*, 5; of the quack, the narrator notes, 'two out of three died of those that he doctored, though he was a conjuror beside'.

94. Beddoes, *The History of Isaac Jenkins*, 37.

95. Beddoes, *The History of Isaac Jenkins*, 40.

96. Beddoes, *The History of Isaac Jenkins*, 43.

97. Thomas Beddoes, *Extract of a Letter on Early Instruction, Particularly that of the Poor* (1792); for education, see Dorothy A. Stansfield, 'Thomas Beddoes and Education'.

98. Beddoes, *Extract of a Letter on Early Instruction.*

99. Beddoes, *Extract of a Letter on Early Instruction*, 7. On Barbauld and Trimmer, see Samuel F. Pickering, *John Locke and Children's Books in Eighteenth Century England*; V.E. Neuburg, *Popular Literature*; David Vincent, *Literacy and Popular Culture. England 1750–1914.*

100. Thomas Beddoes, *Good Advice for the Husbandman in Harvest* (1808).

101. Thomas Beddoes, *Good Advice for the Husbandman in Harvest.*

102. Thomas Beddoes, *A Guide for Self Preservation, and Parental Affection; or Plain Directions for Enabling People to Keep Themselves and their Children Free from Several Common Disorders* (1793).

103. Thomas Beddoes, *Rules of the Medical Institution, for the Benefit of the Sick and Drooping Poor; with an Explanation of its Peculiar Design and Various Necessary Instructions* (1804); see also *idem, Suggestions Towards Setting on Foot the Projected Establishment for Pneumatic Medicine* (1797); on dispensaries, see I.S.L. Loudon, 'The Origins and Growth of the Dispensary Movement in England'.

104. Beddoes's inventiveness with architectural technology inevitably calls to mind the experiments in discipline discussed in Michel Foucault, *Discipline and Punish.* For specific discussion, see F.F. Cartwright, *The English Pioneers of Anaesthesia*; L.S. Gottlieb, 'Thomas Beddoes M.D. and the Pneumatic Institution at Clifton 1798–1801'; T.H. Levere, 'Dr Thomas Beddoes and the Establishment of his Pneumatic Institution: a Tale of Three Presidents'; A.H. Miller, 'The Pneumatic Institution of Thomas Beddoes at Clifton, 1798'; W.D.A. Smith, *Under the Influence.*

105. Beddoes, *Rules of the Medical Institution*, 5. One is tempted to see certain parallels, in arrangement and spirit, between Beddoes's Institution and the Peckham Health Centre established in the 1930s. See Jane Lewis and Barbara Brookes, 'The Peckham Health Centre'; Innes Pearse and Lucy H. Crocker, *The Peckham Experiment.*

106. Beddoes, *Rules*, 12, 14, 23, 127. One of many popular errors, Beddoes insisted, was that scrophula, or 'the [King's] evil', was thought 'more disgraceful than consumption' – presumably because it is more visibly disfiguring.

107. Beddoes, *Rules*, 23. For Beddoes's views on tuberculosis, see the discussion in Roy Porter, 'Consumption: Disease of the Consumer Society?'.

108. Beddoes, *Rules*, 33.

109. Beddoes, *Rules*, 128.

110. Beddoes, *Rules*, 42. It is not clear that Beddoes subjected them to physical examination. For the limits of hands-on examinations see Roy Porter, 'The Rise of Physical Examination'.

111. Beddoes, *Rules*, 50.

112. Beddoes, *Rules*, 49.

113. Beddoes, *Rules*, 56.

114. Beddoes, *Rules*, 76.

115. Beddoes, *Rules*, 81.

116. Beddoes, *Rules*, 56.

117. Beddoes, *Rules*, 92–3.

118. Beddoes, *Rules*, 95.

119. Beddoes, *Rules*, 95.

120. Beddoes, *Rules*, 95.

121. Beddoes, *Rules*, 95.

122. Beddoes, *Rules*, 133.

123. Beddoes, *Rules*, 100.

124. Beddoes, *Rules*, 110.

125. Beddoes, *Rules*, 117.

126. Beddoes, *Rules*, 118.

127. Beddoes, *Rules*, 119.

128. Beddoes, *Rules*, 119. Beddoes goes on to attack opponents of dissection: 251; compare Beddoes's condemnation of 'prejudices so generally prevalent especially among the lower classes, against the examination of the bodies of the dead', mentioned in J.E. Stock, *Memoirs of the Life of Thomas Beddoes MD*, 327. There is a good discussion in M.R. Neve, 'Natural Philosophy, Medicine and the Culture of Science in Provincial England'.

129. Beddoes, *Rules*, 146.

130. Beddoes, *Rules*, 251.

131. Stock, *Memoirs of the Life of Thomas Beddoes MD*, 308.

132. W. Buchan, *Observations Concerning the Prevention and Cure of the Venereal Disease*, xxiii, xxvi.

10

Conclusion

> Hatred – revenge – misanthropy . . . . Hm. This is the morbid anatomy of black bile.
>
> (Peacock, *Nightmare Abbey*)

Beddoes believed in the progressive powers of free speech, and he thought with his pen. He wrote about the great topics that agitated his age and involved him directly: political reform and revolution; the obstacles and opportunities for individual fulfilment; poverty and injustice, education, science and progress; disease, health, and the role of medicine. He viewed himself as a doctor to his own age, hearing its complaints, feeling its pulse, examining its symptoms, assessing its constitution, recommending regimes and treatments.

Beddoes was acutely aware of the problematic nature of consciousness. Words, language, discourse, reason – all should be engines of inquiry, torches of truth. But the putatively isomorphic relations between words and things – so crucial to any espousal of empiricism – were in reality more tantalizing. Sometimes words were simply wanting. 'The hypochondria sufferer', he noted, 'always finds language fails him, when he gives vent to his complaints'.[1] Despite the patient's efforts to find the words, they all sounded inadequate or anti-climactic: 'He tells you he has heart-burn, dreadful flatulence', and so forth, but these are at best distant approximations to his actual feelings. And so, 'after vain and unsatisfactory efforts, his conclusion generally is, "In short you see before you, the most miserable wretch upon the face of the earth".'[2] One is tempted to substitute 'Everyman' for the hypochondriac.

Thus the doctor discovered the obliquities between malaise, pain, and the words articulating them. Representations were opaque, reality always at a remove, held at bay.[3]

> Language has not yet been adjusted with any degree of exactness, to our inward feelings. Hence medical reports, where these feelings come in question, stand a double chance of inaccuracy. The invalid, with whom the representation must originate, may express himself ill [*sic!*]; and the physician may misconceive him if he takes him simply at his word, or by trying to help him out, may substitute his own ideas. How little then can we depend upon generalisation of such obscure data!

Medicine, putatively a science, thus had dreadful difficulties in expressing itself well. Its semantic problems could not be resolved by waving any logical positivist magic wand. For one thing, symptoms had no rigid boundaries, and diseases themselves no fixed abode. How easy the diagnostic art would have been, were it possible to frame disease nosologies rather as Linnaeus had pencilled in the classification of plants. Certain authors had indeed 'laboured, so much in vain, to give *definitions* of diseases, similar to those which occur in books of botanical nomenclature': the labour, however, was abortive.[4] Dismissing the taxonomic nomenclature of his erstwhile mentor, the great Edinburgh professor, William Cullen, Beddoes curtly concluded that his 'definitions of diseases have perhaps more authority than value'.[5]

Would, then, medical language grow more exact and stable with the advancement of science? Probably not; for those very forces of change actually produced the opposite effect. The 'progress of knowledge', Beddoes confessed, 'renders stability of language impossible'.[6] He reflected upon his own experience, as a champion in England of the new Lavoisierian chemistry, with its expressly revolutionary vocabulary: 'Whether I have abused this privilege by disoxygenated and other terms of "learned length", persons, skilled alike in the philosophy of things and words, may decide'.[7]

Thus there were representations, and misrepresentations. The short-breathed Beddoes was rarely short of words. But – as is shown by his perennial reflections upon the subterfuges and ambushes of language, he knew how often, how easily, words served as alibis for clear thinking. He endlessly drew attention to the seductions of forms of speech, to the obfuscating work of clichés, proverbs, and catchphrases. He exposed authority's use of newspeak to deceive, occlude, legitimate, brainwash. He knew the sick in particular often used, maybe needed, language to protect them from reality.[8]

As any reader of Beddoes will be aware – and it is both the strength and weakness of his prose and the thinking behind it – he was habitually self-referential. He was fascinated by literary forms. His own writings compulsively incorporate the speech and sayings of others; he is continually alluding, appropriating, and quoting, sometimes with, sometimes without acknowledgement. He wrote poetry and polemic, and his prose moves from addresses to the barely literate to entertainments for sophisticates, and always with a glance over his shoulder at his intellectual peers or other implied audiences. If rather a fustian stylist, he was preoccupied with style, with form and the formulaic. He can be a mimic, parodist, a satirist; a creator of Peacockian comedy of opinions; a caricaturist, and a dramatist.[9] He wrote for effect, for pleasure, for vengeance, and just to let off steam; he enjoyed literary experiments, winding up his readers, being seriously playful and playfully serious, a Doubting Thomas, a Tom o'Beddoes. As every reader of this study will be aware, it is at one's peril that one takes his observations *au pied de la lettre. Caveant lectores.*

He was moreover, an eavesdropper (good doctors must be good listeners). Apparently quiet in company, he was fascinated by the voices of others. He was acutely attuned (in ways today's deconstructionists might appreciate) to the power of language to think, write, and reproduce itself; he could hear and see contemporary actors sleepwalking their way through parts dictated by role and custom, fashion and prejudice. In Beddoes's anthropological understanding of society as 'scripted', even those who landed eligible parts in high society were also victims, condemned to vacant enjoyments, insatiable desires, sick dreams.

Swift satirized such vanities with a misanthropic delight in levelling man's pride. Samuel Johnson's sombre broodings on man's shortcomings, on the fictions necessary to make life bearable, were the work of a Christian moralist. There were elements of Swift and Johnson in Beddoes;[10] but the part he assumed above all was that of a *philosophe*-doctor.[11] In his more optimistic moods, chiefly earlier in his career, Beddoes used his pen to probe, to diagnose, to prescribe a healthier future. Later, he grew more preoccupied with socio- and psycho-pathology, individual delusion and collective self-deception, more resigned perhaps to the chronic, even terminal, nature of the human condition.

Who can doubt that the times turned Beddoes pessimist? If it was bliss to be alive, and better still, to be a young, clever male graduate, around 1790, by the turn of the century, it was hard for a radical to avoid embitterment. Jacobin antics had wrecked revolution abroad and given reactionaries at home the chance of a lifetime to delay the age of improvement for a generation. Beddoes of course did not merely witness this putting out of the lights all over Europe as a bystander. He was one of the *illuminati* extinguished. After a dazzling start, he passed the remainder of his life in frustrating private practice, scraping to finance a laboratory of his own, which, in the event, produced no significant scientific breakthroughs.

In explaining Beddoes's jaundiced attitudes towards society, the sick, and his own profession, a biographer might make much of personal disappointments and disenchantments. Some of his closest friends – Giddy, Southey, Coleridge – turned Tory. Beddoes probably had very mixed feelings about the meteoric rise of Humphry Davy, who got out almost as soon as he got on, and displayed precisely that simpering sycophancy as a youthful Royal Institution professor that the old ironside in Beddoes detested in courtier doctors. Something went wrong with Beddoes's own marriage. Though apparently a dedicated domestic and family man, he had a brusque and taciturn demeanour, holding himself at a distance; and this perhaps explains why his passionate wife, Anna, grew disconsolate and depressed, eventually growing infatuated with Giddy, his closest friend. Giddy seems to have behaved honourably, but the impact of the affair on Beddoes – a man who could write at such length and with such urgency about the importance of happy families – must have been devastating. And what of this educator's own children? As with Freud, we know tantalizingly little about how this paterfamilias got on with his own offspring. But one wonders whether something in the domestic scene was responsible for the profound isolation, eccentricity, and morbid imagination which blighted the adult life of his son, Thomas Lovell, skewing his very considerable poetic talents, making him more than half in love with easeful death, and driving him finally to suicide.[12]

Finally, if we are looking in the circumstances of his own life for explanations of Beddoes's increasing concern with socio-pathology, there is the question of his health. He early grew fat, and developed respiratory problems. From his mid-forties, he easily became fatigued, and his physique deteriorated; he died at forty-eight. Did he neglect his health? Did poor health undermine his temper? Was his worsening health psychosomatic, or (as enemies gleefully suggested) Providence's punishment for his rash and dangerous medico-chemical self-experimentation? How far did Beddoes believe his diagnoses of the ills and complaints of educated society applied to himself? Were they drawn from self-examination?

These are intriguing questions. I have no answers to them. They are probably unanswerable, since we possess no diaries or similarly intimate materials which would contain clues. One may of course speculate that, as with a variety of other sick and medically-qualified or -interested authors – Sterne comes to mind – writing itself must have been for Beddoes both pathological and therapeutic, an irritant and an analgesic.[13]

The personal interrogation could be taken further: his prejudices and passions, his last letter to Humphry Davy, in which he describes himself as 'one who has scattered abroad the Avena Fatua [wild oats] of knowledge, from which neither branch nor blossom nor fruit has resulted'[14] – all these would be meat and drink to a Freudian psycho-historical sleuth. I shall leave these entertainments to others. Rather, by way of conclusion, I wish to suggest that Beddoes's lasting interest lies in the fact that the dialectic of his medical life and times produced a penetrating socio-political critique of a somewhat different stamp from those advanced by most of his contemporaries.

Of course, Beddoes may, in the broadest sense, be called a typical philosophical radical.[15] He tracked the evils of present society to the root. Through his investigations into cognitive psychology and the philosophy of education, through his attempts to lay bare their techniques of persuasion and mental control, and to understand the force of habit, custom, and the empire of language, he exposed the ideological foundations of the Establishment. He took principled stands on personal freedoms; he stood for the individual against the institution, for freedom against arbitrary government, for opportunity against privilege, for equality against hierarchy. He subjected the *ancien régime* to withering criticism. He traced its affinities with war, imperialism, corruption, and ecclesiastical dominion. In all such commitments he shared much with Paine, Holcroft, Godwin, the early Coleridge, Bentham and other utilitarians, the leaders of the London Corresponding Society, including James Parkinson, with Thelwall, Cobbett, and many other free-thinking friends of liberty.[16]

Yet his medical interests also imparted a somewhat distinctive slant to this familiar socio-political critique. Unlike many of the radical orators of his day, Beddoes was not primarily concerned with abstract rights, common law precedent, the Revolution of 1688, or the principles of representation. Through being a practising doctor, he was led to emphasize the politics of health in the widest sense, the well-being of bodies, and to scrutinize the positive responsibilities of government for the good of its people in such departments as the distribution of wealth, taxation policy, food supply, education provision, the standard of living, the relief of poverty and hunger, and of course, the prevention and cure of disease. His most indignant and effective protests of the mid-1790s conveyed his outrage that Englishmen were starving and sick, as a result not of natural dearth but of Treasury-induced scarcity and penury.

More broadly, Beddoes repeatedly analysed the ills of ignorance, prejudice, false information, false expectations, and false consciousness. His diagnostics and diatribes exposed the folly of waste, of misdirected energies, erroneous dogmatism, the strategies to which people had recourse to render life bearable. The poor drowned their sorrows in drink, the rich took refuge in the fantasies money could buy, in false delicacy and refinement, and in unwieldy, complex, and counter-productive cultural superstructures – including invalidism, valetudinarianism, and hypochondria. Rationality had been uprooted by the gusts of fashion. There must be a better way. Simple modes of existence would ensure better health, happiness, and effective expenditure of effort. Beddoes flayed folly, not, as traditionally, in the guise of the moralist, but as a physician, appalled at the psychopathology of addiction. Health had to be the touchstone of radicalism.

So what role was there for the 'doctor to society'? As this book has documented, Beddoes believed that, as then constituted, medicine was a disgrace, reduced to quackery, as the political establishment had been reduced to corruption. Doctors had prostituted their art for gain. Clearly, medicine must cease to be a racket. Above all, it had to cease to be a trade. It had to escape from the market, for medicine had a higher mission.

Beddoes lived at a time when the first treatises upon medical ethics were being written in Britain. In Scotland, John Gregory, and in Manchester, Thomas Percival, attempted to raise medicine's standing and sights. But Gregory's *Observations on the Duties of a Physician* (1770) and Percival's *Medical Ethics* (1803) were largely concerned with prescribing an emollient etiquette to ensure well-lubricated relations between physicians and patients, and above all, amongst the various ranks of practitioners themselves.[17] Beddoes went much further. As we have seen, he offered a radical critique which suggested that the pressures governing the practice of medicine in Britain – the laws of supply and demand, the axiom that the customer was always right (tempered by *caveat emptor*) did not provide an ethical platform for healing the sick. And this mattered to Beddoes. Medicine had to be ethical, because medicine was indispensable for something much more fundamental.

Medicine itself – or at least the biomedical understanding of life – should rightly be the cornerstone of ethics as a whole. Chemist, physiologist, and, perhaps, atheist, Beddoes was disposed, like his French contemporaries, the *idéologues*, to take a materialist perspective upon the entire panorama of animated existence.[18] Beddoes ridiculed the attempts of Cartesian dualists to draw sharp divides between mind and brain, spirit and flesh – such sciolists overlooked 'the inseparable connection between moral and medical topics'.[19] Through advancing numerous clinical demonstrations of psychosomatic and somatopsychic complaints, Beddoes denied the rigid ontological differentiation between the physical and the moral. Hair-splitting metaphysicians he held in utter contempt. For all his admiration for *Sturm und Drang*, Beddoes rarely had a good word to say for Kant.

No moral system – or, more broadly, no code of living, no value-system, or even life style – could hold any real value, could be *moral*, unless grounded upon, and conducive to, the permanent well-being of man as an organic being. Physiology was the basis, and test, of all sound morals, for 'the science of human nature is altogether incapable of division into independent branches':[20]

> Every code of morals must ground its precepts on a comprehensive view of the laws that regulate feeling, and deliver the conditions of an offensive and defensive league, having for its object the well-being of individuals. Without accurate ideas therefore of the causes that affect the personal condition of mankind, how is it possible to conceive any progress in genuine morality? And will not every addition to this branch of knowledge necesarily tend to purify morals – that is, to introduce into the social compact covenants more beneficial to the parties? Without reference to the body, it is equally impossible to unfold the nature of the mind. Physiology therefore – or, more strictly, *biology* – by which I mean the doctrine of the living system in all its states, appears to be the foundation of ethics and pneumatology.

Thus there was an ethics of medicine; but, more importantly still, medicine itself must be the measure for all valid ethics. The physician thereby became the legislator of the new moral world. The doctor's duty was to instruct the people in the lessons of living, because without understanding these, how could they possibly make the wider choices of life? Here his friendship with Coleridge was surely no accident.[21] For Beddoes's vision of the doctor as intellectual guru parallels Coleridge's ideal of the new intelligentsia, the clerisy, called to serve as moral leaders of the future. No servile tradesman, no sycophantic courtier, no technocratic fixer, the Beddoesian doctor would be the humanist physician become priest and preceptor to humanity. Beddoes thus formulated a new, upstanding vocational vision for medicine as a modern profession.

Thus Beddoes perceived the interconnectedness of knowledge, science, medicine and ethics, while investing unswerving faith in experimental science as the engine of advance. He clearly intended that a breed of intellectuals, committed to truth and progress, to inquiry and experiment, should sway the destiny of nations. Once freed from the counter, doctors could take their rightful place amongst such an élite. They would be able to pursue national improvement. They would succour the people. In a manner almost presaging Virchow, the Beddoesian doctor would be the natural attorney of the poor.[22]

It is noteworthy, however, how little Beddoes translated this vision into institutional terms. Hardly surprising, perhaps. By contrast, say, to *Kameradwissenschaft* in Central Europe, England had no tradition of the physician as public functionary within a system of medical police.[23] Beddoes, in any case, entertained profound suspicions of government and its extension. Hence his vision of the medical man as a force for progress focused upon books and lectures, education and example, and small-scale, face-to-face, private 'clinics' such as the Pneumatic Institute.

Beddoes had no doubts as to medicine's benign potential. But an essential tension also clave his thought. If, as a political and social animal, he was a libertarian, egalitarian, and a democrat, how were these to be squared with the models and metaphors which medicine presupposed? For the fundamental relations of clinical medicine, Beddoes insisted, must hinge upon a hierarchy of expert authority (active physician, passive patient) based, not, of course, as then, on wealth, rank, patronage or pull, but on science and skill. Two incommensurable images thus clashed in Beddoes's projections of a good society. On the one hand, a heartfelt *liberté* and *égalité*. On the other hand, the protocols of the technocrat.[24]

In this tension lies, of course, the essence, and the contradictions, of so many reforming movements, radical and socialist, ever since, not least those to which medical practitioners have subscribed; simultaneously espousing some sort of liberationist faith in the people, and a more *dirigiste* notion that the people need to be saved from their own follies, and guided to a better future by enlightened sanitarians, utilitarians, social engineers, social scientists, St Simonians, Comtian positivists, Fabians, the Party, or whoever, in the name of public health, progress and order, national efficiency, the public good, the dictatorship of the proletariat, or whatever.[25]

Beddoes's ambiguities register the ambiguities of the Enlightenment towards the people – epitomized in Voltaire's supposed anxiety that, were the servants ever freed from their false consciousness, one would have to count the spoons.[26] Classically, the tension implicit between '*for* the people' and '*by* the people' was to be resolved through the medium of education: the wise pedagogue would help the people effect the transition from passive and grateful recipients of good to agencies of good in themselves. It is no accident that Beddoes was an ardent campaigner for education. Yet, when he looked at the educated classes, could he really maintain his faith?

In any case, the debate never got put to the test. In Britain, the kind of alliance that might have been forged between political and medical radicals did not cohere. Medics won their concessions out of the early-Victorian state and retreated into professional conservatism. In Third Republic France, physicians achieved a sizeable representation in Parliament, but used their muscle-power mainly to protect entrenched interests.[27] Over the last century, it has mainly been in the Third World that the natural alliance between doctors, radicals and revolutionaries has come to the fore, notably in our own day in Salvadore Allende and Che Guevara.

There was one fire-cracker in post-Beddoesian England: the somewhat unlikely, yet nevertheless potent figure of Thomas Wakley, libellous medical journalist, radical MP, and democrat, and a man, like Beddoes, consumed by hostility to the traditional medical oligarchy.[28] But the politics of medical change became atomized. As Adrian Desmond has recently shown, reformist currents within the profession were concerned mainly with occupational change (the career open to talent), without a strong commitment to radical social change.[29] And for their part, such leaders of the sanitarian and public health movements as Edwin Chadwick, while enthusiastic about the national utility of hygienic improvement, tended to be bureaucrats rather than democrats.[30] By the close of the nineteenth century, the English medical profession had grown entrenched and sleek, having carved out for itself a new set of professional restrictive practices that masqueraded as ethics and seemed to elevate it above the vulgarities of trade and the ignominy of subservience.

It is little wonder that Beddoes himself soon became just a historical footnote.

Notes

1. Thomas Beddoes, *Hygëia: or Essays Moral and Medical, on the Causes Affecting the Personal State of our Middling and Affluent Classes* (1802–3), vol. 2, Essay viii, p.78. [henceforth references will appear thus: 2 viii 78.].

2. Beddoes, *Hygëia*, 2 viii 78.
3. Beddoes, *Hygëia*, 3 ix 40.
4. Beddoes, *Hygëia*, 2 vi 13.
5. Beddoes, *Hygëia*, 3 ix 21.
6. T. Beddoes, *Manual of Health: or, the Invalid Conducted Safely Through the Seasons* (1806), 47.
7. Beddoes, *Manual of Health*, 47.
8. For further discussion of the radicalism of late eighteenth-century semantic analysis see H. Cunningham, 'The Language of Patriotism, 1750–1914'; Iain McCalman, *Radical Underworld*; James T. Boulton, *The Language of Politics in the Age of Wilkes and Burke*; Olivia Smith, *The Politics of Language*; Raphael Samuel (ed.), *Patriotism*; Peter Burke and Roy Porter (eds), *The Social History of Language*; *idem* (eds), *Language, Self and Society*.
9. None of this should be surprising, given Beddoes's immense familiarity with European literature and his close associations with literary men such as Coleridge. It is further not surprising that his own son became a distinguished poet: Sir Edmund Gosse (ed.), *The Complete Works of Thomas Lovell Beddoes*; Brian Hill, 'Father and Son: Thomas Beddoes and Thomas Lovell Beddoes'; James R. Thompson, *Thomas Lovell Beddoes.*
10. There is maybe more of Swift than Beddoes liked. Beddoes was certainly fascinated by Swift, and by the psychopathology of his misanthropy and his descent into chronic nervous disease (which Beddoes attributed to habitual masturbation). See discussion in Roy Porter, '"Expressing Yourself Ill": The Language of Sickness in Georgian England'.
11. For discussion of this notion, see Daniel Roche, 'Talent, Reason, and Sacrifice: The Physician during the Enlightenment'; Charles Paul, *Science and Immortality: The Eloges of the Paris Academy of Sciences (1699–1799)*; and Roy Porter, 'Medicine in the Enlightenment'.
12. Brian Hill, 'Father and Son: Thomas Beddoes and Thomas Lovell Beddoes'; James R. Thompson, *Thomas Lovell Beddoes.*
13. On Sterne, see D. Furst, 'Sterne and Physick'; Roy Porter, 'Against the Spleen'.
14. Quoted in F.F. Cartwright, *The English Pioneers of Anaesthesia*, 157.
15. Elie Halévy, *The Growth of Philosophical Radicalism.* By using this term, I do not mean to imply that Beddoes was a utilitarian in the Benthamite mould.
16. Iain McCalman, *Radical Underworld: Prophets, Revolutionaries and Pornographers in London, 1795–1840*; E.P. Thompson, *The Making of the English Working Class.*
17. See the Introduction to, and the essays in, Robert Baker, Dorothy Porter and Roy Porter (eds), *The Codification of Medical Morality in the Eighteenth and Nineteenth Centuries*, vol. 1.
18. On the *idéologues*, see M. Staum, *Cabanis*; S. Moravia, 'The Enlightenment and the Sciences of Man'.
19. Beddoes, *Hygëia*, 1 iii 83.

20. T. Beddoes, *Contributions to Physical and Medical Knowledge, Principally from the West of England* (1799), 3, 4.

21. See Richard Holmes, *Coleridge: Early Visions*. For the Romantic vision of the scientist as seer, see T.H. Levere, *Poetry Realised in Nature*; Andrew Cunningham and Nicholas Jardine (eds), *Romanticism and the Sciences*. For the rise of the professional ethic in a new middle-class ideal see H.J. Perkin, *The Origins of Modern English Society 1780–1880*.

22. On Virchow, see Karl Figlio and Paul Weindling, 'Was Social Medicine Revolutionary? Rudolf Virchow and the Revolutions of 1848'. See also Jack D. Ellis, *The Physician-Legislators of France*.

23. George Rosen, *A History of Public Health*, 161–6: *idem*, *From Medical Police to Social Medicine*.

24. On experts, see J.A. Passmore, *The Perfectibility of Man*; H. Armytage, *The Rise of the Technocrats*.

25. For medicine, the St Simonians and the politics of medical expertise in France see Frank Manuel, *The Prophets of Paris*; K. Baker, 'The Early History of the Term "Social Science"'; *idem*, *Condorcet: From Natural Philosophy to Social Mathematics*; J.V. Pickstone, 'Bureaucracy, Liberalism and the Body in Post-Revolutionary France'; W. Coleman, *Death is a Social Disease*; Dorinda Outram, 'Science and Political Ideology, 1790–1848'; Theodore M. Porter, 'Natural Science and Social Theory'; B. Haines, 'The Inter-relations between Social, Biological and Medical Thought, 1750–1850: Saint-Simon and Comte'.

26. H.C. Payne, *The Philosophes and the People*; see the closing discussion in Roy Porter, *The Enlightenment*.

27. Jack D. Ellis, *The Physician-Legislators of France*.

28. S.S. Sprigge, *The Life and Times of Sir Thomas Wakley*.

29. Adrian Desmond, *The Politics of Evolution*.

30. Note Bentham's own advocacy of a 'health minister' to perform functions such as controlling dangerous exhalations, registering changes in the air, and so forth. See Benjamin Spector, 'Jeremy Bentham, his Influence upon Medical Thought and Legislation'. Bentham believed that 'the art of legislation is but the art of healing practised upon a large scale': M. Mack, *Jeremy Bentham*, 264.

Bibliography

Abraham, J.J., *Lettsom: His Life, Times, Friends and Descendants* (London: Heinemann, 1933).

Ackerknecht, Erwin H., *Medicine at the Paris Hospital, 1794–1848* (Baltimore: Johns Hopkins University Press, 1967).

Adair, J.M., *Essays on Fashionable Diseases* . . . (London: Bateman, 1790).

Allan, D.G.C. and Schofield, R.E., *Stephen Hales: Scientist and Philanthropist* (London: Scolar Press, 1980).

Andrews, C.B., (ed.), *The Torrington Diaries*, 4 vols (London: Eyre & Spottiswoode, 1954).

Anstey, C., *The New Bath Guide*, ed. by Peter Wagner (Hildesheim/Zürich/New York: Georg Olms Verlag, 1989).

Appleby, A., 'Nutrition and Disease: The Case of London, 1550–1750', *Journal of Interdisciplinary History*, vi (1975), 1–22.

Appleby, A., *Famine in Tudor and Stuart England* (Stanford: Stanford University Press, 1978).

Appleby, Joyce, 'Ideology and Theory: The Tension between Political and Economic Liberalism in Seventeenth Century England', *American Historical Review*, lxxxi (1976), 499–515.

Appleby, Joyce, *Economic Thought in Seventeenth-Century England* (Princeton, N.J.: Princeton University Press, 1978).

Arbuthnot, J., *An Essay Concerning the Nature of Aliments* (London: J. & R. Tonson, 1731).

Arbuthnot, J., *An Essay Concerning the Effects of Air on Human Bodies* (London: J. & R. Tonson & S. Draper, 1733).

Ariès, P., *The Hour of our Death* (London: Allen Lane, 1981).

Armytage, W.H.G., *The Rise of the Technocrats; A Social History* (London: Routledge & Kegan Paul, 1965).

Arnold-Forster, Kate and Tallis, Nigel, *The Bruising Apothecary: Images of Pharmacy and Medicine in Caricature* (London: The Pharmaceutical Press, 1989).

Aronson, J.K., *An Account of the Foxglove and its Medicinal Uses, 1785–1985* (London: Oxford University Press, 1985).

Austen, Jane, *Sanditon*, ed. by M. Drabble (Harmondsworth: Penguin, 1974).

Baglivi, G., *De Praxi Medica* (Rome: Typis D.A. Herculis, 1696).

Baker, K., 'The Early History of the Term "Social Science"', *Annals of Science*, xx (1964), 211–26.

Baker, K., *Condorcet: From Natural Philosophy to Social Mathematics* (Chicago: Chicago University Press, 1975).

Baker, Robert, Porter, Dorothy and Porter, Roy (eds), *The Codification of Medical Morality in the Eighteenth and Nineteenth Centuries*, vol. i (Dordrecht: Kluwer, 1991).

Bambrough, J.B., *The Little World of Man* (London: Longman, Green & Co., 1952).

Barbeau, A., *Life and Letters at Bath in the Eighteenth Century*, ed. by A. Dobson (London: Heinemann, 1904).

Barkan, L. *Nature's Work of Art: The Human Body as Image of the World* (New Haven, Conn.: Yale University Press, 1975).

Barker, F., *The Tremulous Private Body* (London: Methuen, 1984).

Barnes, B. and Shapin, S. (eds), *Natural Order: Historical Studies of Scientific Culture* (London: Sage, 1979).

Barrell, John, *The Idea of Landscape and the Sense of Place, 1730–1840: An Approach to the Poetry of John Clare* (Cambridge: Cambridge University Press, 1972).

Barrell, John, *The Dark Side of the Landscape. The Rural Poor in English Painting, 1730–1840* (Cambridge: Cambridge University Press, 1983).

Barrell, John, *English Literature in History, 1730–80: An Equal, Wide Survey* (London: Hutchinson; New York: St Martin's Press, 1983).

Barry, J., 'The Cultural Life of Bristol, 1640–1775' (D.Phil. thesis, Oxford University, 1986).

Baur, S., *Hypochondria: Woeful Imaginings* (Princeton, N.J.: Princeton University Press, 1988).

Beddoes, Thomas (ed. and trans.), T. Bergman, *A Dissertation on Elective Attractions. Translated by the translator of Spallanzani's Dissertations* (London: J. Murray, 1785).

Beddoes, Thomas (ed. and trans.), *The Chemical Essays of C.W. Scheele Translated . . . with Additions* (London: J. Murray, 1786).

Beddoes, Thomas, *A Memorial Concerning the State of the Bodleian Library, and the Conduct of the Principal Librarian. Addressed to the Curators of that Library, by the Chemical Reader* (Oxford: University Press, 1787).

Beddoes, Thomas (ed.), L. Spallanzani, *Dissertations Relative to the Natural History of Animals and Vegetables*, 2nd edn. (London: J. Murray, 1789).

Beddoes, Thomas (ed.), *Chemical Experiments and Opinions; Extracted from a Work Published in the Last Century* (Oxford: Clarendon Press, 1790).

Beddoes, Thomas, *Extract of a Letter on Early Instruction, Particularly that of the Poor* (Madeley: J. Edmunds, 1792).

Beddoes, Thomas, *Alexander's Expedition down the Hydaspes and the Indus to the Indian Ocean* (Madeley: J. Edmunds, 1792).

Beddoes, Thomas, *The History of Isaac Jenkins, and of the Sickness of Sarah his Wife, and Their Three Children* (Madeley: J. Edmunds, 1792).

Beddoes, Thomas, *Observations on the Nature and Cure of Calculus, Sea Scurvy, Consumption, Catarrh, and Fever: Together with Conjectures upon*

Several Other Subjects of Physiology and Pathology (London: J. Murray, 1793).

Beddoes, Thomas, *A Guide for Self Preservation, and Parental Affection; or Plain Directions for Enabling People to Keep Themselves and their Children Free from Several Common Disorders* (Bristol: Bulgin & Rosser, 1793).

Beddoes, Thomas, *A Letter to Erasmus Darwin, M.D., on a New Method of Treating Pulmonary Consumption and Some Other Diseases Hitherto Found Incurable* (Bristol: Bulgin & Rosser, 1793).

Beddoes, Thomas, *Considerations on the Medicinal Use of Factitious Airs and on the Manner of Obtaining Them in Large Quantities.* Part I by Thomas Beddoes, Part II by James Watt, 2 parts (Bristol: Bulgin & Rosser; London: J. Johnson, 1794).

Beddoes, Thomas, *A New Method of Treating Pulmonary Consumption* (London: J. Pridden, 1794).

Beddoes, Thomas, *Where would be the Harm of a Speedy Peace?* (Bristol: N. Biggs, 1795).

Beddoes, Thomas, *A Word in Defence of the Bill of Rights against Gagging Bills* (1795).

Beddoes, Thomas, *An Essay on the Public Merits of Mr Pitt* (London: J. Johnson, 1796).

Beddoes, Thomas, *A Letter to the Right Hon William Pitt, on the Means of Relieving the Present Scarcity, and Preventing the Diseases that Arise from Meagre Food* (London: J. Johnson, 1796).

Beddoes, Thomas, *Alternatives Compared: or, What Shall the Rich Do to be Safe?* (London: J. Debrett, 1797).

Beddoes, Thomas, *A Lecture Introductory to a Course of Popular Instruction on the Constitution and Management of the Human Body* (Bristol: Joseph Cottle, 1797).

Beddoes, Thomas, *Suggestions Towards Setting on Foot the Projected Establishment for Pneumatic Medicine* (Bristol: Biggs and Cottle, 1797).

Beddoes, Thomas, *Suggestions Towards an Essential Improvement in the Medical and Surgical Departments of the Bristol Infirmary* (Bristol: Biggs & Cottle, 1798).

Beddoes, Thomas (ed.), *Contributions to Physical and Medical Knowledge, Principally from the West of England* (London: T.N. Longman & O. Rees, 1799).

Beddoes, Thomas, *Essay on the Causes, Early Signs, and Prevention of Pulmonary Consumption for the Use of Parents and Preceptors* (Bristol: Biggs & Cottle, 1799).

Beddoes, Thomas, *Observations on the Medical and Domestic Management of the Consumptive; on the Powers of Digitalis Purpurea; and on the Cure of Scrophula* (London: Longman, 1801).

Beddoes, Thomas, *Hygëia: or Essays Moral and Medical, on the Causes Affecting the Personal State of our Middling and Affluent Classes*, 3 vols (Bristol: J. Mills, 1802–3).

Beddoes, Thomas, *Rules of the Medical Institution, for the Benefit of the Sick and Drooping Poor; with an Explanation of its Peculiar Design and Various Necessary Instructions* (Bristol: J. Mills, 1804).

Beddoes, Thomas, *A Manual of Health: or, the Invalid Conducted Safely Through the Seasons* (London: J. Johnson, 1806).

Beddoes, Thomas, *Researches Anatomical and Practical Concerning Fever, as Connected with Inflammation* (London: Longman, Hurst, Rees & Orme, 1807).

Beddoes, Thomas, *Good Advice for the Husbandman in Harvest* (Bristol: Mills & Co., 1808).

Beddoes, Thomas, *A Letter to the Right Honourable Sir Joseph Banks . . . on the Causes and Removal of the Prevailing Discontents, Imperfections, and Abuses, in Medicine* (London: Richard Phillips, 1808).

Beddoes, Thomas, 'Considerations on Infirmaries', appendix 3 to J.E. Stock, *Memoir of the Life of Thomas Beddoes, M.D.* (London: Murray, 1811).

Beier, L.M., *Sufferers and Healers. The Experience of Illness in Seventeenth-Century England* (London: Routledge & Kegan Paul, 1987).

Bell, R.M., *Holy Anorexia* (Chicago: University of Chicago Press, 1985).

Benjamin, Marina, 'Medicine, Morality and the Politics of Berkeley's Tar-water', in Andrew Cunningham and Roger French (eds), *The Medical Enlightenment of the Eighteenth Century* (Cambridge: Cambridge University Press, 1990), 165–93.

Bennet, Christopher, *Theatrum Tabidorum, or the Nature and Cure of Consumptions, Whether A Phthisick, an Atrophy or an Hectick* (London: W. & J. Inny, 1720).

Benthall, J. and Polhemus, T. (eds), *The Body as a Medium of Expression* (London: Allen Lane, 1975).

Berg, Maxine, *The Age of Manufactures, 1700–1820* (London: Fontana, 1985).

Berman, M., '"Hegemony" and the Amateur Tradition in British Science"', *Journal of Social History*, viii (1974), 30–50.

Berridge, V. and Edwards, G., *Opium and the People* (London: Allen Lane, 1981).

Bishop, P.J., 'Blackmore on Consumption', *Tubercle*, xl (1958), 118–21.

Bishop, P.J., 'Thomas Young and his "Practical and Historical Treatise on Consumptive Disorders"', *Tubercle*, liv (1973), 159–64.

Bloch, M., *The Royal Touch: Sacred Monarchy and Scrofula in England and France* (London: Routledge & Kegan Paul, 1973).

Boissier de Sauvages, François, *Dissertatio Medica de Motuum Vitalium Causa* (Montpellier, 1740).

Booth, Christopher, *Doctors in Science and Society. Essays of a Clinical Scientist* (London: British Medical Journal, 1987).

Borsay, Peter, *The English Urban Renaissance* (Oxford: Clarendon Press, 1989).

Borsay, Peter (ed.), *The Eighteenth Century Town. A Reader in English Urban History 1688–1820* (London: Longman, 1990).

Bottomley, F., *Attitudes to the Body in Western Christendom* (London: Lepus Books, 1979).

Boucé, P.-G., 'Les Jeux Interdits de l'Imaginaire: Onanism et Culpabilisation Sexuelle au XVIIIe Siècle', in J. Céard (ed.), *La Folie et le Corps* (Paris: Presses de l'Ecole Normale Supérieure, 1985), 223–43.

Boulton, James T., *The Language of Politics in the Age of Wilkes and Burke* (London: Routledge & Kegan Paul, 1963).

Bourdieu, Pierre, *Distinction. A Social Critique of the Judgement of Taste* (Cambridge, Mass.: Harvard University Press, 1984).
Braudy, Leo, *The Frenzy of Renown* (Oxford: Oxford University Press, 1987).
Brewer, John, 'Commercialization and Politics', in N. McKendrick, John Brewer and J.H. Plumb, *The Birth of a Consumer Society: The Commercialization of Eighteenth-Century England* (London: Europa, 1982), 197–264.
Brewer, John and Porter, Roy (eds), *Consumption and the World of Goods* (London: Routledge, forthcoming).
Broadbent, J., 'The Image of God or Two Yards of Skin', in J. Benthall and T. Polhemus (eds), *The Body as a Medium of Expression* (London: Allen Lane, 1975), 305–26.
Brock, C.H., 'The Happiness of Riches', in W.F. Bynum and R. Porter (eds), *William Hunter and the Eighteenth-Century Medical World* (Cambridge: Cambridge University Press, 1985), 35–56.
Brody, H., *Stories of Sickness* (New Haven, Conn.: Yale University Press, 1987).
Brown, Theodore, 'From Mechanism to Vitalism in Eighteenth Century English Physiology', *Journal of the History of Biology*, vii (1974), 179–216.
Brown, T., 'Descartes, Dualism and Psychosomatic Medicine', in W.F. Bynum, Roy Porter and M. Shepherd (eds), *The Anatomy of Madness*, vol. 1 (London: Tavistock, 1985), 151–65.
Brumberg, J.J., *Fasting Girls: The Emergence of Anorexia Nervosa as a Modern Disease* (Cambridge, Mass.: Harvard University Press, 1988).
Bryder, L., *Below the Magic Mountain. A Social History of Tuberculosis in Twentieth-Century Britain* (Oxford: Clarendon Press, 1988).
Bryson, G., *Man and Society* (Princeton, N.J.: Princeton University Press, 1945).
Buchan, W., *Domestic Medicine, or a Treatise on the Prevention and Cure of Diseases by Regimen and Simple Medicines* (Edinburgh: Balfour, Auld & Smellie, 1769).
Buchan, W., *Observations Concerning the Prevention and Cure of the Venereal Disease* (London: Chapman, 1796).
Burke, Peter, *Popular Culture in Early Modern Europe* (London: Temple Smith, 1978).
Burke, Peter, 'Popular Culture between History and Ethnology', *Ethnologi Europaea*, xiv (1984), 5–13.
Burke, Peter, *'Revolution in Popular Culture'*, in Roy Porter and M. Teich (eds), Revolution in History (Cambridge: Cambridge University Press, 1986), 206–25.
Burke, Peter and Porter, Roy (eds), *The Social History of Language* (Cambridge: Cambridge University Press, 1987).
Burke, Peter and Porter, Roy (eds), *Language, Self and Society: The Social History of Language* (Cambridge: Polity Press, 1991).
Burke, R.M., *A Historical Chronology of Tuberculosis* (Springfield, Ill.: Thomas, 1955).
Burnby, J.G.L., *A Study of the English Apothecary from 1660 to 1760*

(*Medical History*, Supplement no. 3, London: Wellcome Institute, 1983).

Burtt, E.A., *The Metaphysical Foundations of Modern Science* (London: Kegan Paul, Trench, 1925).

Butler, Marilyn, *Romantics, Rebels and Reactionaries: English Literature and its Background 1760–1830* (Oxford: Oxford University Press, 1981).

Butterfield, Herbert, *The Origins of Modern Science, 1300–1800* (London: Bell, 1949).

Butterfield, L.H. (ed.), *The Letters of Benjamin Rush*, 2 vols (Princeton, N.J.: Princeton University Press, 1951).

Bynum, W.F., 'Chronic Alcoholism in the First Half of the 19th Century', *Bulletin of the History of Medicine*, xlii (1968), 160–85.

Bynum, W.F., 'Health, Disease and Medical Care', in G.S. Rousseau and R. Porter (eds), *The Ferment of Knowledge* (Cambridge: Cambridge University Press, 1980), 211–54.

Bynum, W.F., 'Cullen and the Study of Fevers in Britain 1760–1820', in W.F. Bynum and V. Nutton (eds), *Theories of Fever from Antiquity to the Enlightenment* (*Medical History*, Supplement No. 1, London: Wellcome Institute for the History of Medicine, 1981), 135–48.

Bynum, W.F. and Porter, Roy (eds), *William Hunter and the Eighteenth-Century Medical World* (Cambridge: Cambridge University Press, 1985), 323–42.

Bynum, W.F. and Porter, Roy (eds) *Brunonianism in Britain and Europe* (*Medical History*, Supplement 8, London: Wellcome Institute, 1989).

Byrne, Muriel St Clare (ed.), *The Lisle Letters*, vol. 5 (Chicago and London: The University of Chicago Press, 1981).

Campbell, C., *The Romantic Ethic and the Spirit of Modern Consumerism* (Oxford: Basil Blackwell, 1987).

Campbell, R., *The London Tradesman* (London: David & Charles, 1969, 1st edn. 1747).

Cannadine, David, 'The Present and the Past in the English Industrial Revolution, 1880–1980', *Past and Present*, 103 (1984), 131–72.

Carpenter, K., *The History of Scurvy and Vitamin C* (Cambridge: Cambridge University Press, 1986).

Cartwright, F.F., *The English Pioneers of Anaesthesia (Beddoes, Davy and Hickman)*, (Bristol: J. Wright, 1952).

Cartwright, F.F., 'The Association of Thomas Beddoes, M.D. with James Watt, F.R.S.', *Notes and Records of the Royal Society of London*, xxii (1967), 131–43.

Castel, Françoise, Castel, Robert and Lovell, Anne, *The Psychiatric Society* (New York: Columbia University Press, 1981).

Castiglioni, A., *History of Medicine* (New York: Knopf, 1941).

Caton, Hiram, *The Politics of Progress. The Origins and Development of the Commercial Republic, 1600–1835* (Gainesville: University of Florida Press, 1988).

Cave, K. (ed.), *The Diary of Joseph Farington*, vols 7–16 (New Haven, Conn.: Yale University Press, 1982–84).

Chalke, H.D., 'Some Historical Aspects of Tuberculosis', *Public Health,* lxxiv (1959), 83–95.
Chamberlain, M., *Old Wives' Tales: Their History, Remedies and Spells* (London: Virago, 1981).
Chambers, E., *Cyclopaedia, Or an Universal Dictionary of Arts and Sciences,* 2nd edn., 2 vols (London: Midwinter, 1738).
Chambers, J.D., *Population, Economy, and Society in Pre-Industrial England* (Oxford: Oxford University Press, 1972).
Chancellor, V. (ed.), *Master and Artisan in Victorian England* (London: Evelyn, Adams & MacKay, 1969).
Chapman, R.W. (ed.), *The Letters of Samuel Johnson,* 3 vols (Oxford: Clarendon Press, 1984).
Cheyne, G., *The English Malady; or, A Treatise of Nervous Diseases* (London: G. Strahan, 1733).
Cheyne, G., *An Essay on Regimen* (London: C. Rivington, 1740).
Cheyne, G., *The Natural Method of Cureing* (London: G. Strahan, 1742).
Cheyne, G., *The Method of Cureing Diseases of the Body and the Disorders of the Mind* (London: G. Strahan, 1742).
Childs, F., 'Prescriptions for Manners in Eighteenth Century Courtesy Literature' (University of Oxford, D.Phil. thesis, 1984).
Clark, P., *The English Ale-House* (London: Longman, 1983).
Clarke, D., *The Ingenious Mr Edgeworth* (London: Oldbourne, 1965).
Clarkson, L., *Death, Disease and Famine in Pre-Industrial England* (Dublin: Gill & Macmillan, 1975).
Coffey, T.G., 'Beer Street: Gin Lane: Some Views of 18th Century Drinking', *Quarterly Journal for the Study of Alcoholism,* xxxiv (1966), 662–92.
Cohen, I. Bernard, *Revolution in Science* (Cambridge, Mass.: Belknap Press, 1985).
Cohen, P.C., *A Calculating People: The Spread of Numeracy in Early America* (Chicago: University of Chicago Press, 1982).
Coleman, W., 'Health and Hygiene: A Medical Doctrine for the Bourgeoisie', *Journal of the History of Medicine,* xxiv (1974), 399–421.
Coleman, W., 'The People's Health: Medical Themes in Eighteenth Century French Popular Medicine', *Bulletin of the History of Medicine,* li (1977), 55–74.
Coleman, W., *Death is a Social Disease. Public Health and Political Economy* (Madison, Wisc.: University of Wisconsin Press, 1982).
Colley, Linda, 'The Apotheosis of George III: Loyalty, Royalty and the English Nation', *Past and Present,* cii (1984), 94–129.
Colley, Linda, 'Whose Nation? Class and National Consciousness in England, 1750–1830', *Past and Present,* cxiii (1986), 96–117.
Cone, C.B., *The English Jacobins: Reformers in Late 18th Century England* (New York: Scribner, 1968).
Cooter, R., 'The Power of the Body: the Early Nineteenth Century', in B. Barnes and S. Shapin (eds), *Natural Order: Historical Studies of Scientific Culture* (London and Beverly Hills: Sage Publications, 1979), 73–92.
Cooter, Roger, 'Interpreting the Fringe: Brief Comments on a Broad

Topic', *Society for the Social History of Medicine Bulletin*, xxix (1981), 32–6.

Cooter, R. (ed.), *Studies in the History of Alternative Medicine* (London: Macmillan, 1988).

Copeland, Edward, 'Jane Austen and the Consumer Revolution', in David Grey, A. Walton Litz and Brian Southam (eds), *The Jane Austen Companion* (New York: Macmillan, 1986), 77–92.

Copeland, Edward, 'Fictions of Employment: Jane Austen and the Woman's Novel', *Studies in Philology*, lxxxv (1988), 114–24.

Copeland, Edward, 'Money Talks: Jane Austen and the *Lady's Magazine*', in J. David Grey (ed.), *Jane Austen's Beginnings: The Juvenilia and Lady Susan*, foreword by Margaret Drabble (Ann Arbor, Mich., and London: U.M.I. Research Press, 1989), 153–71.

Cottle, J., *Reminiscences of Samuel Taylor Coleridge and Robert Southey* (Highgate: Lime Tree Bower Press, 1970; 1st edn., London: Houlston & Stoneman, 1847).

Coulter, H.L., *Divided Legacy* (Washington, DC: Ehawken Book Co., 1977).

Craddock, P., *Young Edward Gibbon* (Baltimore: Johns Hopkins University Press, 1982).

Crawford, P., 'Printed Advertisements for Women Medical Practitioners in London, 1670–1710', *Society for the Social History of Medicine Bulletin*, xxxv (1984), 66–70.

Crook, N. and Guiton, D., *Shelley's Venomed Melody* (Cambridge: Cambridge University Press, 1986).

Cross, S.J., 'John Hunter, the Animal Economy, and Late Eighteenth Century Physiological Discourse', *Studies in the History of Biology*, v (1981), 1–110.

Cross, W., *The Life and Times of Laurence Sterne* (New York: Macmillan, 1930).

Csikszentmihalyi, Mihaly and Rochberg-Halton, Eugene, *The Meaning of Things: Domestic Symbols and the Self* (New York: Cambridge University Press, 1981).

Cummins, S.L., *Tuberculosis in History from the 17th Century to our Own Times* (London: Baillière, Tindall & Cox, 1949).

Cunningham, Andrew, 'William Harvey: The Discoverer of the Circulation of the Blood', in Roy Porter (ed.), *Man Masters Nature* (London: BBC Publications, 1987), 65–76.

Cunningham, Andrew, 'Thomas Sydenham: Epidemics, Experiment and the "Good Old Cause"', in Roger French and Andrew Wear (eds), *The Medical Revolution of the Seventeenth Century* (Cambridge: Cambridge University Press, 1989), 164–90.

Cunningham, Andrew, 'Medicine to Calm the Mind: Boerhaave's Medical System, and Why it was Adopted in Edinburgh', in Andrew Cunningham and Roger French (eds), *The Medical Enlightenment of the Eighteenth Century* (Cambridge: Cambridge University Press, 1990), 40–66.

Cunningham, Andrew and French, Roger (eds), *The Medical Enlightenment of the Eighteenth Century* (Cambridge: Cambridge University Press, 1990).

Cunningham, Andrew and Jardine, Nicholas (eds), *Romanticism and the Sciences* (Cambridge: Cambridge University Press, 1990).

Cunningham, H., 'The Language of Patriotism, 1750–1914', *History Workshop Journal*, xii (1981), 8–33.

Curry, Patrick (ed.), *Astrology, Science and Society: Historical Essays* (Woodbridge: Suffolk, 1987).

Curry, Patrick, *Prophecy and Power. Astrology in Early Modern England* (Cambridge: Polity Press, 1989).

Darlington, Anne Carol, 'The Royal Academy and its Anatomical Teachings; with an Examination of Art-Anatomy Practices During the Eighteenth and Early Nineteenth Centuries in Britain' (Ph.D. thesis, University of London, 1991).

Darwin, E., *Zoonomia; or, the Laws of Organic Life*, 2 vols (London: J. Johnson, 1794–6).

Darwin, E., *The Temple of Nature or the Origin of Society: A Poem with Philosophical Notes* (London: J. Johnson, 1803).

Davidoff, L. and Hall, C., *Family Fortunes. Men and Women of the English Middle Classes* (London: Hutchinson, 1987).

Deane, Seamus, *The French Revolution and Enlightenment in England 1789–1832* (Cambridge, Mass.: Harvard University Press, 1989).

Desmond, Adrian, *The Politics of Evolution. Morphology, Medicine and Reform in Radical London* (Chicago: University of Chicago Press, 1990).

Dewhurst, K., *Thomas Willis as a Physician* (Berkeley, Cal.: University of California Press, 1964).

Dewhurst, K., *Dr Thomas Sydenham 1624–1689* (Berkeley, Cal.: University of California Press, 1966).

Dijksterhuis, E.J., *The Mechanisation of the World Picture* (Oxford: Clarendon Press, 1961).

Dobson, M.J., 'Population, Disease and Mortality in Southeast England, 1600–1800' (University of Oxford, D.Phil. thesis, 1982).

Dobson, M.J., 'A Chronology of Epidemic Disease and Mortality in Southeast England, 1601–1800' (*Historical Research Series*, 19, 1987).

Dobson, M.J., *From Old England to New England: Changing Patterns of Mortality* (Oxford: School of Geography, University of Oxford, Research Paper 38, 1987).

Donzelot, Jacques, *The Policing of Families*, trans. by Robert Hurley (New York: Pantheon, 1979).

Doughty, O., 'The English Malady of the Eighteenth Century', *Review of English Studies*, ii (1929), 257–69.

Dubos, René and Dubos, Jean, *The White Plague. Tuberculosis, Man and Society* (London: Gollancz, 1953).

Duchesneau, François, 'Vitalism in Late Eighteenth-Century Physiology: the Cases of Bordeu, Blumenbach and John Hunter', in W.F. Bynum and Roy Porter (eds), *William Hunter and the Eighteenth-Century Medical World* (Cambridge: Cambridge University Press, 1985), 259–295.

Eagleton, Terry, *The Function of Criticism: From the Spectator to Post-Structuralism* (London: Verso, 1984).

Eagleton, Terry, *The Ideology of the Aesthetic* (Oxford: Basil Blackwell, 1990).

Earle, Peter, *The Making of the English Middle Class: Business, Society and Family Life in London, 1660–1730* (London: Methuen, 1989).

Elias, Norbert, *The Civilizing Process*, vol. 1: *The History of Manners* (New York: Pantheon, 1978); vol. 2: *Power and Civility* (New York: Pantheon, 1982); vol. 3: *The Court Society* (New York: Pantheon, 1984).

Ellis, Jack D., *The Physician-Legislators of France. Medicine and Politics in the Early Third Republic, 1870–1914* (Cambridge: Cambridge University Press, 1990).

Emch-Deriaz, A., 'Towards a Social Conception of Health in the Second Half of the Eighteenth Century: Tissot (1728–1797) and the New Preoccupation with Health and Well-Being' (Ann Arbor, Mich.: University Microfilms, 1984).

Ernst, W., *Mad Tales from the Raj. The European Insane in British India* (London: Routledge, 1990).

Eversley, D.E.C., 'The Home Market and Economic Growth in England 1750–1800', in E.L. Jones and C.E. Mingay (eds), *Land, Labour and Population in the Industrial Revolution* (London: Edward Arnold, 1967), 206–59.

Ewing, E., *Dress and Undress. A History of Women's Underwear* (London: Batsford, 1978).

Faber, Knud, *Nosography: A History of Clinical Medicine* (New York: Hoeber, 1930).

The Family Companion for Health (London: F. Fayram & Leake, 1729).

The Family Guide to Health (London: J. Fletcher, 1767).

Farr, A.D., 'Medical Developments and Religious Belief, with Special Reference to the Eighteenth and Nineteenth Centuries' (Ph.D. thesis, Open University, 1977).

Fielding, H., *A Voyage to Lisbon* (London: Dent, 1901).

Figlio, Karl M., 'Theories of Perception and the Physiology of the Mind in the Late Eighteenth Century', *History of Science*, xiii (1975), 177–212.

Figlio, K., 'Chlorosis and Chronic Disease in Nineteenth-Century Britain: The Social Constitution of Somatic Illness in a Capitalist Society', *Social History*, iii (1978), 167–97.

Figlio, Karl and Weindling, Paul, 'Was Social Medicine Revolutionary? Rudolf Virchow and the Revolutions of 1848', *Bulletin of the Society for the Social History of Medicine*, xxxiv (1984), 10–18.

Fildes, V., *Breasts, Bottles and Babies. A History of Infant Feeding* (Edinburgh: Edinburgh University Press, 1986).

Fildes, V., *Wetnursing* (Oxford: Basil Blackwell, 1988).

Fildes, V. (ed.), *Women as Mothers in Early Modern England* (London: Routledge, 1989).

Finer, S.E., *The Life and Times of Sir Edwin Chadwick* (London: Methuen, 1952).

Fischer-Homberger, E., 'Hypochondriasis of the Eighteenth Century – Neurosis of the Present Century', *Bulletin of the History of Medicine*, xlvi (1972), 391–401.

Fissell, M.E., 'The Physic of Charity: Health and Welfare in the West Country, 1690–1834' (Philadelphia, University of Pennsylvania Ph.D. thesis, 1988).

Fissell, Mary E., *The Physic of Charity: Health and Welfare in the West Country, 1690–1810* (Cambridge: Cambridge University Press, 1991).

Flick, L.F., *Development of our Knowledge of Tuberculosis* (Philadelphia: the author, 1925).

Flinn, M., 'Stabilization of Mortality in Pre-Industrial Western Europe', *Journal of European Economic History*, iii (1974), 285–318.

Flynn, Carol Houlihan, 'Running out of Matter. The Body Exercised in Eighteenth Century Fiction', in G.S. Rousseau (ed.), *Mind and Body in the Enlightenment* (Berkeley: University of California Press, 1990).

Forgan, S. *et al.* (eds), *Science and the Sons of Genius: Studies on Humphry Davy* (London: Science Reviews Ltd, 1980).

Forty, A., *Objects of Desire. Design and Society 1750–1980* (London: Thames & Hudson, 1986).

Foucault, M., *The Birth of the Clinic*, trans. A.M. Sheridan Smith (London: Tavistock, 1973).

Foucault, Michel, *Histoire de la sexualité*: vol. 1. *La volonté de savoir* (Paris: Gallimard, 1976); transl. *The History of Sexuality: Introduction* (London: Allen Lane, 1978).

Foucault, Michel, *Discipline and Punish: The Birth of the Prison* (Harmondsworth: Allen Lane, 1979).

Frängsmyr, Tore, Heilbron, J.L. and Rider, Robin E. (eds), *The Quantifying Spirit in the Eighteenth Century* (Berkeley: University of California Press, 1990).

Frank, J.P., *A System of Complete Medical Police*, trans. Erna Lesky (Baltimore: Johns Hopkins University Press, 1976).

Frank, Robert G., *Harvey and the Oxford Physiologists: Scientific Ideas and Social Interaction* (Berkeley: University of California Press, 1980).

French, R., *Robert Whytt, the Soul and Medicine* (London: Wellcome Institute for the History of Medicine, 1969).

French, Roger, 'Sickness and the Soul: Stahl, Hoffman and Sauvages on Pathology', in Andrew Cunningham and Roger French (eds), *The Medical Enlightenment of the Eighteenth Century* (Cambridge: Cambridge University Press, 1990), 88–110.

French, Roger and Wear, Andrew (eds), *The Medical Revolution of the Seventeenth Century* (Cambridge: Cambridge University Press, 1989).

Fruman, N., *Coleridge, the Damaged Archangel* (London: Allen & Unwin, 1971).

Furst, D., 'Sterne and Physick: Images of Health and Disease in *Tristram Shandy*' (Ph.D. dissertation, Columbia University, 1974).

Gabbay, J., 'Asthma Attacked? Tactics for the Reconstruction of a Disease Concept', in P. Wright and A. Treacher (eds), *The Problem of Medical Knowledge* (Edinburgh: Edinburgh University Press, 1982), 23–48.

Gallagher, Catherine, 'The Body Versus the Social Body in the Works of Thomas Malthus and Henry Mayhew', in C. Gallagher and T. Laqueur (eds), *The Making of the Modern Body: Sexuality and Society in the Nineteenth Century* (Berkeley: University of California Press, 1987), 83–106.

Garfinkle, N., 'Science and Religion in England, 1790–1800', *Journal of the History of Ideas*, xvi (1955), 376–88.

Garnett, D., (ed.), *The Novels of Thomas Love Peacock* (London: Rupert Hart-Davis, 1948).

Garrison, Fielding H., *An Introduction to the History of Medicine* (Philadelphia and London: Saunders, 1917).

Gascoigne, John, *Cambridge in the Age of the Enlightenment: Science, Religion and Politics from the Restoration to the French Revolution* (Cambridge: Cambridge University Press, 1989).

Gay, P., 'The Enlightenment as Medicine and as Cure', in W.H. Barber (ed.), *The Age of the Enlightenment. Studies Presented to Theodore Besterman* (Edinburgh: St Andrews University Publications, 1967), 375–86.

Gay, Peter, *The Enlightenment*, 2 vols (New York: Knopf, 1967–9).

Gay, Peter, *The Party of Humanity: Essays in the French Enlightenment* (New York: Norton, 1971).

Gelfand, Toby, *Professionalizing Modern Medicine. Paris Surgeons and Medical Science and Institutions in the Eighteenth Century* (Westport, Conn.: Greenwood Press, 1980).

George, D.M., *London Life in the Eighteenth Century* (Harmondsworth: Penguin, 1966).

Geyer-Kordesch, Johanna, 'The Cultural Habits of Illness: The Enlightened and the Pious in Eighteenth-Century Germany', in R. Porter (ed.), *Patients and Practitioners* (Cambridge: Cambridge University Press, 1985), 177–204.

Geyer-Kordesch, Johanna, 'Passions and the Ghost in the Machine: Or What Not to Ask about Science in Seventeenth- and Eighteenth-Century Germany', in Roger French and Andrew Wear (eds), *The Medical Revolution of the Seventeenth Century* (Cambridge: Cambridge University Press, 1989), 145–63.

Geyer-Kordesch, Johanna, 'Georg Ernst Stahl's Radical Pietist Medicine and its Influence in the German Enlightenment', in Andrew Cunningham and Roger French (eds), *The Medical Enlightenment of the Eighteenth Century* (Cambridge: Cambridge University Press, 1990), 67–88.

Gibbs, F.W. and Smeaton, W., 'Thomas Beddoes at Oxford', *Ambix*, ix (1961), 417–49.

Gigerenzer, Gerd, Swijtink, Zeno, Porter, Theodore, Daston, Lorraine, Beatty, John and Kruger, Lorenz, *The Empire of Chance* (Cambridge: Cambridge University Press, 1989).

Gillispie, C.C., *The Edge of Objectivity: An Essay in the History of Scientific Ideas* (Princeton, N.J.: Princeton University Press, 1960).

Gittings, C., *Death, Burial and the Individual in Early Modern England* (London: Croom Helm, 1984).

Glatt, M.M., 'The English Drink Problem: its Rise and Decline Through the Ages', *British Journal of Addiction*, iv (1958), 51–67.

Glyster, Gregory [pseud.], *A Dose for the Doctors; or the Aesculapian Labyrinth Explored* (London: Kearsley, 1789).

Goellnicht, D.C., *The Poet-Physician, Keats and Medical Science* (Pittsburgh, Pa.: University of Pittsburgh Press, 1984).

Golby, J.M. and Purdue, A.W., *The Civilization of the Crowd: Popular Culture in England, 1750–1900* (London: Batsford, 1984).

Golinski, Jan, *Science as Public Culture: Chemistry and Enlightenment in Britain, 1760–1820* (Cambridge: Cambridge University Press, 1991).

Goodfield-Toulmin, June, 'Some Aspects of English Physiology, 1780–1840', *Journal of the History of Biology*, ii (1969), 283–320.

Goodwin, Albert, *The Friends of Liberty: The English Democratic Movement in the Age of the French Revolution* (London: Hutchinson, 1979).

Gosse, Sir Edmund (ed.), *The Complete Works of Thomas Lovell Beddoes* (London: The Canfrolico Press, 1928).

Gottlieb, L.S., 'Thomas Beddoes M.D. and the Pneumatic Institution at Clifton 1798–1801', *Annals of Internal Medicine*, lxiii (1965), 530–3.

Goubert, J.-P., *La Médicalisation de la Société Française 1770–1830* (Waterloo, Ontario: Historical Reflections Press, 1982).

Goubert, J.-P., 'Twenty Years On: Problems of Historical Methodology in the History of Health', in R. Porter and A. Wear (eds), *Problems and Methods in the History of Medicine* (London: Croom Helm, 1987), 40–56.

Graham, H.G., *The Social Life of Scotland in the Eighteenth Century* (London: Black, 1969).

Greenacre, F., *The Bristol School of Artists: Francis Danby and Painting in Bristol 1810–1840* (Catalogue: Bristol: The Gallery, 1973).

Greenleaf, W.J., *Order, Empiricism and Politics. Two Traditions of English Political Thought, 1500–1700* (London: Oxford University Press, 1964).

Gregory, J., *Observations on the Duties of a Physician* (London: Strahan & Cadell, 1770).

Griggs, E.L. (ed.), *Collected Letters of Samuel Taylor Coleridge*, 6 vols (Oxford: Clarendon Press, 1956–1968).

Grosvenor Myer, Valerie, 'Tristram and the Animal Spirits', in *idem* (ed.), *Laurence Sterne: Riddles and Mysteries* (London: Vision Press, 1984), 99–112.

Grundy, Isobel, *Samuel Johnson and the Scale of Greatness* (Leicester: Leicester University Press, 1986).

Guerrini, Anita, 'James Keill, George Cheyne, and Newtonian Physiology, 1690–1740', *Journal of the History of Biology*, xviii (1985), 247–66.

Guerrini, Anita, 'Isaac Newton, George Cheyne and the *Principia Medicinae*', in Roger French and Andrew Wear (eds), *The Medical Revolution of the Seventeenth Century* (Cambridge: Cambridge University Press, 1989), 222–45.

Guthrie, Douglas, *A History of Medicine* (London: Nelson, 1960).

Guthrie, L., 'The Lady Sedley's Receipt Book, 1686, and other

Seventeenth-century Receipt Books', *Proceedings of the Royal Society of Medicine*, vi (1913), 150–70.

Habermas, Jürgen, *Knowledge and Human Interests*, trans. by J. Shapiro (Boston, Mass.: Beacon Press, 1971).

Hacking, Ian, *The Taming of Chance* (Cambridge: Cambridge University Press, 1990).

Haigh, Elizabeth, 'Vitalism, the Soul and Sensibility: the Physiology of Théophile Bordeu', *Journal of the History of Medicine*, xxxi (1976), 30–41.

Haigh, Elizabeth, 'The Vital Principle of Paul Joseph Barthez: the Clash Between Monism and Dualism', *Medical History*, xxi (1977), 1–14.

Haines, B., 'The Inter-relations between Social, Biological and Medical Thought, 1750–1850: Saint-Simon and Comte', *The British Journal for the History of Science*, xi (1978), 19–35.

Halévy, Elie, *The Growth of Philosophical Radicalism* (London: Faber & Faber, 1924).

Haley, B., *The Healthy Body and Victorian Culture* (Cambridge, Mass.: Harvard University Press, 1978).

Hall, A.R., *The Scientific Revolution, 1500–1800* (London: Longman, 1954).

Hare, E.H., 'Masturbatory Insanity: the History of an Idea', *Journal of Mental Science*, cviii (1962), 1–25.

Harley, David, 'A Sword in a Madman's Hand: Professional Opposition to Popular Consumption in the Waters Literature of Southern England and the Midlands, 1570–1870', in Roy Porter (ed.), *The Medical History of Waters and Spas* (*Medical History*, Supplement 10, London: Wellcome Institute, 1990), 48–55.

Harrison, E., *Remarks on the Ineffective State of the Practice of Physic in Great Britain* (London: R. Bickerstaff, 1806).

Harrison, Mark, *Crowds and History: Mass Phenomena in English Towns, 1790–1835* (Cambridge, New York: Cambridge University Press, 1988).

Harvey, Gideon, *Morbus Anglicus, or a Theoretick and Practical Discourse of Consumptions and Hypochondriack Melancholy* (London: Thackeray, 1672).

Harvey, Gideon, *The Disease of London, or a New Discovery of the Scorvey* (London: Thackeray, 1675).

Haygarth, J., *Of the Imagination, as a Cause and as a Cure of Disorders of the Body* (Bath: Cadell & Davies, 1800).

Heberden, Ernest, *The Life of William Heberden* (London: Royal Society of Medicine, 1989).

Heberden, W., *Medical Commentaries* (London: T. Payne, 1802).

Hembry, Phyllis, *The English Spa, 1560–1815. A Social History* (London: Athlone, 1990).

Hill, Brian, 'Father and Son: Thomas Beddoes and Thomas Lovell Beddoes', *Practitioner*, clxxxiv (1960), 513–18.

Hill, J., *Hypochondriasis* (London: for the author, 1756).

Hirsch, J., 'Enlightened Eighteenth Century Views of the Alcohol Problem', *Journal of the History of Medicine*, iv (1949), 230–6.

Hirschman, A.O., *The Passions and the Interests. Political Arguments for Capitalism before its Triumph* (Princeton, N.J.: Princeton University Press, 1977).

Hodgson, J.E., 'James Sadler of Oxford, Aeronaut, Chemist, Engineer and Inventor', *Newcomen Society Transactions*, viii (1927–8), 66–82.

Holloway, S.W.F., 'Medical Education in England, 1830–1858: A Sociological Analysis', *History*, il (1964), 299–32.

Holmes, G., *Augustan England: Profession, State and Society, 1680–1730* (London: George Allen & Unwin, 1982).

Holmes, Richard, *Coleridge: Early Visions* (London: Hodder & Stoughton, 1989; Harmondsworth: Penguin, 1990).

Hoppit, Julian, 'The Use and Abuse of Credit in Eighteenth-Century England', in N. McKendrick and R.B. Outhwaite (eds), *Business Life and Public Policy* (Cambridge: Cambridge University Press, 1986).

Howe, G.M., *Man, Environment and Disease in Britain. A Medical Geography Through the Ages* (New York: Barnes & Noble Books, 1972).

Hunt, Thomas (ed.), *The Medical Society of London 1773–1973* (London: Heinemann, 1972).

Illich, I., *Limits to Medicine. The Expropriation of Health* (Harmondsworth: Penguin, 1977).

Inglis, B., *The Diseases of Civilisation* (London: Hodder & Stoughton, 1981).

Jacob, Margaret C., *The Radical Enlightenment: Pantheists, Freemasons and Republicans* (London: George Allen & Unwin, 1981).

Jacyna, L.S., 'Images of John Hunter in the Nineteenth Century', *History of Science*, xxii (1983), 85–108.

Jarcho, Saul (trans. and ed.), *The Clinical Consultations of Giambattista Morgagni* (Boston: Countway Library of Medicine, 1984).

Jennings, H., *Pandaemonium. The Coming of the Machine as Seen by Contemporary Observers, 1660–1886* (New York: Free Press, 1985).

Jewson, N., 'Medical Knowledge and the Patronage System in Eighteenth Century England', *Sociology*, viii (1974), 369–85.

Jewson, N., 'The Disappearance of the Sick Man from Medical Cosmology, 1770–1870', *Sociology*, x (1976), 225–44.

Jones, E.L., 'The Fashion Manipulators: Consumer Tastes and British Industries, 1660–1800', in L.P. Cain and P.J. Uselding (eds), *Business Enterprise and Economic Change* (Kent State, Ohio: Kent State University Press, 1973), 198–226.

Jordanova, L.J., 'The Popularisation of Medicine: Tissot on Onanism', *Textual Practice*, i (1987), 68–80.

Keers, R.Y., 'Richard Morton (1637–98) and his "Physiologia"', *Thorax*, xxxvii (1982), 26–31.

Kelly, Gary, *The English Jacobin Novel, 1780–1805* (Oxford, New York: Clarendon Press, 1976).

Kilpatrick, R., '"Living in the Light": Dispensaries, Philanthropy and Medical Reform in Late-Eighteenth Century London', in Andrew Cunningham and Roger French (eds), *The Medical Enlightenment of the Eighteenth Century* (Cambridge: Cambridge University Press, 1990), 254–80.

King, Lester S., *The Medical World of the Eighteenth Century* (Chicago: University of Chicago Press, 1958).

King, Lester S., *The Road to Medical Enlightenment, 1650–1695* (London: Macdonald, 1970).

King, Lester S., *The Philosophy of Medicine: The Early Eighteenth Century* (Cambridge, Mass.: Harvard University Press, 1978).

King, L.S., *Medical Thinking. A Historical Preface* (Princeton, N.J.: Princeton University Press, 1982).

King-Hele, D., *Erasmus Darwin* (London: Macmillan, 1963).

King-Hele, D., *Doctor of Revolution: The Life and Genius of Erasmus Darwin* (London: Faber, 1977).

King-Hele, D., *The Letters of Erasmus Darwin* (Cambridge: Cambridge University Press, 1981).

Kleinman, A., *Patients and Healers in the Context of Culture: An Exploration of the Borderline between Anthropology, Medicine, and Psychiatry* (Berkeley: University of California Press, 1980).

Kleinman, A., *Social Origins of Distress and Disease: Depression, Neurasthenia, and Pain in Modern China* (New Haven, Conn.: Yale University Press, 1986).

Kleinman, A., *The Illness Narratives: Suffering, Healing and the Human Condition* (New York: Basic Books, 1988).

Kleinman, A. and Good, B. (eds), *Culture and Depression: Studies in the Anthropology and Cultural Psychiatry of Affect and Disorder* (Berkeley: University of California Press, 1985).

Klingender, F.D., *Art and the Industrial Revolution*, ed. A. Elton (St Albans: Paladin, 1968).

Knapp, L.M., *Tobias Smollett: Doctor of Men and Manners* (Princeton, N.J.: Princeton University Press, 1949).

Knight, D.M., 'Science and Professionalism in England, 1770–1830', *Proceedings of the XIV International Congress of the History of Science*, i (1974), 53–67.

Knox, R.A., *Enthusiasm* (London: Oxford University Press, 1950).

Kondratas, R.A., 'Joseph Frank (1771–1842) and the Development of Clinical Medicine' (Ph.D. thesis, Harvard University, 1977).

Lain Entralgo, P., *Doctor and Patient*, trans. by Frances Partridge (London: Weidenfeld & Nicolson, 1969).

Lane, J., 'The Provincial Practitioner and his Services to the Poor 1750-1800', *Society for the Social History of Medicine Bulletin*, xxviii (1981), 10–14.

Lane, J., 'The Medical Practitioners of Provincial England in 1783', *Medical History*, xxviii (1984), 353–71.

Lane, J., 'The Role of Apprenticeship in Eighteenth-Century Medical Education in England', in W.F. Bynum and R. Porter (eds), *William Hunter and the Eighteenth-Century Medical World* (Cambridge: Cambridge University Press, 1985), 57–104.

Lane, J., '"The Doctor Scolds Me": The Diaries and Correspondence of Patients in Eighteenth-Century England', in Roy Porter (ed.), *Patients and Practitioners* (Cambridge: Cambridge University Press, 1985), 207–14.

Lane, J., 'A Provincial Surgeon and his Obstetric Practice: Thomas W. Jones of Henley-in-Arden, 1764–1846', *Medical History*, xxxi (1987), 333–48.

Langford, Paul, *A Polite and Commercial People: England, 1727–1783* (Oxford: Oxford University Press, 1989).

Latour, Bruno, *The Pasteurization of France* (Cambridge, Mass.: Harvard University Press, 1988).

Lawrence, C.J., 'William Buchan: Medicine Laid Open', *Medical History*, xix (1975), 20–35.

Lawrence, C.J., 'The Nervous System and Society in the Scottish Enlightenment', in B. Barnes and S. Shapin (eds), *Natural Order: Historical Studies of Scientific Culture* (London: Sage Publications, 1979), 19–40.

Lawrence, C.J., 'Medicine as Culture: Edinburgh and the Scottish Enlightenment' (University of London, Ph.D. thesis, 1984).

Lawrence, C.J., 'Cullen, Brown and the Poverty of Essentialism', in W.F. Bynum and Roy Porter (eds.), *Brunonianism in Britain and Europe* (*Medical History*, Supplement 8, London: Wellcome Institute, 1988), 1–21.

Lawrence, S., 'Science and Medicine at the London Hospitals. The Development of Teaching and Research 1750–1815' (Ph.D. thesis, University of Toronto, 1985).

Lawrence, S., 'Entrepreneurs and Private Enterprise: The Development of Medical Lecturing in London, 1775–1820', *Bulletin of the History of Medicine*, lxii (1988), 171–92.

Lawrence, S., 'Educating the Senses. Students, Teachers and Medical Rhetoric in Eighteenth-Century London', in W.F. Bynum and R. Porter (eds), *Medicine and the Five Senses* (Cambridge: Cambridge University Press, forthcoming).

LeFanu, W. (ed.), *Betsy Sheridan's Journal* (London: Eyre & Spottiswoode, 1960).

LeFanu, W.R., 'The Lost Half Century in English Medicine, 1700–1750', *Bulletin of the History of Medicine*, xlvi (1972), 319–48.

Lefebure, M., *Samuel Taylor Coleridge: A Bondage of Opium* (London: Victor Gollancz, 1974).

Levere, T.H., 'Dr Thomas Beddoes and the Establishment of his Pneumatic Institution: a Tale of Three Presidents', *Notes and Records of the Royal Society of London*, xxxii (1977), 41–9.

Levere, T.H., *Poetry Realised in Nature: Samuel Taylor Coleridge and Early Nineteenth-Century Science* (Cambridge: Cambridge University Press, 1981).

Levere, T.H., 'Dr Thomas Beddoes at Oxford: Radical Politics in 1788–93, and the Fate of the Regius Chair in Chemistry', *Ambix*, xxviii (July 1981), 61–9.

Levere, T.H., 'Thomas Beddoes, The Interaction of Pneumatic and Preventative Medicine with Chemistry', *ISR: Interdisciplinary Science Reviews*, vii (1982), 137–47.

Levere, T.H., 'Dr Thomas Beddoes (1760–1808): Science and Medicine in Politics and Society', *The British Journal for the History of Science*, xvii (1984), 187–204.

Levine, David, *Family Formation in an Age of Nascent Capitalism* (New York: Academic Press, 1977).

Levine, David, *Reproducing Families: The Political Economy of English Population History* (Cambridge: Cambridge University Press, 1984).

Levine, H.G., 'The Discovery of Addiction: Changing Conceptions of Habitual Drunkenness in America', *Journal of the Study of Alcoholism*, xxxix (1978), 143–74.

Lewis, Jane and Brookes, Barbara, 'The Peckham Health Centre, PEP, and the Concept of General Practice during the 1930s and 1940s', *Medical History*, xxvii (1983), 151–61.

Lewis, Judith S., *In the Family Way: Childbearing in the British Aristocracy 1760–1860* (New Brunswick, N.J.: Rutgers University Press, 1986).

Lindeboom, G.A., *Hermann Boerhaave: The Man and his Work* (London: Methuen, 1968).

Lingo, Alison, 'Empirics and Charlatans in Early Modern France: The Genesis of the Classification of the "Other" Medical Practice', *Journal of Social History*, xix (1986), 583–604.

Litchfield, R.B., *Tom Wedgwood, the First Photographer: an Account of his Life, his Discovery and his Friendship with Samuel Taylor Coleridge, including the Letters of Coleridge to the Wedgwoods and an Examination of Accounts of Alleged Earlier Photographic Discoveries* (London: Duckworth, 1903).

Little, D. and Kahrl, G. (eds), *The Letters of David Garrick*, 3 vols (London: Oxford University Press, 1963).

Lobo, Francis M., 'John Haygarth, Smallpox and Religious Dissent in Eighteenth-Century England', in Andrew Cunningham and Roger French (eds), *The Medical Enlightenment of the Eighteenth Century* (Cambridge: Cambridge University Press, 1990), 217–53.

Long, E.R., 'Tuberculosis in Modern Society', *Bulletin of the History of Medicine*, xxvii (1953), 301–19.

Loudon, I.S.L., 'Chlorosis, Anaemia and Anorexia Nervosa', *British Medical Journal*, ii (1980), 1669–87.

Loudon, I.S.L., 'The Origins and Growth of the Dispensary Movement in England', *Bulletin of the History of Medicine*, lv (1981), 322–42.

Loudon, I.S.L., 'The Origins of the General Practitioner' (The James Mackenzie Lecture of the Royal College of General Practitioners for 1982), *Journal of the Royal College of General Practitiioners*, xxxiii (1983), 13–18.

Loudon, I.S.L., 'The Nature of Provincial Medical Practice in Eighteenth-Century England', *Medical History*, xxix (1985), 1–32.

Loudon, Irvine, '"The Vile Race of Quacks With Which This Country is Infested"', in W.F. Bynum and Roy Porter (eds), *Medical Fringe and Medical Orthodoxy, 1750–1850* (London: Croom Helm, 1986), 106–28.

Loudon, I.S.L., *Medical Care and the General Practitioner 1750–1850* (Oxford: Clarendon Press, 1986).

Lustig, J.S. and Pottle, F.A. (eds), *Boswell: The Applause of the Jury, 1782–85* (London: Heinemann, 1982).

McCalman, Iain, *Radical Underworld: Prophets, Revolutionaries and Porno-*

graphers in London, 1795–1840 (Cambridge: Cambridge University Press, 1988).

McCulloch, L., 'John Gregory's Medical Ethics and Humean Sympathy: A Closer Look', in Robert Baker, Dorothy Porter and Roy Porter (eds), *The Codification of Medical Morality in the Eighteenth and Nineteenth Centuries*, vol. i (Dordrecht: Kluwer, 1991).

MacDonald, R.H., 'The Frightful Consequences of Onanism', *Journal of the History of Ideas*, xxviii (1967), 423–41.

Macdonald, V.M. (ed.), *The Letters of Eliza Pierce (Eliza Taylor) 1751–1775* (London: F. Etchells & H. Macdonald, 1927).

Macfarlane, Alan, *The Culture of Capitalism* (Oxford: Basil Blackwell, 1987).

Mack, M., *Jeremy Bentham: An Odyssey of Ideas, 1748–1792* (London: Heinemann, 1962).

McKee, Francis, 'The Earlier Works of Bernard Mandeville, 1685–1715' (Ph.D. thesis, University of Glasgow, 1991).

McKendrick, N., 'Home Demand and Economic Growth: A New View of the Role of Women and Children in the Industrial Revolution', in N. McKendrick (ed.), *Historical Perspectives: Studies in English Thought and Society* (London: Europa, 1974), 152–210.

McKendrick, N., Brewer, John and Plumb, J.H., *The Birth of a Consumer Society: The Commercialization of Eighteenth-Century England* (London: Europa, 1982).

McKeown, Thomas, *The Role of Medicine: Dream, Mirage or Nemesis?* (London: Nuffield Provincial Hospitals Trust, 1976).

MacLaren, A., *Reproductive Rituals: The Perception of Fertility in England from the 16th Century to the 19th Century* (London and New York: Methuen, 1984).

McManners, J., *Death and the Enlightenment: Changing Attitudes Towards Death Among Christians and Unbelievers in Eighteenth-Century France* (Oxford: Clarendon Press, 1981).

McNeil, M., *Under the Banner of Science* (Manchester: Manchester University Press, 1987).

Macpherson, C.B., *The Political Theory of Possessive Individualism: Hobbes to Locke* (London: Oxford University Press, 1962).

Malcolmson, R., *Popular Recreations in English Society 1700–1850* (Cambridge: Cambridge University Press, 1973).

Mandeville, B., *A Treatise of the Hypochondriack and Hysterick Diseases* (2nd edn., London: Tonson, 1730; reprinted by George Olms Verlag, Hildesheim, 1981).

Manuel, F., *The Eighteenth Century Confronts the Gods* (Cambridge, Mass.: Harvard University Press, 1959).

Manuel, Frank, *The Prophets of Paris* (Cambridge, Mass.: Harvard University Press, 1962).

Marcovich, A., 'Concerning the Continuity between the Image of Society and the Image of the Human Body: An Examination of the Work of the English Physician J.C. Lettsom (1746–1815)', in P. Wright and A. Treacher (eds), *The Problem of Medical Knowledge* (Edinburgh: Edinburgh University Press, 1982), 69–87.

Marten, Benjamin, *A New Theory of Consumptions, More Especially of a Phthisis, or Consumption of the Lungs* (London: Knaplock, 1720).

Martin, Julian, 'Explaining John Freind's *History of Physick*', *Studies in History and Philosophy of Science*, xix (1988), 399–418.

Martin, Julian, 'Sauvages's Nosology: Medical Enlightenment in Montpellier', in Andrew Cunningham and Roger French (eds), *The Medical Enlightenment of the Eighteenth Century* (Cambridge: Cambridge University Press, 1990), 111–37.

Mason, Stephen, *A History of the Sciences* (London: Routledge & Kegan Paul, 1953).

Meachen, G.N., *A Short History of Tuberculosis* (London: Bale, 1936).

Mennell, S., *All Manners of Food: Eating and Taste in England and France from the Middle Ages to the Present* (Oxford and New York: Basil Blackwell, 1985).

Milkomane, G.A.M., *The Conquest of Tuberculosis* (London: Macdonald, 1946).

Miller, A.H., 'The Pneumatic Institution of Thomas Beddoes at Clifton', *Annals of Medical History*, n.s., iii (1931), 253–60.

Miller, D., *Material Culture and Mass Consumption* (Oxford: Basil Blackwell, 1987).

Miller, G., *The Adoption of Inoculation for Smallpox in England and France* (London: Oxford University Press, 1957).

Miller, G., 'Airs, Waters and Places in History', *Journal of the History of Medicine*, xvii (1962), 129–38.

Miller, G. (ed.), *Letters of Edward Jenner* (Baltimore: Johns Hopkins University Press, 1983).

Mitchell, B. and Penrose, H. (eds), *Letters from Bath 1766–1767 by the Rev. John Penrose* (London: Alan Sutton, 1983).

Money, John, *Experience and Identity: Birmingham and the West Midlands 1760–1800* (Manchester: Manchester University Press, 1977).

Moravia, S., 'From *Homme Machine* to *Homme Sensible*: Changing Eighteenth-Century Models of Man's Image', *Journal of the History of Ideas*, xxxix (1978), 45–60.

Moravia, S., 'The Enlightenment and the Sciences of Man', *History of Science*, xviii (1980), 247–58.

Morris, A.D., *James Parkinson, His Life and Times* (Boston: Birkhauser, 1989).

Morton, Richard, *Phthisiologia, or a Treatise of Consumptions, Wherein The Difference, Nature, Causes, Signs and Cure of all Sorts of Consumptions are Explained* (London: Smith & Walford, 1694).

Muchembled, R., *Popular Culture and Elite Culture in France, 1400–1750* (Baton Rouge: Louisiana State University Press, 1985).

Murphy, Terence, 'Medical Culture under the Old Regime', *Historical Reflections/Réflexions Historiques*, xvi (1989), 307–50.

Musson, A.E. and Robinson, E., *Science and Technology in the Industrial Revolution* (Manchester: Manchester University Press, 1969).

Neuburg, V.E., *Popular Literature: A History and Guide from the Beginning of Printing to the Year 1897* (Harmondsworth: Penguin, 1977).

Neve, M.R., 'The Young Humphry Davy: or John Tonkin's Lament', in S. Forgan *et al.* (eds), *Science and the Sons of Genius: Studies on*

Humphry Davy (London: Science Reviews Ltd, 1980), 1–33.
Neve, M.R., 'Natural Philosophy, Medicine and the Culture of Science in Provincial England: the Cases of Bristol, 1790–1850, and Bath' (University of London, Ph.D. thesis, 1984).
Newman, Charles, *The Evolution of Medical Education in the Nineteenth Century* (London: Oxford University Press, 1957).
Newman, Gerald, *The Rise of English Nationalism: A Cultural History, 1740–1830* (New York: St Martin's Press; London: Weidenfeld & Nicolson, 1987).
Niebyl, P., 'Old Age, Fever, and the Lamp Metaphor', *Journal for the History of Medicine*, xxvi (1971), 351–68.
Niebyl, P., 'The Non-Naturals', *Bulletin of the History of Medicine*, vl (1971), 486–92.
Nutton, Vivian (ed.), *Medicine at the Courts of Europe, 1500–1837* (London: Routledge, 1989).
Onania; or, the Heinous Sin of Self-Pollution, and All Its Frightful Consequences, 15th edn. (London: J. Isted, 1730).
O'Neill, J., *Five Bodies. The Human Shape of Modern Society* (Ithaca, New York: Cornell University Press, 1985).
Outram, Dorinda, 'Science and Political Ideology, 1790–1848', in R.C. Olby, G.N. Cantor, J.R.R. Christie and M.J.S. Hodge (eds), *Companion to the History of Modern Science* (London: Routledge, 1990), 1008–23.
Pagel, W., 'Humoral Pathology: A Lingering Anachronism in the History of Tuberculosis', *Bulletin of the History of Medicine*, xxix (1955), 299–308.
Park, K. and Daston, L., 'Unnatural Conceptions: The Study of Monsters in Sixteenth-Century France and England', *Past and Present*, xcii (1981), 20–54.
[Parkinson, James], *A Sketch by Old Hubert* (London: Burks, 1795).
Parkinson, James, *Medical Admonitions to Families Respecting the Preservation of Health, and the Treatment of the Sick, also a Table of Symptoms Serving to Point out the Degree of Danger, and to Distinguish One Disease from Another* (4th edn., London: C. Whittingham for H.D. Symonds, 1801).
Parkinson, James, *The Way to Health, Extracted from the Villager's Friend and Physician* (London: C. Whittingham for H.D. Symmonds, 1802).
Parkinson, James, *The Villager's Friend and Physician, or a Familiar Address on the Preservation of Health and the Removal of Disease on its First Appearance, Supposed to be Delivered by a Village Apothecary, with Cursory Observations on the Treatment of Children, on Sobriety, Industry, etc, Intended for the Promotion of Domestic Happiness*, 2nd edn. (London: C. Whittingham, 1804).
Parry, N. and Parry, J., *The Rise of the Medical Profession. A Study of Collective Mobility* (London: Croom Helm, 1978).
Parsons, T., *The Social System* (London: Routledge & Kegan Paul, 1951).
Passmore, J.A., *The Perfectibility of Man* (London: Duckworth, 1970).
Paul, Charles, *Science and Immortality: The Eloges of the Paris Academy of Sciences (1699–1799)* (Berkeley: University of California Press, 1980).

Payne, H.C., *The Philosophes and the People* (New Haven, Conn.: Yale University Press, 1976).

Pearse, Innes and Crocker, Lucy H., *The Peckham Experiment* (Edinburgh: The Scottish Academic Press, 1985).

Percival, T., *Medical Ethics; or, a Code of Institutes and Precepts Adapted to the Professional Conduct of Physicians and Surgeons* (Manchester: J. Johnson & R. Bickerstaff, 1803).

Perkin, H.J., *The Origins of Modern English Society 1780–1880* (London: Routledge, 1969).

Peter, J.-P and Revel, J., 'Le Corps: L'Homme malade et son Histoire', in J. Le Goff and P. Nora (eds), *Faire de l'Histoire,* vol. 3 (Paris: Gallimard, 1974), 169–90.

Peterson, M.J., *The Medical Profession in Mid-Victorian London* (Berkeley: University of California Press, 1978).

Pickering, Samuel F., *John Locke and Children's Books in Eighteenth Century England* (Knoxville: University of Tennessee Press, 1981).

Pickstone, J.V., 'Bureaucracy, Liberalism and the Body in Post-Revolutionary France: Bichat's Physiology and the Paris School of Medicine', *History of Science,* xix (1981), 115–42.

Pimlott, J.A.R., *The Englishman's Holiday. A Social History* (London: Faber, 1947).

Plumb, J.H., 'The New World of Children in Eighteenth-Century England', *Past and Present,* lxvii (1975), 64–95.

Pocock, J.G.A., *Virtue, Commerce and History* (Cambridge: Cambridge University Press, 1985).

Pollock, Linda, *Forgotten Children: Parent-Child Relations from 1500 to 1900* (Cambridge: Cambridge University Press, 1983).

Pollock, Linda, *A Lasting Relationship: Parents and Children over Three Centuries* (London: Fourth Estate, 1987).

Porter, Dorothy and Porter, Roy, *Patient's Progress: Doctors and Doctoring in Eighteenth Century England* (Cambridge: Polity Press, 1989).

Porter, Ian, 'Thomas Trotter, M.D., Naval Physician', *Medical History,* vii (1963), 155–64.

Porter, Roy, *The Making of Geology: Earth Science in Britain, 1660–1815* (Cambridge: Cambridge University Press, 1977).

Porter, Roy, 'Science, Provincial Culture and Public Opinion in Enlightenment England', *British Journal for Eighteenth Century Studies,* iii (1980), 20–46.

Porter, Roy, 'The Enlightenment in England', in Roy Porter and Mikuláš Teich (eds), *The Enlightenment in National Context* (Cambridge: Cambridge University Press, 1981), 1–18.

Porter, Roy, 'Was There a Medical Enlightenment in Eighteenth Century England?', *British Journal for Eighteenth Century Studies,* v (1982), 46–63.

Porter, Roy, 'The Rage of Party: A Glorious Revolution in English Psychiatry?', *Medical History,* xxviii (1983), 35–50.

Porter, Roy, 'Against the Spleen', in V. Grosvenor Myer (ed.), *Laurence Sterne: Riddles and Mysteries* (London and New York: Vision Press, 1984), 84–99.

Porter, Roy, 'The Patient's View: Doing Medical History from Below', *Theory and Society*, xiv (1985), 175–98.

Porter, Roy (ed.), *Patients and Practitioners. Lay Perceptions of Medicine in Pre-Industrial Society* (Cambridge: Cambridge University Press, 1985).

Porter, Roy, 'William Hunter: a Surgeon and a Gentleman', in W.F. Bynum and Roy Porter (eds), *William Hunter and the Eighteenth-Century Medical World* (Cambridge: Cambridge University Press, 1985), 7–34.

Porter, Roy, 'Lay Medical Knowledge in the Eighteenth Century: the Evidence of the *Gentleman's Magazine*', *Medical History*, xxix (1985), 138–68.

Porter, Roy, 'The Drinking Man's Disease: The "Pre-History" of Alcoholism in Georgian Britain', *British Journal of Addiction*, lxxx (1985), 385–96.

Porter, Roy, '"Under the Influence": Mesmerism in England', *History Today* (Sept., 1985), 22–9.

Porter, Roy, 'Laymen, Doctors and Medical Knowledge in the Eighteenth Century: The Evidence of the *Gentleman's Magazine*', in R. Porter (ed.), *Patients and Practitioners* (Cambridge: Cambridge University Press, 1985), 283–314.

Porter, Roy, 'Medical Education in England Before the Teaching Hospital: Some Recent Revisions', in J. Wilkes (ed.), *The Professional Teacher* (London: History of Education Society, 1986), 29–44.

Porter, Roy, 'Love, Sex and Madness in Eighteenth-Century England', *Social Research*, liii (1986), 212–42.

Porter, Roy, 'Medicine and the Decline of Magic', *Strawberry Fayre* (Autumn 1986), 88–94.

Porter, Roy, 'Medicine and Religion in Eighteenth-Century England: A Case of Conflict?', *Ideas and Production: Issue Seven – History of Science* (Cam- bridge: Cambridgeshire College of Arts and Technology, 1987), 4–17.

Porter, Roy, 'Monsters and Madmen in Eighteenth-Century France', in D. Fletcher (ed.), *The Monstrous* (Durham: Durham French Colloquies, Number 1, 1987), 83–103.

Porter, Roy, *Mind Forg'd Manacles. A History of Madness from the Restoration to the Regency* (London: Athlone, 1987).

Porter, Roy, *Health for Sale. Quackery in England 1650–1850* (Manchester: Manchester University Press, 1989).

Porter, Roy, 'The Gift Relation: Philanthropy and Provincial Hospitals in Eighteenth-Century England', in L. Granshaw and R. Porter (eds), *The Hospital in History* (London: Routledge, 1989), 149–78.

Porter, Roy, '"The Whole Secret of Health": Mind, Body and Medicine in *Tristram Shandy*', in John Christie and Sally Shuttleworth (eds), *Nature Transfigured* (Manchester: Manchester University Press, 1989), 61–84.

Porter, Roy, 'Introduction', to Thomas Trotter, *An Essay on Drunkenness* (London: Routledge Reprint, 1989; 1st edn., 1804).

Porter, Roy, 'Erasmus Darwin: Doctor of Evolution?', in James R.

Moore (ed.), *History, Humanity and Evolution* (Cambridge: Cambridge University Press, 1989), 39–69.

Porter, Roy, 'The Early Royal Society and the Spread of Medical Knowledge', in Roger French and Andrew Wear (eds), *The Medical Revolution of the Seventeenth Century* (Cambridge: Cambridge University Press, 1989), 272–93.

Porter, Roy, 'Introduction' to G. Cheyne, *The English Malady* (London: Routledge Reprint, 1990; 1st edn., 1734).

Porter, Roy, 'Barely Touching', in G.S. Rousseau (ed.), *The Languages of Psyche. Mind and Body in Enlightenment Thought* (Berkeley: University of California Press, 1990), 45–80.

Porter, Roy (ed.), *The Medical History of Waters and Spas* (*Medical History*, Supplement 10, London: Wellcome Institute, 1990).

Porter, Roy, 'Female Quacks in the Consumer Society', *History of Nursing Journal*, iii (1990), 1–25.

Porter, Roy, *The Enlightenment* (London: Macmillan, 1990).

Porter, Roy, 'Civilization and Disease: Medical Ideology in the Enlightenment', in J. Black and J. Gregory (eds), *Culture, Politics and Society in Britain 1660–1800* (Manchester: Manchester University Press, 1991), 154–83.

Porter, Roy, 'Thomas Gisborne: Physicians, Christians, and Gentlemen', in Roger French, Johanna Geyer-Kordesch and Andrew Wear (eds), *A History of Medical Ethics* (Forthcoming).

Porter, Roy, '"Expressing Yourself Ill": The Language of Sickness in Georgian England', in P. Burke and R. Porter (eds), *Language, Self and Society: The Social History of Language* (Cambridge: Polity Press, 1991).

Porter, Roy, 'Bodies of Thought: Thoughts about the Body in Eighteenth Century England', in J. Pittock Wesson and Andrew Wear (eds), *Interpretation and Cultural History* (London: Macmillan, 1991), 82–108.

Porter, Roy, 'Commerce and Disease in Eighteenth Century England', in S. Halini (ed.), *Commerces en Grande Bretagne au xviiie siecle* (Paris: Publications de la Sorbonne, 1990), 55–73.

Porter, Roy, 'Body Politics: Approaches to the Cultural History of the Body', in P. Burke (ed.), *Historiography Today* (Cambridge: Polity Press, forthcoming).

Porter, Roy, 'Reforming the Patient in the Age of Reform: Thomas Beddoes and Medical Practice', in Roger French and Andrew Wear (eds), *Medicine in the Age of Reform* (London: Routledge, forthcoming).

Porter, Roy, 'Plutus or Hygeia? Thomas Beddoes and Medical Ethics', in Robert Baker, Dorothy Porter and Roy Porter (eds), *The Codification of Medical Morality in the Eighteenth and Nineteenth Centuries*, vol. i (Dordrecht: Kluwer, 1991).

Porter, Roy, 'Consumption: Disease of the Consumer Society?', in John Brewer and Roy Porter (eds), *Consumption and the World of Goods* (London: Routledge, forthcoming).

Porter, Roy, 'Introduction', to John Brewer and Roy Porter (eds),

Consumption and the World of Goods (London: Routledge, forthcoming).

Porter, Roy, 'Medicine in the Enlightenment', in J. Buickerood, C. Fox and R. Porter (eds), *The Human Sciences in the Enlightenment* (Berkeley: University of California Press, forthcoming).

Porter, Roy, 'The People's Health in Georgian England', in Tim Harris (ed.), *Popular Culture in Early Modern England* (London: Macmillan, forthcoming).

Porter, Roy, 'The Rise of Physical Examination', in W.F. Bynum and Roy Porter (eds), *Medicine and the Five Senses* (Cambridge: Cambridge University Press, forthcoming).

Porter, Roy, 'Body and Mind', in G.S. Rousseau and Roy Porter (eds), *Hysteria* (Berkeley: University of California Press, forthcoming).

Porter, Roy, 'The Patient in the Eighteenth Century', in Andrew Wear (ed.), *The Social History of Medicine* (Cambridge: Cambridge University Press, forthcoming).

Porter, Roy, 'Medical Journals to 1800', in W.F. Bynum, Stephen Lock and Roy Porter (eds), *The History of Medical Journalism* (London: Routledge, forthcoming).

Porter, Roy, 'Addicted to Modernity: Nervousness in the Early Consumer Society', in J. Barry and J. Melling (eds), *Production, Consumption and Culture* (Exeter: Exeter Studies in History, forthcoming).

Porter, Roy and Porter, Dorothy, *In Sickness and in Health. The British Experience, 1650–1850* (London: Fourth Estate, 1988).

Porter, Roy and Rousseau, G.S. 'Introduction: Toward a Natural History of Mind and Body', in G.S. Rousseau (ed.), *The Languages of Psyche. Mind and Body in Enlightenment Thought* (Berkeley: University of California Press, 1990), 3–44.

Porter, Theodore M., 'Natural Science and Social Theory', in R.C. Olby, G.N. Cantor, J.R.R. Christie, and M.J.S. Hodge (eds), *Companion to the History of Modern Science* (London: Routledge, 1990), 1024–43.

Poynter, F.N.L. and Keele, K.D., *A Short History of Medicine* (London: Mills & Boon, 1961).

Ramsey, M., 'The Repression of Unauthorized Medical Practice', *Eighteenth Century Life*, vii (1982), 118–35.

Ramsey, M., 'Property Rights and the Right to Health. The Regulation of Secret Remedies in France, 1789–1815', in W.F. Bynum and Roy Porter (eds), *Medical Fringe and Medical Orthodoxy* (London: Croom Helm, 1987), 79–105.

Ramsey, M., *Professional and Popular Medicine in France, 1770–1830* (New York: Cambridge University Press, 1988).

Razzell, P., *The Conquest of Smallpox* (Firle: Caliban Books, 1977).

Rees, G., *Francis Bacon's Natural Philosophy: A New Source* (Chalfont St Giles: British Society for the History of Science, 1984).

Rhodes, Philip, *An Outline History of Medicine* (Sevenoaks: Butterworth, 1985).

Richardson, R., *Death, Dissection and the Destitute: A Political History of the Human Corpse* (London: Routledge & Kegan Paul, 1987).

Richardson, S., *Familiar Letters on Important Occasions*, ed. B.W. Downs (London: Routledge, 1928; 1st edn., 1741).

Riley, James C., *Sickness, Recovery and Death: A History and Forecast of Ill Health* (London: Macmillan, 1989).

Risse, G., *Hospital Life in Enlightenment Scotland: Care and Teaching at the Royal Infirmary of Edinburgh* (Cambridge: Cambridge University Press, 1986).

Risse, G., 'Hospital History: New Sources and Methods', in R. Porter and A. Wear (eds), *Problems and Methods in the History of Medicine, 1750–1850* (London: Croom Helm, 1987), 175–203.

Robinson, Eric, 'Eighteenth Century Commerce and Fashion. Matthew Boulton's Marketing Techniques', *Economic History Review*, xvi (1963–4), 39–60 .

Roche, Daniel, 'Talent, Reason, and Sacrifice: The Physician during the Enlightenment', in R. Forster and O. Ranum (eds), *Medicine and Society in France* (Baltimore: Johns Hopkins University Press, 1980), 66–88.

Rolleston, Sir Humphry, 'Thomas Trotter, M.D.', in *Contributions to Medical and Biological Research Dedicated to Sir William Osler, In Honour of His Seventieth Birthday, by His Pupils and Co-Workers* (New York: Hoeber, 1919), 153–65.

Romano, John, 'Early Contributions to the Study of *Delirium Tremens*', *Annals of Medical History*, iii (1941), 128–39.

Rosen, George, *A History of Public Health* (New York: MD Publications, 1958).

Rosen, George, *From Medical Police to Social Medicine* (New York: Science History Publications, 1974).

Rosenberg, C., 'The Therapeutic Revolution', in M. Vogel and C. Rosenberg (eds), *The Therapeutic Revolution* (Philadelphia: University of Pennsylvania Press, 1979), 3–25.

Rosenberg, C., 'Medical Text and Medical Context; Explaining William Buchan's *Domestic Medicine*', *Bulletin of the History of Medicine*, lvii (1983), 22–4.

Rousseau, G.S., 'John Wesley's *Primitive Physick* (1747)', *Harvard Library Bulletin*, xvi (1968) 242–56.

Rousseau, G.S., 'Science and the Discovery of the Imagination in Enlightenment England', *Eighteenth-Century Studies*, iii (1969–70), 108–35.

Rousseau, G.S., 'Nerves, Spirits and Fibres: Towards Defining the Origins of Sensibility; with a Postscript', *The Blue Guitar*, ii (1976), 125–53.

Rousseau, G.S., 'Psychology', in G.S. Rousseau and Roy Porter (eds), *The Ferment of Knowledge* (Cambridge: Cambridge University Press, 1980), 143–210.

Rousseau, G.S., *Tobias Smollett. Essays of Two Decades* (Edinburgh: T. & T. Clark, 1982).

Rousseau, G.S., 'Mysticism and Millennialism: "Immortal Dr Cheyne"', in R.H. Popkin (ed.), *Millenarianism and Messianism in English Literature and Thought 1650–1800* (Leiden: E. J. Brill, 1988), 81–126.

Samuel, Raphael (ed.), *Patriotism. The Making and Unmaking of British National Identity*, 3 vols (London: Routledge, 1989).
Schaffer, Simon, 'Natural Philosophy', in G.S. Rousseau and R. Porter (eds), *The Ferment of Knowledge* (Cambridge: Cambridge University Press, 1980), 55–91.
Schaffer, Simon, 'Natural Philosophy and Public Spectacle in the Eighteenth Century', *History of Science*, xxi (1983), 1–43.
Schaffer, Simon, 'Measuring Virtue: Eudiometry, Enlightenment and Pneumatic Medicine', in Andrew Cunningham and Roger French (eds), *The Medical Enlightenment of the Eighteenth Century* (Cambridge: Cambridge University Press, 1990), 281–318.
Schofield, Robert E., *The Lunar Society of Birmingham: A Social History of Provincial Science and Industry in Eighteenth-Century England* (Oxford: Oxford University Press, 1963).
Schofield, R.E., *Mechanism and Materialism. British Natural Philosophy in an Age of Reason* (Princeton, N.J.: Princeton University Press, 1970).
Schwab, R.N., 'The History of Medicine in Diderot's *Encyclopédie*', *Bulletin of the History of Medicine*, xxxii (1958), 216–23.
Schwab, R.N., 'The Chevalier de Jaucourt, Physician and Encyclopaedist', *Journal of the History of Medicine*, xxxii (1958), 256–59.
Schwartz, Hillel, *Never Satisfied: A Cultural History of Diets, Fantasies and Fat* (New York: Free Press, 1986).
Sekora, John, *Luxury: The Concept in Western Thought, Eden to Smollett* (Baltimore: Johns Hopkins University Press, 1977).
Sena, J.F., 'The English Malady: The Idea of Melancholy from 1700 to 1760' (Princeton University, Ph.D. thesis, 1967).
Shammas, Carole, *The Pre-Industrial Consumer in England and America* (Oxford: Clarendon Press, 1990).
Shorter, E., *A History of Women's Bodies* (Harmondsworth: Penguin, 1983).
Shorter, Edward, 'The Management of Normal Deliveries and the Generation of William Hunter', in W.F. Bynum and Roy Porter (eds), *Wiliam Hunter and the Eighteenth-Century Medical World* (Cambridge: Cambridge University Press, 1985), 371–84.
Shorter, E., *Bedside Manners: The Troubled History of Doctors and Patients* (New York: Simon & Schuster, 1986).
Shortland, Michael, 'The Body in Question; Some Perceptions, Problems and Perspectives of the Body in Relation to Character, 1750–1850' (Ph.D. thesis, University of Leeds, 1985).
Shortland, Michael, 'Skin Deep: Barthes, Lavater and the Visible Body', *Economy and Society*, xiv (1985), 273–312.
Shortland, Michael, 'The Figure of the Hypocrite: Some Contours of an Historical Problem', *Studies in the History of Psychology and the Social Sciences*, iv (1987), 256–74.
Showalter, E., *The Female Malady: Women, Madness, and English Culture, 1830–1980* (New York: Pantheon Press, 1986).
Simon, A.L., *Bottlescrew Days. Wine Drinking in England During the Eighteenth Century* (London: Duckworth, 1926).
Singer, Charles, *A Short History of Medicine* (Oxford: Clarendon Press, 1928).

Slack, Paul, 'Medical Practitioners and Treasures of Poor Men: The Use of the Vernacular Medical Literature of Tudor England', in C. Webster (ed.), *Health, Medicine and Mortality in the Sixteenth Century* (Cambridge: Cambridge University Press, 1979), 165–235.

Smith, F.B., *The Retreat of Tuberculosis 1850–1950* (London: Croom Helm, 1988).

Smith, Ginnie, 'Prescribing the Rules of Health: Self-Help and Advice in the Late Eighteenth-Century England', in Roy Porter (ed.), *Patients and Practitioners: Lay Perceptions of Medicine in Pre-industrial Society* (Cambridge and New York: Cambridge University Press, 1985), 249–82.

Smith, Ginnie, 'Cleanliness: the Development of an Idea and Practice in Britain 1770–1850' (University of London, Ph.D. thesis, 1985).

Smith, J.R., *The Speckled Monster. Smallpox in England 1670–1970, with Particular Reference to Essex* (Chelmsford: Essex Record Office, 1987).

Smith, Olivia, *The Politics of Language* (Oxford: Clarendon Press, 1984).

Smith, W.D.A., *Under the Influence: A History of Nitrous Oxide and Oxygen Anaesthesia* (London: Macmillan, 1982).

Smollett, Tobias, *The Expedition of Humphry Clinker*, ed. by A. Ross (Harmondsworth: Penguin, 1982).

Sontag, S., *Illness as Metaphor* (New York: Farrar, Straus & Giroux, 1978; London: Allen Lane, 1979).

Sontag, S., *AIDS as Metaphor* (Harmondsworth: Allen Lane, 1989).

Sournia, J.-C., *Histoire de l'Alcoolisme* (Paris: Flammarion, 1986).

Spadafora, David, *The Idea of Progress in Eighteenth Century Britain* (New Haven, Conn.: Yale University Press, 1990).

Spector, Benjamin, 'Jeremy Bentham, his Influence upon Medical Thought and Legislation', *Bulletin of the History of Medicine*, xxxvii (1963), 25–42.

Spillane, J., *The Doctrine of the Nerves* (London: Oxford University Press, 1981).

Sprigge, S.S., *The Life and Times of Sir Thomas Wakley* (London: Longmans, 1897).

Spring, J.A. and Buss, D.H., 'Three Centuries of Alcohol in the British Diet', *Nature*, ccxix (1977), 567–72.

Stallybrass, P. and White, A., *The Politics and Poetics of Transgression* (Ithaca, New York: Cornell University Press, 1986).

Stansfield, D.A., 'Thomas Beddoes and Education', *History of Education Society Bulletin*, xxiii (Spring 1979), 7–14.

Stansfield, Dorothy A., *Thomas Beddoes M.D. 1760–1808, Chemist, Physician, Democrat* (Dordrecht: Reidel, 1984).

Stansfield, Dorothy A. and Stansfield, Ronald G., 'Dr Thomas Beddoes and James Watt: Preparatory Work 1794–96 for the Bristol Pneumatic Institute', *Medical History*, xxx (1986), 276–302.

Staum, M., *Cabanis. Enlightenment and Medical Philosophy in the French Revolution* (Princeton, N.J.: Princeton University Press, 1980).

Steele, R., *The Tatler*, 24 Oct., 1710.

Stengers, J. and Neck, A. Van, *Histoire d'une Grande Peur: La Masturbation* (Brussels: University of Brussels Press, 1984).

Sterne, L., *The Life and Opinions of Tristram Shandy*, ed. C. Ricks (Harmondsworth: Penguin, 1967).
Stevenson, L., '"New Disease" in the Seventeenth Century', *Bulletin of the History of Medicine*, xxxix (1965), 1–2.
Stewart, W.A. Campbell and McCann, W.A., *The Educational Innovators, 1750–1880*, 2 vols (London: Macmillan; New York: St. Martin's Press, 1967, 1968).
Stock, J.E., *Memoirs of the Life of Thomas Beddoes MD* (London: J. Murray, 1811).
Stone, L., *The Family, Sex and Marriage in England 1500–1800* (London: Weidenfeld & Nicolson, 1977).
Sultana, D., *Samuel Taylor Coleridge in Malta and Italy* (Oxford: Basil Blackwell, 1969).
Temkin, O., *Galenism: Rise and Decline of Medical Philosophy* (Ithaca, New York: Cornell University Press, 1973).
Temkin, O., 'Health and Disease', in P.P. Wiener (ed.), *Dictionary of the History of Ideas*, 4 vols (New York: Scribner's Sons, 1973), ii, 395–407.
Temkin, O., 'The Scientific Approach to Disease; Specify Entity and Individual Sickness', in A.L. Caplan, H.T. Engelhardt, Jr, and J.J. McCartney (eds), *Concepts of Health and Disease: Interdisciplinary Perspectives* (Reading, Mass.: Addison-Wesley Publishing Co., 1981), 247–63.
Thackrah, C.T., *The Effects of Arts, Trades, and Professions . . . on Health and Longevity* (London: Longman, 1832).
Thomas, E.G., 'The Old Poor Law and Medicine', *Medical History*, xxiv (1980), 1–19.
Thomas, K.V., *Religion and the Decline of Magic* (London: Weiden- feld & Nicolson, 1971).
Thomas, K.V., *Man and the Natural World* (Harmondsworth: Penguin, 1984).
Thompson, E.P., *The Making of the English Working Class* (Harmondsworth: Penguin, 1963).
Thompson, James R., *Thomas Lovell Beddoes* (Boston: Twayne Publishers, 1985).
Thomson, Ann, *Materialism and Society in the Mid-Eighteenth Century: La Mettrie's Discours Préliminaire* (Genève: Librairie Droz, 1981).
Thornton, R.D., *James Currie, The Entire Stranger and Robert Burns* (Edinburgh and London: Oliver & Boyd, 1963).
Tillyard, E.M.W., *The Elizabethan World Picture* (London: Chatto & Windus, 1943).
Todd, A.C., *Beyond the Blaze, A Biography of Davies Gilbert (Giddy)* (Truro: D. Bradford Barton, 1967).
Todd, Janet, *Sensibility, An Introduction* (London: Methuen, 1986).
Trail, R.R., 'Richard Morton (1637–98)', *Medical History*, xiv (1970), 166–74.
Trillat, E., *Histoire de l'Hystérie* (Paris: Seghers, 1986).
Trinder, B., *The Industrial History of Shropshire* (Chichester: Phillimore, 1973).
Tröhler, U., 'Quantification in British Medicine and Surgery 1750–

1830; with Special Reference to its Introduction into Therapeutics' (University of London, Ph.D. thesis, 1978).

Trotter, Thomas, *De Ebrietate, Eiusque Effectibus in Corpus Humanum* (M.D. degree, Edinburgh, 1788).

Trotter, Thomas, *An Essay, Medical, Philosophical and Chemical, on Drunkenness and its Effects on the Human Body* (London: Longman, Hurst, Rees & Orme, 1804).

Trotter, Thomas, *A View of the Nervous Temperament. A Practical Enquiry into the Increasing Prevalence, Prevention, and Treatment of those Diseases Commonly Called Nervous, Bilious, Stomach and Liver Complaints; Indigestion; Low Spirits; Gout etc.* (London: Longman, 1807).

Trumbach, R., *The Rise of the Egalitarian Family* (London & New York: Academic Press, 1978).

Turner, B.S., *The Body and Society: Explorations in Social Theory* (Oxford and New York: Blackwell, 1984).

Turner, B.S., *Medical Power and Social Knowledge* (London: Sage Publications, 1987).

Veith, I., *Hysteria. The History of a Disease* (Chicago: University of Chicago Press, 1965).

Vess, D., *Medical Revolution in France, 1789–1796* (Gainesville: University Presses of Florida, 1975).

Viets, H.R., 'George Cheyne, 1673–1743', *Bulletin of the Institute for the History of Medicine*, xxiii (1949), 435–52.

Vincent, David, *Literacy and Popular Culture. England 1750–1914* (Cambridge: Cambridge University Press, 1989).

Vyverberg, Henry, *Historical Pessimism in the French Enlightenment* (Cambridge, Mass.: Harvard University Press, 1958).

Waddington, I., 'The Struggle to Reform the Royal College of Physicians, 1767–1771: A Sociological Analysis', *Medical History*, xvii (1973), 107–26.

Waddington, I., 'The Role of the Hospital in the Development of Modern Medicine: A Sociological Analysis', *Sociology*, vii (1973), 211–24.

Waddington, I., 'The Development of Medical Ethics – A Sociological Analysis', *Medical History*, xix (1975), 36–51.

Waddington, I., 'General Practitioners and Consultants in Early Nineteenth Century England: The Sociology of an Intra-Professional Conflict', in J. Woodward and D. Richards (eds), *Health Care and Popular Medicine in Nineteenth Century England: Essays in the Social History of Medicine* (London: Croom Helm, 1977), 164–88.

Waddington, I., *The Medical Profession in the Industrial Revolution* (Dublin: Gill & Macmillan, 1984).

Waldinger, Renée, 'Voltaire and Medicine', in Theodore Besterman (ed.), *Studies on Voltaire and the Eighteenth Century*, lviii (Genève, 1967).

Watney, J., *Mother's Ruin* (London: Peter Owen, 1976).

Wear, Andrew, 'Medical Practice in Late Seventeenth-Century and Early Eighteenth-Century England: Continuity and Union', in Roger French and Andrew Wear (eds), *The Medical Revolution of the*

Seventeenth Century (Cambridge: Cambridge University Press, 1989), 294–320.

Wear, Andrew, 'Puritan Perceptions of Illness in Seventeenth-Century England', in R. Porter (ed.), *Patients and Practitioners* (Cambridge: Cambridge University Press, 1985), 55–99.

Wear, Andrew, 'Historical and Cultural Aspects of Pain', *Bulletin of the Society for the Social History of Medicine*, xxxvi (1985), 7–21.

Wear, Andrew, 'Interfaces: Perceptions of Health and Illness in Early Modern England', in R. Porter and A. Wear (eds), *Problems and Methods in the History of Medicine, 1750–1850* (London: Croom Helm, 1987), 230–55.

Wear, Andrew (ed.), *William Harvey: The Circulation of the Blood and Other Writings* (London: Dent, 1990).

Wear, A., 'Caring for the Sick Poor in St Bartholomew's Exchange: 1580–1676', in W.F. Bynum and Roy Porter (eds), *Living and Dying in London* (*Medical History*, Supplement 11, London: Wellcome Institute, 1991).

Weatherill, Lorna, 'Consumer Behaviour and Social Status in England', *Continuity and Change*, ii (1986), 191–216.

Weatherill, Lorna, 'A Possession of One's Own: Women and Consumer Behaviour in England, 1660–1740', *Journal of British Studies*, xxv (1986), 131–56.

Weatherill, Lorna, *Consumer Behaviour and Material Culture, 1660–1760* (London: Routledge, 1988).

Webster, C., 'The Medical Faculty and the Physic Garden', in *The History of the University of Oxford*, vol. v, *The Eighteenth Century*, L.S. Sutherland and L.G. Mitchell (eds) (Oxford: Oxford University Press, 1986), 683–724.

Wedgwood, B. and Wedgwood, H., *The Wedgwood Circle* (London: Studio Vista, 1980).

Welles, A., *An Account of the Discovery and Operation of a New Medicine for Gout* (London: J. Johnson, 1804).

Wellman, Kathleen, 'Medicine as a Key to Defining Enlightenment Issues: The Case of Julien Offray de la Mettrie', in John Yolton and Leslie Brown (eds), *Studies in Eighteenth Century Culture*, xvii (Colleagues Press-ASECS, 1987), 75–89.

Wesley, J., *Primitive Physick: Or, an Easy and Natural Method of Curing Most Diseases* (London: T. Trye, 1747).

Williams, Raymond, *Culture and Society: Coleridge to Orwell* (London: Chatto & Windus, 1958).

Williams, Raymond, *The Long Revolution* (London: Chatto & Windus, 1961).

Williams, Raymond, *The Country and the City* (London and New York: Chatto & Windus, 1973).

Williams, Raymond, *Keywords: A Vocabulary of Culture and Society* (London: Fontana, 1976).

Willich, A.F.M., *Lectures on Diet and Regimen* (London: Longman & Rees, 1799).

Wilson, A., 'Participant or Patient?', in R. Porter (ed.), *Patients and*

Practitioners (Cambridge: Cambridge University Press, 1985), 129–44.

Wilson, A., 'William Hunter and the Varieties of Man-midwifery', in W.F. Bynum and Roy Porter (eds), *William Hunter and the Eighteenth-Century World* (Cambridge: Cambridge University Press, 1985), 343–69.

Wiltshire, John, *Jane Austen and the Body* (Cambridge: Cambridge University Press, 1991).

Wintrobe, M.M., *Blood, Pure and Eloquent. A Story of Discovery of People, and of Ideas* (New York: McGraw-Hill Book Company, 1980).

Wise, M. Norton, with the collaboration of Crosbie Smith, 'Work and Waste; Political Economy and Natural Philosophy in Nineteenth Century Britain', *History of Science*, xxvii (1989), 263–301; 391–449; xxviii (1990), 221–61.

Woodward, J., *To Do The Sick No Harm. A Study of the British Voluntary Hospital System to 1875* (London and Boston: Routledge & Kegan Paul, 1974).

Wrigley, E.A., 'No Death Without Birth: the Implications of English Mortality in the Early Modern Period', in Roy Porter and A. Wear (eds), *Problems and Methods in the History of Medicine, 1750–1850* (London: Croom Helm, 1987), 133–50.

Wrigley, E.A. and Schofield, R.S., *The Population History of England 1541–1971: A Reconstruction* (London: Edward Arnold, 1981).

Wyman, A.L., 'The Surgeoness. The Female Practitioner of Surgery, 1400–1800', *Medical History*, xxvii (1984), 22–41.

Yolton, J., *John Locke and the Way of Ideas* (Oxford: Oxford University Press, 1956).

Yolton, John, *Thinking Matter* (Minneapolis: University of Minnesota Press, 1984).

Young, Robert M., 'Association of Ideas', in P.P. Wiener (ed.), *Dictionary of the History of Ideas*, 4 vols (New York: Scribner's Sons, 1973), vol.1, 111–18.

Index

Académie Royale des Sciences, Paris 23
Acts of Parliament (Great Britain)
  'Gagging Acts' (1795) 16, 168
  Habeas Corpus, suspension of (1793) 16, 168
Adair, James Makittrick (1728–1802) 8
  critical of Buchan 165
  on hypochondria 107, 108
addiction 109–11, 188
  sedatives 96–7, 109
  stimulants 95, 98, 99, 109
  see also drunkenness; opiates
Addison, Joseph (1672–1719) 67, 102, 105
ague 164
airs *see* pneumatic chemistry
alcohol abuse *see* drunkenness
Alexander III, the Great (356–323 BC), king of Macedon (336–323 BC) 15, 166–7
Allende, Salvadore (1908–73), Chilean statesman 192
America, North, medical profession in 24–5
anatomy 30, 43
  Beddoes proposes public lectures 76–7
  private anatomy schools 12, 30, 43
anatomy, morbid 26, 42, 47–8
Ancients/Antiquity 95, 96
  Beddoes's lack of esteem for 37, 46
  medicine of 90
  view of the human body 99–100
Anglo-French wars (1793–1815) 17, 168
animism 26
Anstey, Christopher (1724–1805), *New Bath Guide* (1757) 119
Anti-Jacobin Review 49
apothecaries 41, 109
  mercenariness of 142
asthma 124
astrology 154
asylums 30
Austen, Jane (1775–1817) 119, 134
  Persuasion 119
  Sanditon 119–22, 129

Bacon, Francis, 1st baron Verulam (1561–1626) 23, 86, 88
  theory of four idols 51–2
Baer, Carl Ernst von (1792–1876), Estonian embryologist 22
Baglivi, Giorgio (1668–1707), Italian anatomist 25,
  De Praxi Medica (1699) 25
Banks, Sir Joseph (1743–1820) 44, 144
Barbauld, Mrs Anna Letitia (1743–1825), writer for children 171
Barrell, John 9
Bath, hydrotherapy at 119, 123, 132, 143
Beddoes, Thomas (1760–1808) 1, 31, 32, 94, 99, 111, 120
  life 5, 6, 11–19
    childhood 11–12
    education
      Oxford (BA and MD) 12, 37
      Great Windmill Street Anatomy School, London 12, 13
      Edinburgh Medical School 12–13
    marriage to Anna Edgeworth 16, 18, 186

children 186–7
character/personality 7, 12, 18, 19, 186
health 187
views on philosophy/religion 5, 15, 18, 37–8, 39, 189–90
death 19
as scientist/physician 4, 37–53, 190
interest in chemistry 9, 12, 13, 37–9, 40, 52–3, 88, 184
experiments on gases 13, 17–18, 105, 110, 125, 128
urges experimental method 13, 18, 45, 48–51, 106, 190
self-experimentation 45, 110, 187
medical practice in Bristol (Pneumatic Institute) 15–19, 37, 44, 60, 61, 191
relationship with patients 45–6, 51, 58–85
treatment of tuberculosis 102–4, 105–7, 125, 128, 133
on reform of medical profession 4, 22, 140–53, 189–91
on physician's role in society 3, 6, 169–70
on medical ethics 189–90
criticizes state of clinical medicine/medical education 40–4, 58–9, 189
criticizes fellow practitioners 46, 50, 59, 109–10, 130, 131–2, 141–2, 143–4, 146–8
on importance of preventive medicine 47, 51, 75
advocates health education for laity 75–8, 154–75
abhors quacks/lay practitioners 69–73, 74–5, 162
debunks medical meteorology/spas 125–55
as medico-political radical 2, 3, 6, 12, 14–15, 16–17, 18, 157, 158, 164–72, 183, 187–92
anger about socio-political events 16–19, 168–9, 186
supports French Revolution 6, 14, 168
but deplores extremism 16, 168, 186
views on Enlightenment society 2–3, 6–7, 102–11
upper classes
condemns fashionable life-style 62–8, 86, 96, 103–4, 166–7
on evils of capitalism 59–62
criticizes child-rearing and education 39–40, 79, 103–5, 126, 165, 191–2
writes health-care manuals 58–80
lower classes (poor)
commitment to help 18, 191
advocates health education 165–7, 169–75
advises on nutrition 102–3, 169, 171
founds Medical Institution for the Sick and Drooping Poor 172–4
writes improving literature 15, 58, 170–5
writings 5, 7, 8, 46, 183–5
medical 6, 58–80, 170–5
political 16, 168–9
edits John Brown's works 26
edits *Contributions to Physical and Medical Knowledge* (1799) 46
republishes John Mayow's work on gases 38
reviews *Wilhelm Meister* 5
translates Continental naturalists' books 13
Alexander's Expedition ... (1792) 15, 166–7
Alternatives Compared (1797) 17
Chemical Experiments and Opinions (1790) 38
Considerations on the Medicinal Use of Factitious Airs (1794) 18
Extract of a Letter on Early Instruction ... of the Poor (1792) 15, 171
Good Advice for the Husbandman in Harvest (1808) 171
Guide for Self Preservation and Parental Affection ... (1793) 172
The History of Isaac Jenkins ... (1792) 15, 58, 170–1
Hygëia (1802–03) 18, 58–9, 60, 79
Letter to Erasmus Darwin (1793) 88
Manual of Health (1806) 18, 58–9, 127
Observations on the Consumptive (1801) 106

Observations on ... Sea Scurvy, Consumption ... (1793), 17–18
Rules of the Medical Institution ... of the Sick and Drooping Poor (1804) 172–4
Beddoes, Mrs Thomas (née Anna Edgeworth; b.1773) 16, 19
Beddoes, Thomas Lovell (1803–49), poet/physiologist 186–7
Bedford, 5th duke of *see* Russell, Francis
Bennet, Christopher (1617–55), on consumptions 101, 102
Bentham, Jeremy (1748–1832), utilitarianism 9, 11, 188
Bergman, T.O. (1735–84), Swedish chemist/physician 13, 51
Bernard, Claude (1813–78) 22
Bichat, Marie François Xavier (1771–1802), French physiologist 22
Bills of Mortality 28, 50, 74, 102
biomedical sciences
in eighteenth century 22–36 *passim*
nineteenth-century 'revolution' 22
Birmingham Riots (1791) 15
Black, Joseph (1728–99), friendship with Beddoes 13, 38
Blake, William (1757–1827) 11
Boerhaave, Herman (1668–1738), Dutch physician/chemist 86, 87
mechanical conceptualization of the body 26
Boissier de Sauvages *see* Sauvages de la Croix
Bordeu, Théophile de (1722–76), Montpellier vitalist 26
Boswell, James (1740–95), hypochondria of 107
Boulton, Matthew (1728–1809), friendship with Beddoes 11, 49
Boyle, Hon. Robert (1627–91) 22, 23, 38, 50
Bristol 143
Beddoes in 15–18, 37, 60, 61
as centre of intellectual radicalism 8, 16–17, 19
commercial centre 16, 60, 61
Hotwells 133
see also Pneumatic Institute
Bristol Gazette 171
Brown, John (1735–88) 26
Brunonianism 13, 29, 105
Buchan, William (1729–1805)
on consumptions 101–2
as political radical/medical reformer 8, 78, 88–9, 157, 158, 160–1, 164
as popularizer 108, 157, 165
Domestic Medicine (1769) 73, 157, 158–9, 161, 164
Observations Concerning ... the Venereal Disease (1796) 157, 158–61
Burke, Edmund (1729–97) 9, 11
Burton, Robert (1577–1640) 78
Butler, Samuel (1612–80)
Erewhon 5
Miscellaneous Thoughts 58
Butterfield, Herbert 23
Byron, George Gordon, 6th baron (1788–1824) 11

Cabanis, Pierre Jean Georges (1757–1808), on medicine and society 8
Calvinism 28
Cambridge University, medical education at 149–50
Campbell, Robert, *London Tradesman* (1747) 93
capitalism 6, 9, 59–67, 144
Carlyle, Thomas (1795–1881) 2
Cartesians *see* Descartes, R.
Cartwright, F.F. 1
Chadwick, Sir Edwin (1800–90) 192
Chambers' Cyclopaedia, 'Medicine' 24
charities *see* hospitals; Preventive Institution
chemistry 4, 8–9, 19
eighteenth-century advances 38
see also Beddoes, Thomas; pneumatic chemistry
Cheyne, George (1671–1743), physician 62
on healthy diet 102, 104, 105
on nervous disorders 89–93, 100
English Malady (1722) 92
childbirth 87
child-rearing 87, 155, 172
unhealthy 67, 103–5
children, literature for 68, 103
chlorosis 59, 104
Christianity, Beddoes's attitude to 37–8
civilization, as cause of sickness 61, 89, 90–2, 95–102, 107–10
Clarke [Clerke], John (1682–1757), dean of Salisbury 122

classification *see* taxonomy
Clerke *see* Clarke
Clifton *see* Pneumatic Institute
clinical medicine, lack of progress in eighteenth century 40–4, 46
see also hospitals
Cobbett, William (1762–1835), radical reformer 11, 15, 188
Coleridge, James (1760–1836) 134
Coleridge, Samuel Taylor (1772–1834)
advocates travel for health 134–5
associated with Pneumatic Institute 44
edits *The Watchman* 17
experiments with drugs 110
friendship with Beddoes 5, 6, 8, 11, 186
ideal of the new intelligentsia 190
opiate addiction 72, 133
radical campaigner 16, 17, 188
Comte, Auguste (1798–1857), French positivist philosopher 5
Condorcet, M.J.A.N., marquis de (1743–94) 24, 37
Esquisse (1794) 88
consumerism/consumption 86, 94–5, 110
role in spread of tuberculosis 102–3, 105
see also capitalism
consumption *see* tuberculosis, pulmonary
'consumptions', the *see* wasting diseases
Cooter, Roger 165
Cottle, Joseph (1770–1853), radical campaigner 16
cowpox 50, 155
Cullen, William (1710–90), Scottish physician/chemist 12, 26, 131
taxonomy 28, 29, 184
Culpeper, Nicholas (1616–54), *Herbal* 154, 155
Currie, James (1756–1805), physician/reformer 32
Curry, Patrick 154

Darwin, Erasmus (1731–1802), physician/friend of Beddoes 1, 3, 5, 11, 13, 39, 46, 49
medico-social reformer 8
poetry of 15, 166
on pulmonary tuberculosis 102
overdosing causes T. Wedgwood's addiction 110
Zoonomia 29
Daston, Lorraine 27
Davy, Sir Humphry (1778–1829) 5, 8, 134, 187
researches at Pneumatic Institute 18, 44, 45
at Royal Institution 19, 186
Day, Thomas (1748–89), on education 39, 171
death 87
demography 28, 63, 87
Descartes, René (1596–1650) 23, 86
Cartesian dualists 189
Desmond, Adrian 192
diabetes 93
diarrhoeas 93
diet *see* nutrition
digestive disorders 59, 60, 95, 97, 101
digitalis 106, 155
Dijon, Beddoes's visit to 13
disease, concepts of 26–7
see also pathology; taxonomy
diseases, fashionable 107, 108
see also hypochondria
dispensaries 30, 87, 155, 172
doctor/patient relationships 45–6, 189
effect of affluence on 60
see also medical profession; patients
domestic medicine 69–73, 74–5, 88–9, 109, 145, 154
literature, self-help 15, 18–19, 58–80, 72–3, 109, 122, 127, 145, 154–75
dropsy 65, 93, 124
drug abuse *see* addiction
drunkenness 15, 62, 94–5, 98–9, 100, 101–2, 111, 162–3, 170, 171, 188
dysentery 41–2

Eagleton, Terry 8
economics *see* capitalism
Edgeworth, Anna *see* Beddoes, Mrs Thomas
Edgeworth, Richard Lovell (1744–1817), friend of Beddoes 11, 16
on education 39
Edinburgh University medical school 12–13, 26, 30, 94, 95, 184, 189
Beddoes's criticisms of 12–13, 90, 148–9, 150

education
  Beddoes's views on 39–40, 44, 165, 191–2
    of upper classes 66, 68, 79, 103
    of working classes 15, 18, 148, 156, 171, 191–2
  Locke/Rousseau's system 39–40
  see also medical education
eighteenth century, medicine in 22–36, 86–118
    scientific medicine 28–9, 37–53
empiricism, philosophical (British school) 25, 39
empirics *see* quacks
'English Malady' *see* nervous disorders
Enlightenment, English 3, 4, 5, 8, 9, 14, 19, 24, 37, 40, 59, 60, 67, 73, 78
  ambiguities 191
  and pathology 86–118
  religion 52
epidemiology 28, 30
ethics, medical 140, 148, 189–90
experimental method, importance to Beddoes 13, 18, 45, 48–51, 106, 190

fashion/fashionable diseases *see* society
Ferriar, John (1751–1815), physician/social reformer 8
fevers 28, 50, 59
Fielding, Henry (1707–54), moves to Ealing for health 124
  Voyage to Lisbon 124
Finch, Mrs William (née Sarah Priestley; d.1803), treated by Beddoes for consumption 106
Fissell, Mary 8
folk cures 106, 154–5
  see also domestic medicine
Fourcroy, Antoine François, comte de (1755–1809), French chemist 38
France 95
  chemistry 38
  medical profession 25, 32, 42
  morbid anatomy 48
  physicians in Third Republic 192
  south, as health resort 124
  wars with Britain (1793–1815) 17, 168
Frank, Johann Peter (1745–1821), German physician/social reformer 5
French Revolution 1, 4, 13, 14, 78, 166, 168
  Terror 6, 16, 64
Freud, Sigmund (1856–1939) 186, 187
Fyfe, Andrew *the elder* (1754–1824), Scottish anatomist 156

Galen (AD 130–200) 24
  Galenic humoralism 92
Galileo Galilei (1564–1642) 23
Garrick, David (1717–79), recommends horse-riding for health 123
gases *see* pneumatic chemistry
Gay, Peter 23, 86–8, 89, 110
general practitioner, evolution of the 30
geology, Beddoes's interest in 15
George III (1738–1820), king of Great Britain 1760–1820 11, 146–7
Gibbon, Edward (1737–94) 12
  travels to Lausanne for health 128
Giddy, Davies *see* Gilbert
Gilbert [formerly Giddy], Davies (1767–1839), friend of Beddoes 14, 16, 168, 186
Gillispie, C.C. 23
Gisborne, Thomas (d.1806), royal physician 146–7
'Glorious Revolution' (1688) 188
gluttony, as cause of illness 62, 65, 92, 100, 101–2, 162–3
Godbold, Nathaniel (d.1799), proprietor of Vegetable Balsam 133
Godwin, William (1756–1836) 11, 188
Goethe, Johann Wolfgang von (1749–1832), *Wilhelm Meister* 5
Golinski, Jan 8–9
gout 59, 65, 69, 94, 119, 124, 128, 134–5, 166
Grainger, Richard Dugard (1801–65), *Elements of General Anatomy* (1829) 156
Gray, Samuel Frederick (fl.1780–1836), *Supplement to the Pharmacopoeia* (1818) 156
Great Windmill Street Anatomy School, London 12
Greece, ancient 24, 90
Gregory, John (1724–73) 140
  Observations on the Duties of a Physician (1770) 189
Guevara, 'Che' (1928–67) 192
Gutenberg, Johann (*c.* 1398–1468) 46
Gutteridge, Joseph (fl.1870), artisan/lay healer 156

Guyton de Morveau, L.B. (1737–1816), French chemist 13, 38

Habermas, Jürgen 8
Hacking, Ian 27
Hales, Stephen (1677–1761), haemostatic experiments 28
Hall, A. Rupert 23
Haller, Albrecht von (1708–77), Swiss physiologist 26
Hamilton, Emma, Lady (1761?–1815) 11
Harrison, Mark 8
Hartley, David *the elder* (1705–57), physician/philosopher 39
  on education 79
Harvey, Gideon *the elder* (1640?–1700?), on scurvy and consumptions 100, 101
Harvey, William (1578–1657) 23, 24
Hastings, Warren (1732–1818) 167
Haygarth, John (1740–1827), medico-social reformer 8, 32
Hazlitt, William (1778–1830) 11
health care, Beddoes's advice to laity 58–85, 165–7, 169–75
  see also domestic medicine
healthy body, model of 99–100
Heberden, William *the elder* (1710–1801) 149
Hill, [Sir] John (1716?–75), on hypochondria 108
Hippocrates of Cos (*c.*460–*c.*370 BC) 24, 122
  Hippocratics 23–4
Hoffmann, Freidrich (1660–1742), clinician of Halle 131
Holcroft, Thomas (1745–1809), dramatist/freethinker 188
Hooke, Robert (1635–1703) 23
hospitals
  charitable 30, 43–4, 47, 87, 155, 172
  clinical education in 30, 43
  clinical experiments in 49, 174
  as 'gateways to death' 31, 87
  role in supplying medical data 46–7
  treatments 127
humane societies 77
Hume, David (1711–76), suffers 'nervous breakdown' 109
humoral theory 92, 122
Hunter, John (1728–93) 4, 50
  anatomical/physiological researches 30
  refutes mechanists 26
Hunter, William (1718–83) 50
  private anatomy school 12, 30, 43
Hutton, James (1726–97), *Theory of the Earth* (1795) 13
hypochondria 59, 60, 69–70, 96, 100, 107–9, 110, 119, 133, 183, 188
  in fiction 120
hysteria 59, 96, 100, 107–9, 110

iatrogenic disorders 4, 8, 97, 110
iatro-mechanists 25–7, 90, 92, 124
idéologues 189
India, history of 167–8
industrialization 5, 9, 32
  effect on workers' health 60, 102–3
  in West Midlands 11
infirmaries 43–4

Jacobins 16, 186
James I (1566–1625), king of Great Britain 1603–25 49
Jenner, Edward (1749–1823) 4, 100
  discoverer of vaccination 154–5
Johnson, Samuel (1709–84) 17, 185
  advises on health 124–5
journalism, medical 30
Jurin, James (1684–1750), physician 28

Kant, Immanuel (1724–1804) 189
Keats, John (1795–1821) 123
Keir, James (1735–1820), chemist/friend of Beddoes 13
King, John (b. Johannes Koenig; 1766–1840), Swiss physician 8
  at Pneumatic Institute 44
Kinglake, Robert (1765–1842), physician at Pneumatic Institute 44
Koch, Robert (1843–1910) 30

La Mettrie, Julien Offray de (1709–51), materialist philosopher 27
language, Beddoes's views on importance of 4, 183–5
Latour, Bruno 22
laudanum *see* opium
laughing-gas *see* nitrous oxide
Lavoisier, Antoine Laurent (1743–94) 38, 51, 184
lay healers 70–3, 154, 156, 162, 173
  see also quacks

laymen *see* domestic medicine; patients
Lefanu, William R. 23
Leiden, University of
iatro-mechanists 90
medical school 26
Leonardo da Vinci (1452–1519) 24
Lettsom, John Coakley (1744–1815), medico-social reformer 8, 32
Levere, Trevor 1, 8
Linnaeus, Carolus (1707–78), taxonomy 28, 184
literary and philosophical societies 44
literature
children's 68, 103
fiction 67–8
health advice for laity *see* domestic medicine
sickness portrayed in satire 31, 119–2
Locke, John (1632–1704), physician/empiricist philosopher 86, 170
on education 39, 40, 79, 97
London 18, 19, 26
Beddoes in 12–13, 148
as commercial centre 61
deaths from pulmonary tuberculosis 102
hospitals, medical education in 30, 43
medical colleges 31
poor in East End 157, 161
London Corresponding Society 157, 188
Loudon, Irvine S.L. 9
Ludwig, Carl Friedrich Wilhelm (1816–95), German physiologist 22
Lunar Society of Birmingham 11, 13, 37, 44
lying-in charities 87

McKeown, T. 87
MacPherson, C.B. 61
Malthus, Thomas Robert (1766–1834) 167
demographic theory 28, 63
Mandeville, Bernard (1670?–1753) 24
Treatise of the Hypochondriack and Hysterick Diseases (1730) 108
Marten, Benjamin (1704–82), theory of consumptions 100, 101, 102
masturbation 68, 104, 111
mathematics *see* statistics
Mayow, John (1640–79), physiologist/pneumatic chemist 38
mechanists *see* iatro-mechanists
medical corporations 31, 42
corrupt 158
medical education 12–13, 26, 30, 42–3, 94, 95, 184, 189
Beddoes's criticisms of 148–50
Medical Institution for the Sick and Drooping Poor *see* Preventive Institution
medical profession 3–4, 22–32, 192
intra-professional rivalries 29, 31
politics of 9
professionalization 30–1, 175
rise of 93–4
role in society 6, 7
need for reform 7, 31–2, 42, 140–53, 160, 175, 189
fashionable treatments/spas 78, 119, 130–2
ineptitude 4, 31, 50–1
lack of organization 143
malpractice 4, 8, 97
mercenariness 40, 41, 50, 51, 52, 59, 78, 109, 119, 130, 142, 143–4, 145, 146–7, 159, 186
overprescribing 41, 96–7, 109, 142
quackery 141–2
secrecy 46, 159–61, 175
unsafe therapeutics 4, 41
Medical Society of London (founded 1773) 30
medicine
in eighteenth century 6, 22–32, 40–4, 46, 86–111
in seventeenth century 23–4, 27
scientific 17–18, 37–53, 87
see also domestic medicine; medical profession
medico-political radicals 2, 3, 6, 8–9, 12, 14–15, 16–19, 157–72, 183, 187–92
meteorological/environmental effects on health 122–30, 134, 135
Mettrie, Julien Offray de la *see* La Mettrie
Middle Ages, lack of scholastic progress in 24, 37–8
healthy diet in 105
midwives 155
Monro, Alexander *secundus* (1733–1817), anatomy lecturer at Edinburgh 12, 148

Montesquieu, Charles-Louis de Secondat, baron (1689–1715) 95, 167
Monthly Review 5
Montpellier
as health resort for consumptives 123
vitalists in 26
morbid anatomy *see* anatomy
More, Hannah (1745–1833), religious writer 58
Morgagni, Giovanni Battista (1682–1771), pioneer of morbid anatomy 26
Morton, Richard (1637–98), *Treatise of Consumptions* (Eng. trans. 1694) 101, 102
Morveau, L.B. Guyton de *see* Guyton de Morveau

Napoleon Bonaparte (1769–1821), emperor of France 1804–15 17, 18
Nash, Richard 'Beau' (1674–1762) 131
Nature, as ideal state 74, 95–6, 166
Nelson, Horatio, viscount Nelson (1758–1805) 11
nervous disorders 59, 66, 86, 89, 92–3, 95–9, 100, 107–9, 110, 119
in fiction 121–2
Neve, Michael 8
Newton, Sir Isaac (1642–1727) 4, 5, 22, 23, 38, 50, 86
Newtonian natural philosophy 27, 39, 90
nineteenth century
medical profession 192
public health movement 192
revolution in biomedical sciences 22, 87
self-improvement campaigns 165
theories of disease 5
nitrous oxide (laughing-gas) 18, 110
nostrum-mongers *see* quacks
nutrition 99–100
Beddoes's views on 169, 171
healthy 102, 126, 163, 171
unhealthy (faddish) 104–5, 166
see also drunkenness; gluttony
nymphomania 111

obstetrics, advances in 30
opiates/opium 30, 72, 88, 95, 98, 110, 133, 160, 169
deleterious effects on poor 180 n90
Oxford University, Beddoes at 12, 13, 14, 15, 16, 37, 148, 150
oxygen, discovery of 17
therapy 45, 59

pain-killers 96–7, 109
see also opiates
Paine, Thomas (1737–1809) 9, 11, 15, 188
palsy 65
Paris 42, 141
hospital reform 44
Parkinson, James (1755–1824) 166
disagrees with Buchan 164, 165
health advice books 157–8, 161–6
idyllic vision of manual labour 162–3
political radical/medical reformer 8, 157, 161, 188
Parsons, Talcott 2
Pasteur, Louis (1822–95) 22, 30
pathology, Enlightenment and 86–118
patients 58–85, 119–39
attitudes to health 60
duped by unscrupulous physicians 50, 159–60
ignorant 3, 52, 68–71, 73–5, 144–5, 146, 159, 163
incoherent/untruthful 159, 183–4
need for education 76–9
patronize quacks 146
role in preventive medicine 51
self-dosing 95, 96–7, 98, 109, 145
'sick role' 2
sickness as status symbol (upper classes) 3, 6, 18–19, 62–7, 91–2, 93, 94, 96, 97–8, 104–5, 109, 131–2, 144–5
working classes (poor) 58, 172–4
see also medical profession
Peacock, Thomas Love (1785–1866) 185
Crotchet Castle 37, 124–5
Gryll Grange 1
Melincourt 22
Nightmare Abbey 11, 86, 119, 140, 183
Pepys, Samuel (1633–1703) 122
Percival, Thomas (1740–1804) 4, 140
Medical Ethics (1803) 189
Perkins, John (fl.1760s), advised on health by Samuel Johnson 124–5
Peruvian bark *see* quinine
pharmaceutics, advances in 30, 88

philanthropy 87
philosophes 3, 15, 23, 37, 52, 78, 87, 88, 89, 110, 185
philosophy, British school of empiricism 39
phrenology 165
physicians *see* medical profession
physics 6, 53
physiology 25–7, 30, 190
  cardiovascular system 24, 26
  education of laity 76–7, 165
  lymphatic system 30
  nervous system 26, 29, 30
  respiration 38
Pickstone, John 9
Pierce, Eliza (fl.1751–75) 155–6
Pitcairn [Pitcairne], Archibald (1652–1713), iatro-mechanist 26
Pitt, William *the younger* (1759–1806) 7, 11
  Beddoes's opposition to 17, 168–9
Plato (*c*.427–*c*.347 BC), Beddoes's opinion of 137
  compares statesman with physician 5
pleurisy 164
pneumatic chemistry 13, 17, 18, 38–9, 88, 105, 110, 125, 128
  discovery of oxygen 17
  John Mayow's work 38
Pneumatic Institute, Clifton, Bristol (founded 1799) 17, 18, 19, 37, 44, 191
  researches/therapy 17, 18, 19, 37, 44–5, 48, 105
political radicalism *see* medico-political radicals
Poole, Thomas (1765–1837), radical activist 16
poor (working classes)
  attitude to sickness 173–4
  charities *see* hospitals
  folklore of health 154, 155–6
  effects of working conditions on health 6, 162–3
  susceptibility to tuberculosis 7, 102–3
  see also domestic medicine; education; patients
Poor Law, medical provision 30, 87, 155
Porter, Theodore 27
Portugal, as health resort 124, 133
Pott, Percivall (1714–88), surgeon 50
Preventive Institution (Medical Institution for the Sick and Drooping Poor), Clifton, Bristol (founded 1802) 18, 37, 172–4
Price, Richard (1723–91), radical reformer 16
Priestley, Joseph (1733–1804) 11, 106
  attacked in Birmingham Riots (1791) 15
  radical opinions 16
Priestley, Sarah *see* Finch, Mrs William
printing/publishing 4, 8, 24, 46
psychology, physiological 39
public health movement 30, 31, 192
  education of laity 76–9
  effects of industrialization 60–1
  medical police 191
Pyle, Revd Edmund (1729–63), prebendary to Salisbury Cathedral 122

quackery/quacks 25, 31, 41–2, 46, 59, 109, 130, 133, 140, 141–2, 145–6, 147, 150, 158, 162, 173, 174, 189
quinine 88, 160

radical physicians *see* medico-political radicals
Ray, John (1627–1705), taxonomy 28
regimen, natural, as cure for most diseases 161, 164
religion
  Beddoes's criticisms 5, 15, 37–8
  Enlightenment analyses 51
  secularization 28
Renaissance/classical revival 24, 48
respiration 38
respiratory diseases *see* Pneumatic Institute; tuberculosis, pulmonary
Reynolds, William (1758–1803), friend of Beddoes 13, 15
Richardson, Samuel (1689–1761), condemns drunkards 100
Risse, G. 87
Robespierre, Maximilien (1758–94) 64
Roget, Peter Mark (1799–1869), physician at Pneumatic Institute 44
Romanticism 9, 11, 19
Rosenberg, Charles 22, 87
Rousseau, Jean Jacques (1712–78) 59, 92, 158, 164
  disparages art/science 66
  on education 39
  on Nature as ideal state 74

Royal College of Physicians of London (founded 1518) 142, 149
Royal Institution of Great Britain (founded 1799) 19, 186
Royal Society of London (royal charter 1662) 22, 23, 28, 38
Rush, Benjamin (1745–1813) 25, 88, 159, 160
Russell, Francis, 5th duke of Bedford (1765–1805) 44

Sanctorius [Santorio], S. (1561–1636), Italian iatro-mechanist 28
Sauvages de la Croix, François Boissier de (1706–67) 26
  Nouvelles Classes des Maladies (1731) 28
Scheele, Carl Wilhelm (1742–86), Swedish chemist 13
Schwann, Theodor (1810–82), German biologist 22
science/scientific revolution 23, 86–7
  see also chemistry
scientific medicine 37–53
  experimental method 13, 17–18, 45, 48–51, 106, 110, 190
Scotland, medicine in 26, 28, 42
scrophula 59, 69, 93, 100, 172, 173
scurvies *see* wasting diseases
sea air, healthy effects of 129
sea-sickness, as treatment for stomach complaints 125
self-help *see* domestic medicine; education
seventeenth century
  medicine in 23–6, 27, 50, 100, 102, 105
  'scientific revolution' 23, 86–7
Sheldon, John (1752–1808), William Hunter's successor at Great Windmill Street Anatomy School 12, 43
Shelley, Percy Bysshe (1792–1822) 11, 123, 167
Sheridan, Mrs Richard Brinsley (née Elizabeth Ann Linley; 1754–92) 123
Shifnal, Shropshire, birthplace of Beddoes 5, 11
Shorter, E. 87
'sickness culture' 119–36, 188
  see also medical profession; patients
Sinclair, Sir John (1754–1835), *Statistical Survey of Scotland* (1791–9) 127
smallpox 28, 31, 155
  inoculation 28, 30, 50, 87, 88, 164
  vaccination 50, 154–5
Smith, Thomas Southwood (1788–1861), *Philosophy of Health* (1835–7) 156
Smollett, Tobias George (1721–71) 123
  travels on Continent for health 124
  Humphry Clinker (1771) 119
'social' disorders *see* drunkenness; hypochondria; nervous disorders
Société Royale de Médecine, Paris 141
societies, medical 30
society (upper classes) 119–39, 188
  life style, Beddoes's criticisms of
    child-rearing practices 103–5
    diet 104–5, 166
    'fashionable diseases' 94, 104–5, 107, 108, 131–2
    fiction (novels) 103
    modish clothes 103, 126
    patronage of fashionable physicians 145–8
    spas 41, 105, 119–22, 123–4, 130–3, 188
    travelling for health 123, 124–5, 128–9, 132, 133–5
  see also hypochondria; patients
Solomon, Samuel (d.1819), Liverpool nostrum-monger 41
  Balm of Gilead 146
Southey, Robert (1774–1843) 8, 11, 134, 135
  modifies views (to High Tory) 186
  radical campaigner 16
Spallanzani, Lazaro (1729–99), Italian biologist 13
spas 41, 105, 123–4, 130–3, 188
  in fiction 119–22
Stahl, Georg Ernst (1660–1743), German biologist/animist 26
Stansfield, Dorothy 1
statistics, as applied to natural philosophy 27–8, 29
  importance in medicine 46, 48
Steele, Sir Richard (1672–1729) 102
Sterne, Laurence (1713–68) 2, 78, 187
  Tristram Shandy (1760–7) 31, 124
Stock, J.E., *Memoir of the Life of Thomas*

Beddoes MD (1811) 19
supernatural explanations of sickness 27—8
superstition/magic 155
surgeon-apothecaries 147
surgery, eighteenth-century advances in 30
Sutton, Daniel (1735–1819), smallpox inoculator 164
Swift, Jonathan (1667–1745) 11, 185
Modest Proposal 169
Switzerland, as health resort 128
Sydenham, Thomas (1624–89), physician 22, 50, 160
natural history of disease 28–9

Tacitus, Publius Cornelius (*c.*AD 55–*c.*116) 96
Tatler 100
taxonomy 28–9
Thelwall, John (1764–1835), radical reformer 16, 188
therapies, unsafe/unsuccessful 4, 41, 59
see also tuberculosis, pulmonary
Tissot, Simon André (1728–97), Swiss physician 128
on diseases of civilization 8
Tooke, Revd John Horne (1736–1812), radical intellectual 16
Tories 17, 186
Tournefort, Joseph Pitton de (1656–1708), French botanist/taxonomist 28
Trimmer, Mrs Sarah (1741–1810), author of children's books 171
Trotter, Thomas (1760–1832), physician
early life/education 94
Essay on Drunkenness (1804) 94–5, 98–9
View of the Nervous Temperament (1807) 89–90, 94, 95, 97–8
tuberculosis, lymphatic *see* scrophula
tuberculosis, pulmonary 7, 16, 17, 31, 38, 59, 99, 101, 102, 124, 172–3
Beddoes's researches 45, 102, 105–6, 125
therapies
cowhouse 106–7, 133
digitalis 106
pneumatic *see* Pneumatic Institute
causes 102–4, 105
as 'fashionable' disease 104–5, 131–2
susceptibility of working classes 7, 102–3
warm climate recommended 123–4, 129
see also spas
twentieth-century medicine 87
Third World problems 192

ulcers, skin 69
universities, role in medical instruction 42, 43
see also under university towns
urbanization *see* civilization
Utilitarianism 9, 110, 188

vegetarianism 104–5
venereal disease 100, 157, 158–61
Vesalius, Andreas (1514–64) 24
Virchow, Rudolf Ludwig Karl (1821–1902), German pathologist 191
vitalism 26–7
vivisection, in Beddoes's researches 48–9
Volney, comte de (Constantin François de Chasseboeuf; 1757–1820), French scholar 166
Voltaire (pseud. of François-Marie Arouet; 1694–1778) 191

Waddington, Ivan 9
Wakley, Thomas (1795–1862), medical reformer 192
Warren, Richard (1731–97), fashionable physician 109, 144
wasting diseases (called the 'consumptions' or scurvies) 100–2, 110
Watchman, The, radical journal 17
Watt, Gregory (1777–1804), friend of Beddoes 16
Watt, James (1736–1819), friendship with Beddoes 5, 11, 13
designs apparatus for Beddoes's gas experiments 17
Watt, James *the younger* (1769–1848), friend of Beddoes 16
wealth *see* capitalism; society
Wedgwood, Thomas (1771–1805) 16
gives financial support to Pneumatic Institute 18

opium addiction 72, 110
Welles, A. (fl.1804), proprietor of gout medicine 135
Wesley, John (1703–91) 123
Primitive Physick (1747) 157, 158
West Midlands Lunar Society *see* Lunar Society of Birmingham
Whytt, Robert (1714–66), physician/vitalist 26
Wilberforce, William (1759–1833), philanthropist 11
Williams, Raymond 8, 9
Willich, Anthony Florian Madinger (fl.1799), on fashionable complaints 94
Willis, Thomas (1621–75), physician 25
on consumptions 101, 102
Withering, William (1741–99), physician 13
medical use of digitalis 106, 155
Wollstonecraft, Mary (1759–97) 11
women
addiction 95
childhood (upper classes) 104–5
diseases 108, 143
education 66, 79, 103
lay practitioners 71, 72, 143
medical lectures for 76
Wordsworth, William (1770–1850) 11
working classes *see* poor